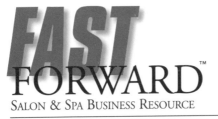

FORWARD ™
SALON & SPA BUSINESS RESOURCE

**THE SALON INDUSTRY'S DEFINITIVE BUSINESS MANAGEMENT
REFERENCE GUIDE FOR OWNERS, MANAGERS AND KEY STAFF**

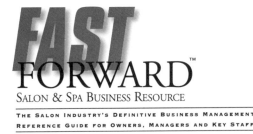

FAST FORWARD™

SALON & SPA BUSINESS RESOURCE

THE SALON INDUSTRY'S DEFINITIVE BUSINESS MANAGEMENT
REFERENCE GUIDE FOR OWNERS, MANAGERS AND KEY STAFF

WRITTEN BY:
Neil Ducoff, President
STRATEGIES PUBLISHING GROUP, INC.

CONTENT DIRECTOR, INDUSTRY MARKETING CONSULTANT
Nancy Flinn, President
NANCY FLINN MARKETING RESOURCES, INC.

CONTRIBUTING WRITERS:
Matthew Cross
LEADERSHIP ALLIANCE

Andrew R. Finkelstein
BEAUTY MATTERS, LTD.

Keri Manuel
SALON BUSINESS STRATEGIES

Larry Oskin
MARKETING SOLUTIONS, INC.

EDITED BY:
Heather Slater, Editor
STRATEGIES PUBLISHING GROUP, INC.

PUBLISHED BY:
STRATEGIES PUBLISHING GROUP, INC.
Centerbrook, CT

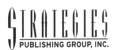

STRATEGIES
PUBLISHING GROUP, INC.

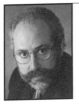

Neil Ducoff, President
STRATEGIES PUBLISHING GROUP, INC.

In 1993, Neil Ducoff founded STRATEGIES PUBLISHING GROUP, INC. for the specific purpose of publishing SALON BUSINESS STRATEGIES, a specialized monthly management magazine for salons and spas. Since the first issue was published in January 1994, the publication has become a recognized and vital resource for salon business information and has rightfully positioned itself as "The Premier Business Resource For Salon & Spa Growth" — all without the financial support of advertising.

Neil and the SALON BUSINESS STRATEGIES team have developed an extensive array of in-salon consulting services and distributor education programs. STRATEGIES' management seminars, including Pay & Performance, The Client Retention Course and the STRATEGIES INCUBATOR, deliver a level of business awareness previously unavailable through traditional salon educational sources.

Neil has also gained respect as the industry "guru" on salon salary systems and team-based incentive compensation programs. His consulting services are the highest-rated in the industry. Participants in STRATEGIES seminars have received, in their own words: "the wings to fly"; "a new lease on life"; and "hope and motivation." STRATEGIES helps salon and spa owners see the light at the end of the tunnel.

Nancy Flinn, President
NANCY FLINN MARKETING RESOURCES, INC.

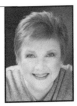

Nancy Flinn is a beauty expert with an industry reputation for new business development, creative problem-solving and an in-depth knowledge of the professional salon segment of the beauty industry.

NANCY FLINN MARKETING RESOURCES, INC. (NFMR) was formed in 1991 to provide the beauty industry with a range of sophisticated services including business and product development, strategic planning, qualitative market research, syndicated and custom quantitative market research, product evaluation, industry sales tracking, database and target marketing, education and communication programs.

In addition to creating unique services such as COSMOPINION PANEL (a 600-member salon panel that evaluates salon products), NFMR has partnered with the best resources outside the beauty industry to create specific services for the beauty industry:

- ■ *MARKET DECISIONS (A.C. NEILSON)…to create a quarterly sales audit program with a panel of salons to measure movement of all hair care products by category.*
- ■ *MULTI-SPONSOR SURVEYS/GALLUP SURVEYS…to provide syndicated exploration of salon professionals and clients, and distributors' attitudes and behaviors.*
- ■ *TARGETRENDS ASSOCIATES…to implement database and target marketing.*

In the ever-changing, competitive and sophisticated business of professional beauty, NFMR takes pride in providing reliable resources of knowledge for innovative and practical business solutions.

Prior to forming NFMR, Nancy Flinn's career at CLAIROL, INC. included vice presidential marketing positions in all divisions: Mass Retail Beauty, Professional Beauty, and Personal Care Appliances.

Published by: STRATEGIES PUBLISHING GROUP, INC.
P.O. Box 296
40 Main Street
Centerbrook, CT 06409
TOLL-FREE: 800.417.4848 USA/Canada
CORPORATE OFFICES: 860.767.2064
Fax: 860.767.2084
WWW.STRATEGIESPUB.COM

ISBN   0-9701028-0-1

Printed in the United States of America
First edition: May 2000
Book production: Shannon Printing Company, Inc., Deep River, CT

Contents

U.S. Salon and Spa Trends
■

Technology
■

Maximizing Your Human Resources

Leadership

■

Front Desk Strategies

■

Moving Towards "TRUE QUALITY"

■

Client Retention

■

Service Marketing & Sales

■

Retailing Like the Pros

■

Public Relations

■

World-Class Customer Service

■

Salon & Spa Numbers Made Easy

■

Compensation Strategies

■

Taxes: A Fact of Business Life

■

Personal and Interpersonal Motivation
■

Acknowledgements & Insights

Publishing a book of the magnitude of Fast Forward has truly been a *team* effort. It began with a phone call in the fall of 1998 from my long-time friend and mentor, Nancy Flinn. She wanted to discuss a very special project that would offer long-term benefits to the advancement of business knowledge in the professional salon and spa industry. The Fast Forward book project was born as we later sat at Nancy's dining room table. In the following months, detailed chapter outlines were finalized, contributing experts were brought on board and the arduous task of writing a definitive business reference guide for the salon and spa industry commenced.

As chapters were completed, we gathered feedback from industry leaders. The comment we heard most often was, "It's a lot to read…there's so much content." That was exactly the response we were looking for. We wanted Fast Forward to be a true reference guide that would offer in-depth solutions to the real issues, problems and frustrations that challenge today's salon and spa owners and managers. Fast Forward has achieved this goal in grand style.

Nancy Flinn has been a true partner on Fast Forward. Her insights and sense of urgency kept the project focused and moving forward. Nancy was "strong" when the project needed her strength, and she was supportive when we needed encouragement.

Our contributing experts were a joy to work with and their generosity must be acknowledged. Andrew Finkelstein, Larry Oskin and Matthew Cross…thank you so much for your energy, knowledge and critical contributions to this important project.

Through it all, no one individual has done more to make Fast Forward a reality than the editor of Strategies, Heather Slater. Her devotion to this project was relentless. Her insights, attention to detail…not to mention the chapters she wrote…gave life and accuracy to Fast Forward. Heather, you came to Strategies right out of college in 1997. Today, you play a vital role in the professional salon/spa industry. You're a cherished friend. Working beside you is an honor. I am so proud of you. Thank you for Fast Forward.

Neil Ducoff

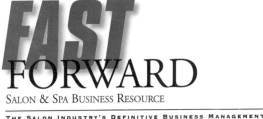

FORWARD

SALON & SPA BUSINESS RESOURCE

THE SALON INDUSTRY'S DEFINITIVE BUSINESS MANAGEMENT
REFERENCE GUIDE FOR OWNERS, MANAGERS AND KEY STAFF

Introduction

BY   NEIL DUCOFF,
PUBLISHER & PRESIDENT
SALON BUSINESS STRATEGIES MAGAZINE

G rowing a salon or day spa today is akin to venturing
through a minefield of historically inefficient business
practices and beliefs. Times have changed. Yesterday's success strategies seem tired and rusty in today's rapid-fire, change-
everything-now business climate.

Simply put, the rules for winning the salon business game have
changed. Commission payrolls have skyrocketed. Staff walkouts
have intensified. Salons talk "teamwork" but staff still cling to the
old "my chair, my client" thinking. Working owners struggle to find
time to meet their management responsibilities. Operating costs

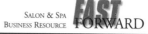
have soared. The labor market has tightened to a point at which many owners are in a scramble for new staff. Many more, lured by the promise of expanded service and gift certificate sales, have invested heavily in day spa expansion…and are finding profits hard to come by.

And the pace of change will only get faster. The labor-intensive and "technically artistic" nature of salons creates a level of management complexity that can challenge even the most experienced business professional. Maintaining consistently high levels of technical execution and quality customer service is a never-ending challenge. Competing for qualified labor while managing payroll costs often translates into an endless quest for the ultimate compensation system. And so goes the business of providing hair, skin, nail and body services — and a bevy of professional products — to the consuming public.

For working owners, growing a dynamic salon business is especially daunting because of the demands placed on their often undeveloped or untested management skills. Every day, working owners with extraordinary technical expertise struggle with the performance, productivity and profitability of their salons. If only they had developed their skills in financial management; cash-flow planning and control; leadership and human relations; marketing, retailing and a host of other critical business skills…But this is the real world, where many working owners and managers are first devoted to their passion: the creative, technical, often *magical*, side of the industry. And their passion not only holds our great industry together, but pushes it forward. Technician or manager, independent owner or franchisee — everyone gets caught up in the wonder, excitement and ever-present madness of salon management.

We wrote FAST FORWARD SALONS & SPAS to offer a comprehensive, friendly, *useable* book to fill the salon business knowledge voids. It speaks the language of business in a style that all individuals responsible for growing a salon business, from those behind the chair to those behind the desk, can learn from.

This book addresses a myriad of business issues and problems confronting today's salon and spa owners, managers, administra-

tors and employees. Readers will discover exciting, no-nonsense…
and easy-to-follow…approaches to salon business. Most importantly, this book will be a reference to which all salon professionals
and business people can turn for fast answers, guidance and insight
into today's real-life salon and day spa growth problems.

Business is a voyage

GET IN TOUCH WITH YOUR SALON'S INHERENT NEEDS. Consider the
exuberance and euphoria of opening day, and the freshness of a
new salon with sparkling equipment and furnishings. As the voyage continues, progress is charted. And as the business and the crew
mature, the voyage may halt at ports of call along the way.

Some salons will settle in at certain stages of the voyage. Perhaps
they're not physically or financially prepared to continue, or perhaps their initial provisions were inadequate. Perhaps they were
unclear on the destination, or simply began questioning their ability to press on. These salons drop anchor; progress stops; the voyage goes on indefinite hold. Leadership gives way to abdication.
The excitement and vision that once captured the crew's imagination fades and their focus shifts to other voyages and opportunities.
As the business stalls, the grip of complacency tightens.
Meanwhile, other brave explorers and competitors press forward to
discover new opportunities and rewards.

The lessons of business success are based on a single tenet:
Forward progress is not an option. A business cannot rest on its lau-
rels, previous achievements or market status. Tom Peters —
forward-thinker, speaker, consultant and author — says it best:
"No longer is it the big eat the small — now the fast eat the slow."
Salons are no exception. You must move your salon business forward or be trampled. *YOU MUST BE FAST.*

Shifting into fast forward

This text may be your map — a pathway through the fog and
confusion of growing a salon business. It may be a collection of
keys to open the doors of productivity, efficiency and performance.
Within these pages, you may discover how to raise the anchor that

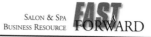
holds you fast to yesterday's achievements at the expense of tomorrow's adventures, opportunities and rewards. (Anchors prevent motion; where there is no motion, there can be no progress.) It may be the catalyst that raises your personal bar of success and challenges you to reach your full potential, igniting the energy and self-confidence to break through the chaos and confusion that are the ever-present partners of change and forward progress.

Where and how quickly your business voyage progresses depends on you. The necessary constant is *knowledge* — a tool kit for navigating a salon and/or day spa business to the highest levels of achievement and success. This text covers a lot of ground on many different fronts, tackling old issues with fresh ideas and strategies. You must put it work. Use it a little, and you'll make a little progress. Use it a lot, and you may travel further and faster than you ever dreamed possible.

We push the envelope of traditional salon business thinking. It's the best of the best.

Exploration and implementation

Your current coordinates on your salon business voyage will determine your pace in implementing the concepts and systems presented here. Just remember, you cannot do it all at once. As you progress, bookmark pages and sections that address problems and/or situations that rank high on your "fix it first" list. When finished, prioritize the list to develop your game plan.

Each chapter contains worksheets to help organize your thoughts and resources.

DO YOU HAVE TO IMPLEMENT EVERYTHING? Absolutely not. FAST FORWARD SALONS & SPAS is a resource guide designed to offer information, strategies, and insight on a vast array of salon and spa business issues, programs and situations. Use what you need. If certain elements intrigue you or seem like a good fit for your business, use the worksheets and chart your progress. You may want to create a comprehensive game plan for implementing a series of strategies over a period of months or years. As always, planning is the foundation for business success. *Don't rush.*

Think outside the box

I have always been entrepreneurial. I have always been intrigued by the inner workings of business and how money is made. I grew up in my parents' dry cleaning business and have been involved in service-based businesses ever since. After college, I explored the opportunities in the beauty salon business and, in 1970, entered Franklin Beauty School. There was never a doubt that I would own a salon. I opened my first in 1973 and a second in 1975.

Those were great times, driven by the precision haircutting boom and the energy of the post-war baby boom generation. Salon retailing also came of age. In those days, if your salon offered great haircuts, blowdrys and curling iron work, you made money. And why not? Rent and overhead expenses were incredibly low compared to today's costs of doing business. There was margin for error. We were having a ton of fun leading the charge and riding the crest of change.

But change is relentless. Just as the wash-and-set salons withered as they clung to yesterday's thinking, modern haircutting salons would also soon feel the challenge of change. The '70s and '80s saw an explosion in salon population. Franchise salons and chains made their presence known. Salons with names like SUPERCUTS, FANTASTIC SAMS and COST CUTTERS offered consumers a value-priced choice. The competitive advantage of precision haircutting was gone. From a service standpoint, salons of this era looked remarkably alike.

But if the '70s and '80s will be remembered as the haircutting boom decades, the '90s will be remembered as the decade of the day spa, from small salon day spas to 15,000 square-foot meccas with 150 staff members. The salon experience now encompasses the total human body — head to toe, inside and out. Salons talk "wellness" and nutrition. Haircutting is now only a piece of the pie.

Today's salon and day spa business environment is complex. The stakes are high, the competition intense. For many independent

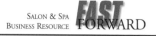
owners, building a true day spa with wet services means "betting the ranch." It's simply the way today's game is played.

But opportunities abound for forward-thinkers — people who regularly think outside the box. These pioneers were the first to invest in point-of-sale computers, pagers and voice mail. They explored and tested new compensation programs and raised the definition of salon professionalism by instituting no-tipping policies. They departmentalized, and moved busy telephone centers away from the front desk and into dedicated booking rooms. Some multi-salon chains are exploring off-site booking centers where one primary database houses all pertinent information (e.g., appointments, client service histories), and serves all locations. Forward-thinkers not only embrace change, they seek it.

Read and explore this book as a forward-thinker. Don't lock yourself into "what is" while unlimited opportunities are waiting to be seized. Don't hesitate. Don't fear the natural progression of business change. Shift your business thinking into fast forward. Absorb the knowledge, data and systems contained in these pages. Challenge yourself. Take your business, and your team, to that next level of business, professional and personal success.

Now it's time to cast off the docklines,
and begin your business voyage.

We're here to help you along the way.

FAST FORWARD Advisory Board

Thank you to the following industry leaders who provided valuable feedback during this endeavor.

Peter DeCaprio
NOËLLE, THE DAY SPA

Gordon Miller
NATIONAL COSMETOLOGY ASSOC.

Debbie Elliott
DEBBIE ELLIOTT SALON & DAY SPA

Edwin Neill
NEILL CORPORATION

Jill Kohler
THE SALON ASSOCIATION

Leo Passage
PIVOT POINT INT'L, INC.

Karen McRann
J GORDON DESIGNS, LTD.

Catherine Renaud
SOFTWARE CREATIONS, INC.

Dennis Marquez
PIZZAZZ HAIR DESIGN

Bob Zupko
ROBERT ANDREW DAYSPA SALON

Max Matteson
SALON ENTERPRISES;
COSMETOLOGY ADVANCEMENT
FOUNDATION

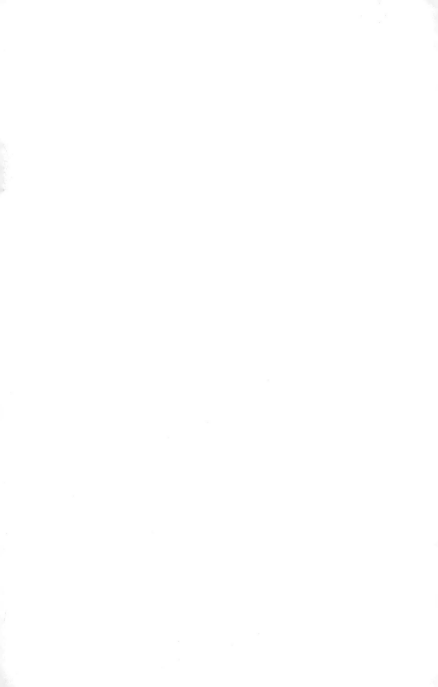

U.S. SALON AND SPA TRENDS

SPECIAL CHAPTER BY:
Nancy Flinn, President
NANCY FLINN MARKETING RESOURCES, INC.

The growth potential of American salons is linked to the demographics of their clientele and the disposable income allowed by the economy. These two factors — further refined by a salon's geographic location, and the lifestyle and psychographic profile of its customers — are a measure of consumer willingness to move beyond traditional services such as hair styling, and create new service and retail sales categories for salons.

Today, consumer confusion about what a salon could or should be limits the potential for growth. To address this customer confusion in the coming decade, we must develop *standards* concerning activity and service expectations…and better define the role of the beauty salon, spa and day spa within the industry.

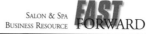
Currently, a majority of salons focus on hair, though segments of the industry are developing skincare, nailcare and other service categories. We are seeing the development of specialty outlets where haircare is a minor service element, if it exists at all. And the salon environment is evolving toward a more personal and caring attitude, with greater service expertise and retail orientation.

Enter: The millennium

The beauty industry is built on style, and style is ever-changing, created as individuals react to an environment in flux. The major salon trends in our current environment will serve as the basis of style for the next generation. They derive from a groundswell that emerged in the recent past: an emphasis on health (of the body and the planet) as the major determinant of physical style; a growing diversity of voices and ideas; and the creation of wealth that fuels the drive for new forms and formulations. These three drivers provide the raw material which energetic and creative salon owners will use to catapult a new kind of style into existence.

As you read the next pages, keep these ideas in mind. They are the determiners of what we are becoming.

A still burgeoning economy

GROWING CONSUMER SOPHISTICATION AND EDUCATION: Demand will grow for higher quality goods, with obvious differentiating qualities. Segmentation and specialization are key, especially as grooming needs are seen as part of the emphasis on health. Products for this group will be touted as "good for me" *and* "good for the environment."

POLARIZATION OF BEAUTY SPENDING: Mid-price brands will suffer as the market regroups around both ends of the spectrum: high-quality premium products and lower-priced private label brands. This polarization will be seen in increased sales of premium products through salons, and of price brands through trade class alternatives such as price clubs and discounters.

Look for an exaggerated separation of the utilitarian versus the cosmetic, and a value-added role for service or consultation efforts.

Women will be willing to pay more for differentiated products which promise superior image or performance.

The new clientele

- AN INCREASING NUMBER OF WOMEN IN THE WORKPLACE, AND DUAL-INCOME HOUSEHOLDS…This market is driven by simplification: the need for added convenience, and lower stress and pressure. *Kids* and *teens* will take on more buying power.
- AN AGING POPULATION…There is huge demand for products and services that help maintain a healthier, fitter and younger appearance of hair, face and body.
- AN INCREASING MALE MARKET…This market is led by younger men for whom personal care is a necessity. Brand positioning and performance claims will focus on male care, including skincare and overall appearance. As they spend more time in salons, men are more likely to buy their own haircare products.
- *Skincare, nailcare and cosmetics will grow if salons make the required environmental and retailing commitments. The consumer has many choices in beauty retailing.*

Product and demographic trends

Changes in American culture are reflected in the demands of haircare consumers. Salon owners must recognize these trends and be prepared to take advantage of them in order to develop their customer base and product mix. The following checklist of societal changes explains how they will affect salon customers, as well as their implications for retail and service businesses.

- MULTI-CULTURALISM AND THE GROWTH OF THE CULTURAL MARKET: Customers are looking for hair formulations specific to their own type of hair — Asian, Latin and African-American — and for stylists skilled with their unique hair type and cultural stylings. Stylists must therefore be knowledgeable about specific haircare needs and regimens.
- FURTHER PRODUCT DIFFERENTIATION: Customers will have higher performance expectations. Technology will lead to product differentiation.

- MARKET GLOBALIZATION: There is a new awareness of products worldwide, and new global brands are developing, along with multi-language packaging. Ingredients are more exotic, drawn from around the world. The growth potential for beauty services and retailing in the U.S. will attract manufacturers from around the world, and result in new opportunities for salons and spas.

- ADDING INDIVIDUALITY: This is the key variable in defining a salon "signature look" for clients. Individuality makes a personal statement and creates an image.

The salon and spa universe: Who, what, where

It's important to understand the salon world…and to know your own place in it.

The salon is the core of the professional beauty industry. Progressive salons and spas study their own market share…as well as observe competitors to ascertain specific benefits their own salons provide, and to measure how their services, pricing and image compare with those in their own geographic base.

Salon owners and the suppliers that serve them need to better understand their potential. By examining their client base and its disposable income, owners can determine how best to reach their customers in order to improve revenues and achieve financial growth. But first, one must look at the demographics of salons and spas themselves, including their size and who works in them.

An overview of the universe

One instructive way to analyze the salon industry, and a particular salon's place in it, is to look at a breakdown of the industry by size. To do this, the employee categories in SALONLINK™ (developed using 1999 DUN & BRADSTREET business activity data) were broken into seven tiers:

- TIER 1: Salons with 15 or more employees…3.7%.
- TIER 2: Salons with 10–14 employees…4.9%.
- TIER 3: Salons with 7–9 employees…5.3%.
- TIER 4: Salons with 4–6 employees…18%.
- TIER 5: Salons with 3 employees…10.4%.
- TIER 6: Salons with 2 employees represent 20% of all salons.
- TIER 7: Individual shop owners…37.7%.

Analysis of salon size by revenue shows that about 70% of salon volume is produced by 30% of the outlets.

These seven tiers were then refined into two groups for comparative purposes in a Multi-sponsor Survey. Larger salons, with four or more operators/employees (31.9%), were compared to salons with three or fewer (68.1%). They were studied together and separately, to compare and contrast their approach to business.

Larger salons are likely to offer more services and retail items. (For example: Almost twice as many offer color cosmetics and skincare products as their smaller counterparts.) Additionally, larger salons are more likely to buy the majority of goods from full-service distributors or directly from the manufacturer, while smaller ones tend to buy through cash-and-carry outlets or mail order, as well as distributors.

How many employees?

- One full-timer: 30% of salons.
- One part-timer: 15% of salons.

- Two full-timers: 20%.
- Two part-timers: 10%.

- Three full-timers: 10%.
- Three part-timers: 6%.

- Four to five full-timers: 17%.
- Four to five part-timers: 4%.

- Six to nine full-timers: 10%.
- Six to nine part-timers: 2%.

- Ten or more full-timers: 8%.
- Ten or more part-timers: 2%.

- Curiously, 4% of salons said they had no full-time employees, and 59% had no part-timers.

Employees and independents

There are about 1,400,000 practicing cosmetologists in the U.S., and 60% say they work full-time. However, not all cosmetologists are employed by their workplaces. One major industry trend is booth rental within a salon. States with the highest number of independent contractors are…

- 76%–90%: Alaska, Arizona, California, Hawaii, Idaho, Kentucky, Montana, New Hampshire, New Mexico, Nevada, Ohio, Oklahoma, Oregon, Texas, Utah, Vermont, West Virginia.
- 51%–75%: Colorado, Georgia, Iowa, Kansas, Minnesota, North Carolina, North Dakota, Nebraska, South Carolina, South Dakota, Virginia, Wyoming.
- 26%–50%: Alabama, Arkansas, Florida, Louisiana, Mississippi, Tennessee, Washington.
- 5%–25%: Connecticut, Illinois, Indiana, Michigan, New York, Wisconsin.
- Less than 5%: Delaware, District of Columbia, Maine, Maryland, Massachusetts, New Jersey, Pennsylvania, Rhode Island.

Salons can be of any size, one-chair or huge establishments, and the professionals that staff them can either be independent contractors or on a payroll. But the key to success for any salon is that its staff serve customers well, and provide the retail goods and services consumers expect to find in a "modern" salon. Currently, there are over 240,000 salon outlets in the U.S.

The chains of industry

The leading salon chains account for about 15,000 outlets of the total SALONLINK™ database…which means an estimated 6% of total salon outlets are chains. Most commonly, a chain is identified as an entity having five or more locations with a common name designation. However, there is a growing segment of smaller chains with two to four locations.

It is estimated (though there is no hard data on this estimate) that chain salon revenues per outlet roughly double the value of their count, due to the fact that they tend to have larger locations with more traffic. Additionally, the service and retail focus of chains which do not offer chemical services (or who are positioning for low-price haircuts) dramatically affects their relative importance.

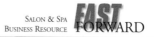
Whom salons and spas serve...and how

Understanding its customers and their needs is the only way for a salon to grow...and control the future.

Given the fact that clients are the lifeblood of salons and spas, it is important to know the clientele they serve, and to be aware of demographic changes that could affect the customer mix. The first step in increasing your client base is to understand your current patrons. Unfortunately, the Multi-sponsor Surveys/Gallup Survey found that many salons — some 28% — were not sure how many clients they served in an average week. However:

- 19% of respondents saw 200 or more.
- 15% saw 100–199.
- 7% saw 61–99.
- 12% saw 41–60.
- 12% saw 21–40.
- 7% saw 20 or fewer.

The Multi-sponsor Surveys/Gallup Survey pegged the average: 144.

Baby Boomers

The American population is aging. This trend, led by the Baby Boomers, will directly impact many salon services, as well as the emergence of spa services. For example: 37% of those aged 50–64 (and 49% of those aged 65 and older) are plagued by thinning hair.

The aging population will provide an opportunity for salons to gain business by spotlighting services such as haircolor and perms; care for aging skin and facial hair removal; and scalp and hair growth consultations and treatments.

Women at the forefront

According to the Census Bureau, the female population as a group is aging. The bureau predicts an overall increase (9.4% from 1998–2010) in women over age eighteen.

Women made an estimated 901 million trips to the beauty salon in 1998, according to the Multi-sponsor Surveys/Gallup Survey, and that number is expected to grow by roughly *125 million* visits over the next twelve years — zooming to over a billion trips per year. Fifty-two percent of the 901 million visits in 1998 were by women aged fifty and over, and the survey estimates that percentage will increase to fifty-seven by 2010. Women of this age are currently salons' most committed customer base, averaging *ten or more* visits per year. The challenge salons currently face is to get the daughters and sons of these women to increase their visits as well.

Making men comfortable

The male market is another customer demographic to focus on. Men are now taking a more active interest in their appearance, and are increasingly turning to hair stylists rather than to barbers for styling and grooming advice and services. The per-visit value of male clients is significantly less than the average multi-service female customer, but they visit more frequently and are proving more susceptible to retail purchases.

As would be expected, younger men are more likely than older ones to visit a stylist. In this demographic, youth rules. While 6% of salons in the Multi-sponsor Surveys/Gallup Survey had only female clients, and 12% had under 10% of male clients, some 25% of salon patrons overall last year were men. What's more, men who visit salons are likely to keep doing so if salons:

- make them feel welcome and comfortable by recognizing the male difference.
- acquaint them with the full range of services available to them.
- offer expert advice about their hair that they did not get from their barbers.

The growing ethnic market

In the current Multi-sponsor Surveys/Gallup Survey, 80% of clients were recorded as white; 9% African-American; 4% Hispanic; 6% other races; and one percent of salon visitors were not differentiated as to race. Those numbers, if they mirror the general population, are expected to change. There is a clear opportunity to staff salons with multi-cultural employees, and serve the beauty needs of a global community.

For example: The urban ethnic market is burgeoning, and shows enormous growth potential. These statistics cannot be overlooked when planning for future client growth.

Consider these U.S. population statistics gathered (and projected) by SEGMENTED MARKETING SERVICES, INC. (SMSi):

■ 1990…
   76%…109 million white residents
   12%…29 million African-Americans
   9%…21 million Hispanics
   3%…7 million Asians

■ 2000…
   72%…198 million white residents
   13%…34 million African-Americans
   11%…31 million Hispanics
   4%…11 million Asians

■ 2020…
   64%…208 million white residents
   13%…42 million African-Americans
   16%…51 million Hispanics
   7%…21 million Asians

■ 2050…
   53%…206 million white residents
   14%…56 million African-Americans
   23%…88 million Hispanics
   10%…38 million Asians

Services demanded by ethnic groups (varying by specific hair requirements) in order of popularity are cutting; coloring; styling; perming and texturizing; hair relaxing; hair treatments; hair removal; nail care; braiding; hair extensions; and pedicures.

Salon and spa services

I t stands to reason that haircuts and hair styling are the reasons most customers flock to traditional salons. In fact, a study by Multi-sponsor Surveys/Gallup Survey found that they remain the most popular services offered, and are available at 97% of salons surveyed. Other services offered include:

- Haircolor: 95%. It is in high demand, and gaining popularity every day. Women who color their hair are almost evenly divided between "do-it-yourselfers" (45%) and those seeking the professional touch (41%), while the remainder do both, depending on the circumstances. Fifty percent of adult women (aged eighteen and older) in the U.S. now use haircolor.
- Permanent waves: 93%. Though they are decreasing in popularity, they are still a cornerstone of the salon industry.
- Hair relaxing and straightening: 68%. This is a service boom for both the general and ethnic markets.
- Hair and scalp treatments and massage — desired by clients looking for a little pampering — are offered by 61%.
- Depilatory work: 54%.
- Manicures and nail treatments: 54%.
- Treatments for thinning hair: 48%.
- Pedicures: 37%.
- Makeup: 33%.
- Tanning services: 18%.

Clearly, customers are merging the need for basic grooming services with a desire to look good, and feel good about themselves…and they are becoming more willing to ask a salon professional for help.

How customers spend their money

Nancy Flinn Marketing Resources (NFMR) studied the salon service dollar, and generated a breakdown of the way consumers have spent money in salons during recent years. The study found

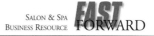
that, in 1997, hair cutting and styling accounted for 43% of the salon service dollar. This changed little in 1998. However, haircolor rose in that period from a little under 18% to an estimated 19.3%. Perming and relaxing services declined from 18% to an estimated 15% of the salon service dollar, reflecting a trend to more natural styles. The nailcare percentage stayed even at 8%, retail sales went from 7% to over 8%, and skincare stayed even at 4%.

In totality, service dollars rose from an average of $41.90 per visit to an estimated $43.50. Clearly, customers are spending more — and expecting more for their hard-earned money. It's up to the savvy salon to provide what they want in hair and spa services, and in product.

Spa services rule

Another growing trend is customers' desire for spa services from their salons. Salons are showing no hesitation in providing them, but there is inconsistency in performance standards…and in which services or type of environment defines a spa versus a salon providing skin or other spa services.

But one thing is clear: *The salon is becoming the place customers go for more than just a hair cut and styling.* In response, salons plan to add still more spa services.

Understanding the required environmental conditions of a "spa," and how it relates to an average or above average hair salon, is key to attracting or upgrading consumers to a spa experience.

Enhancing the spa experience

Consumers are looking for health, beauty and relaxation in more and more places.

Though there is much less information available on this business segment than on traditional salons, spas are definitely taking off. They are in fact booming.

An outlook at spas

A special component of the Multi-sponsor Surveys/Gallup Survey studied 1000 consumers and 300 salons and spas to determine the future of the salon and spa, and who the customer will be. The poll of day spas found that 41% operate within or as part of a hair salon; 32% are independent; and the rest are in hotels or resorts, fitness centers or medical facilities.

Twenty-five percent of customer respondents have been to a spa: 19% of males, and 31% of females. But the *kinds* of spas visited are important. Sixty percent have been to fitness centers or health clubs, and 30% to the salon spa (45% of women and, unfortunately, only 6% of men).

Who goes to spas

According to the Multi-sponsor Surveys/Gallup Survey, the most likely demographic profile of a spa visitor is:

- women.
- persons 25–34 years old.
- Westerners.
- dieters.
- regular exercisers.
- those who devote time to their appearance.
- those who are proactive about wellness.

Sometimes this proactivity in spa-goers is a result of health problems such as physical pain, stress, anxiety, obesity, skin problems, arthritis and depression. This suggests the mature market as a natural one for spas…if health enhancement services are marketed correctly.

What's more, one in three spa-goers visits the spa at least every six months or more. Women are more likely to visit frequently, and indicate a preference for visiting spas in salons and fitness centers. They gravitate to places where they can relax and indulge. Men, however, prefer fitness centers and health clubs — in keeping with their emphasis on physical health and enhancement.

Salon and spa buying and retail selling

…what salons are buying for use and for retail, who they buy it from, and what it means to the bottom line.

An essential element of a successful salon is *product selection:* for use in the salon and to be sold as retail. Taken as a whole, the salon universe's product purchases can tell us a lot about what salons today are doing, and what customers want from them.

What salons buy

In 1999, the salon industry purchased 2.764 billion manufacturer factory dollars in measured categories goods. *(This figure was developed in conjunction with the American Beauty Association, the organization of professional beauty manufacturers and manufacturer representatives.)* Nearly sixty-eight percent (67.5%), or $1.867 billion, was spent on haircare products, according to NFMR. This figure is approximately one percent less than in 1998.

About 60% of hair products purchased are used within the salon, while 40% are retailed.

What salons sell now

Retail sales are vital to a salon's bottom line and growth potential. Recently, according to NFMR, retail grew from about 7% of the client's bill to over 8%. *This is a market worth pursuing through education and staff incentives.*

Currently, the largest part of the client's retail shopping bag is filled with haircare products. But to augment these sales, salons also sell other items. The most popular are styling tools such as combs and brushes (offered by 62% of salons), and products for treating and re-growing thinning hair (offered by 44% of salons). Nailcare products are sold by 40%; skincare products by 33%; and bath and bodycare products by 29%. Color cosmetics are sold at only 24% of salons, and fragrances at 15%.

What salons plan to sell

Salons in general plan to sell new categories of products, such as nail-, skin- and bathcare; fragrances; color cosmetics; styling tools; and products for thinning hair. And 22% of those surveyed plan to add more than one product line. Enhanced manufacturer relationships are helping salons develop retail opportunities.

Salons must look into improving retail sales through innovative merchandising and client education.

Becoming a better retailer

A majority of salons and spas report retail growth due to the wider array of products now available, and most find customers more willing to listen to salon recommendations. In fact, almost three-fourths of initial purchases are based on salon suggestions.

Salons which have trouble retailing attribute it to:
- stylists' reluctance to sell aggressively, or even recommend.
- competitors selling salon products, confusing consumer loyalty.
- customer perception that salon products are more costly.
- clientele are more informed and more demanding.
- mass-marketed haircare is improving, and offering products with professional characteristics.

There *are* ways to overcome these problems: According to the Multi-sponsor Surveys/Gallup Survey, salons must *distinguish* their products in order to compete with non-salon retailers.

Why consumers buy from salons

Salons not only sell products…they also sell the knowledge and expert guidance to help customers buy product for each unique situation, and *use it* to the best advantage. The professional recommendation is the foundation of the relationship with those consumers who value the salon relationship.

CURRENTLY, MOST SALON RETAIL PURCHASES ARE MADE BY WOMEN…
- aged 18–49.
- working full-time.
- who are affluent or college-educated.

THE WOMEN'S MARKET CAN BE BROKEN INTO MAJOR "CONSUMER ATTI-
TUDE SEGMENTS":

- Salon product advocates (6%).
- Forget me's (18%).
- Salon avoiders (22%).
- Cost-conscious salon enthusiasts (34%).
- About 20% of the market, "salon devotees," should be targeted to become better salon retail and service purchasers.

THESE SALON DEVOTEES HAVE THE FOLLOWING ATTRIBUTES:

- They rely on their stylists for advice.
- Their time in a salon is enjoyable, making them feel pampered.
- They like to treat themselves to premium products and experiences.
- They like natural or herbal ingredients.
- They believe salon products are superior.
- They average forty-seven years of age.

Natural product trends

Today's burgeoning interest in herbs, aromatherapy and botanical beauty products is part of the customers' proactive stance toward health, wellness and the environment. Use of herbals and aromatherapy has risen in recent years. And they are a "natural" sell for salons, since they can compete with specialty stores and mass outlets. But the salon which goes in this direction should make sure its overall ambience matches the spirit of the natural lifestyle — with sounds, scents and textures to make clients feel a *visit* is a true *experience.*

Salons should target loyal customers

These patrons trust stylists' advice. Indeed, salons have the greatest retail success by selling the same products they use on clients. It stands to reason that the more services you offer, the more kinds of products you will use and, therefore, the more you are likely to sell. (*Tips for one-to-one selling are in chapter 8. Techniques for calculating inventory turns can be found in chapter 9.*)

Where salons buy

Overall, salon owners are evaluating products more thoroughly before committing, and are becoming more assertive in sharing their needs and wishes with distributors and manufacturers. They are also working harder at retailing: creating displays, educating stylists, conducting product promotions and focusing on solving customer problems in order to create new opportunities.

Salons tend to buy product from full-service distributors (76%) and cash-and-carry chains affiliated with distributors (51%). Some 43% have bought directly from the manufacturer at some time, and 35% choose mail order. Finally, 34% use independent cash-and-carry sources for some products.

But no matter where salons get their supplies, it is important for them to get on the retail bandwagon. *Customers are looking for guidance in product selection, and expertise from people they trust.*

Salons: Which brands they prefer

According to an A.C. NIELSEN'S MARKET DECISIONS study, the top haircare product manufacturers entering 2000 were:

All major haircare categories overall (in alphabetical order):

AVEDA
MATRIX
PAUL MITCHELL
REDKEN
SEBASTIAN

The top lines in salon volume, by category:

Based on equivalent unit calculations of a national salon panel of representative hair salons with three or more employees/staff.

SHAMPOOS

Products	Distribution
AVEDA	GRAHAM WEBB
GRAHAM WEBB	MATRIX
MATRIX	PAUL MITCHELL
PAUL MITCHELL	NEXXUS
REDKEN	REDKEN

CONDITIONERS

Products	Distribution
AVEDA	GRAHAM WEBB
GRAHAM WEBB	MATRIX
MATRIX	PAUL MITCHELL
PAUL MITCHELL	NEXXUS
REDKEN	REDKEN

HAIR SPRAYS

Products	Distribution
AVEDA	MATRIX
MATRIX	PAUL MITCHELL
PAUL MITCHELL	NEXXUS
REDKEN	REDKEN
SEBASTIAN	SEBASTIAN

STYLING AIDS

Products	Distribution
AVEDA	MATRIX
MATRIX	PAUL MITCHELL
PAUL MITCHELL	NEXXUS
REDKEN	REDKEN
TONI & GUY	SEBASTIAN

PERMANENTS/RELAXERS/STRAIGHTENERS

Products	Distribution
ZOTOS	ZOTOS
MATRIX	MATRIX
REDKEN	REDKEN
REVLON	REVLON
TRESSA	GOLDWELL

HAIRCOLOR

Products	Distribution
CLAIROL	CLAIROL
GOLDWELL	L'OREAL
MATRIX	MATRIX
REDKEN	REDKEN
WELLA	WELLA

.

Data sources: 1999 NFMR, A.C. NIELSEN/MARKET DECISIONS, MULTI-SPONSOR SURVEYS

TECHNOLOGY

How fast do you want to go?

The wonders of technology surround us. Orthoscopic surgery has transformed many major surgical procedures with long recuperative periods into out-patient visits and minor inconveniences. On many air flights, LCD monitors are used to show safety instructions and videos while passengers watch DVD movies on laptop computers and plot driving directions on palmtops. Cell phones and beepers abound. Consumer shopping on the internet is now a cause of concern for major department stores and retailers. All it takes is a short power outage to remind us just how much we rely on technology.

In the workplace, the magic of technology is the driving force of change. From communications and data storage to task processing and information reporting, technology allows us to move faster by dramatically increasing efficiency and productivity. A good example is the way in which e-mail has transformed written communications on a level far exceeding the one-time magic of the fax machine. Another is the simple but indispensible credit card processing machine which, with one swipe and a couple of key strokes, processes a charge, retrieves authorization and prints a receipt.

Personal computers continue to be the benchmark for technological change. It wasn't so long ago that a 286 processor running at eight megahertz with 640k of RAM and a 20 megabyte hard drive was state-of-the-art. Today, a 450–500 megahertz processor with 128 meg of RAM and an eight gigabyte hard drive is not only commonplace, but almost a necessity. And the new hot-rod computer you buy today will be out-gunned by an even faster and less expensive one tomorrow.

Technological advances cannot be ignored or underestimated. You either lead the charge or keep pace with the pack. If you settle for anything less, you will be stomped by competitors who do it faster and more efficiently using less time, money and resources.

Technology in salons and spas

As in all other industries, technology is shaping the way salons and day spas conduct business. Driven by the need for maximum efficiency and speed, forward-thinking salon and day spa owners are jumping on the technology bandwagon and reaping big rewards. The three primary areas in which technology shines in salons are *data capture, communications* and *productivity enhancement.*

1. Data capture

Like all service-based businesses, salons generate mountains of vital data that must be processed, retained and regularly evaluated.

THE CUSTOMER DATABASE IS MOST IMPORTANT. In this age of one-to-one relationships, instant access to individual client data is no longer an option — it's a necessity. To fill client needs at a level that far exceeds traditional thinking, salons

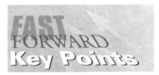

In this age of one-to-one relationships, instant access to individual client data is no longer an option — it's a necessity.

must retain every bit of personal information gathered from clients. This information should reside in a centralized database which will enable each team member to become as knowledgeable as the next on client histories, buying patterns and preferences. *(We'll discuss the concept of one-to-one relationships in chapter 11.)*

Traditional salon thinking often revolves around personal request rates and followings. Yet, this business design prevents the flow of client information into a centralized database that can be shared by the entire team. CONSIDER THIS: When you visit a RITZ-CARLTON Hotel and request a "no tuck" on your bed sheets and a fluffy pillow, this personal preference data is entered into your customer file in the company database. The next time you visit any RITZ-CARLTON, you will automatically get your "no tuck" and fluffy pillow. Never underestimate the power of an information-rich customer database.

Performance monitoring and reporting is another area in which technology shines. In addition to customer preference data, computers can store employee performance data. This includes sales in all service and retail departments and categories, and reaches right down to individual performance. Average service and retail ticket, productivity and client retention rates, percentage each service represents of total sales, and gift certificates sold and redeemed are a handful of the reports and performance statistics technology can provide the astute salon business owner. Performance data is the basis for all business growth decisions.

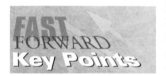

FAST FORWARD Key Points

Performance data is the basis for all business growth decisions.
Accounting and financial software like One-Write Plus, Peachtree and QuickBooks Pro provide instant access to key business information.

Nothing collects and crunches numbers like a computer. Today's point-of-sale software provides almost instant access to all manner of client and employee data. And accounting software such as One-Write Plus, Peachtree and QuickBooks Pro provides instant access to key business information — so much so that the historical dependence on accountants for financial statements is all but gone. With in-house accounting software, owners can run financial statements and reports at the push of a button. Waiting weeks or months for an accountant to process your financials is unnecessary with today's technology.

2. Communications

The internet and World Wide Web can bring new sophistication to both internal and external salon communications. Salons are eagerly exploring and testing web sites for marketing, product sales and appointment scheduling. Breakthroughs in web technology are fast and furious, and there are many possibilities for salons and day spas.

E-mail is lightning-fast and amazingly affordable for all manner of communication. You're missing an opportunity if your salon is not aggressively collecting and adding client e-mail addresses to their personal data records in your computer. Imagine e-mailing your *entire client base* to announce the opening of an expanded day spa facility. The message, complete with special incentive offers, can be delivered in seconds and costs only pennies. E-mail can also confirm appointments quickly and inexpensively.

Phone system capabilities that were once the luxury of large corporations are now available to salons and other small businesses. Sophisticated voice mail eliminates interruptions and message-taking. Menu-driven electronic operators answer phones and direct calls to bookers, information boxes (e.g., for directions to the salon) or service menus. Even message-on-hold offers marketing opportunities.

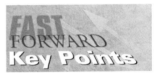

You're missing an opportunity if your salon is not aggressively collecting and adding client e-mail addresses to their personal data records in your computer.

3. Productivity

A major benefit of technology is its positive impact on productivity. Automated front desks and booking rooms have streamlined salon operations to a point at which some are now completely paperless. All tickets, work schedules and client records are automated. The efficiency of the paper appointment book pales beside today's high-powered software, which can book complex days of beauty in seconds. End-of-day closeouts are push-button fast. Even internal paging systems, allowing quick and efficient communication with team members in various departments, can be incorporated into some systems.

Phone systems that organize, sell and inform

Today's phone systems are true marvels of technology. They transmit all forms of communication, from voice, fax and e-mail to data files, pictures and video. Just a few years ago, most salons were happy with a multi-line phone system with "hold" and intercom capabilities. Today, there is a seemingly unquenchable thirst for features and options. And as technology speeds forward, mass distribution drives the cost of once-exotic features into a range affordable for small businesses.

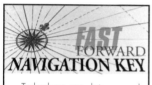

FAST FORWARD NAVIGATION KEY

Technology can bring speed, efficiency, cost-effectiveness and high impact to your salon business. Don't fear technology.

Look for areas in which technology can make your business run smoother and faster, with better use of resources. Use technology to work smarter, not harder.

Full-featured phone systems which include electronic answering, programmable greetings and directories (i.e., press "one" to make an appointment, "two" to purchase a gift certificate), voice mail for all employees, music-on-hold, credit card capture, even customer survey capabilities — are available for around $5,000 to $6,000, depending on the number of phone units required. According to Peter Baron, president of STEVENS COMMUNICATIONS, a Connecticut-based data communications systems reseller and installer for COMDIAL, "Any data device that connects to or works through a computer can be integrated into an affordable phone system." Excellent systems are available from AT&T, COMDIAL, NEC, LUCENT TECHNOLOGIES and other well-known suppliers.

The magic of these powerful and compact phone systems is the computers that drive them. They utilize sophisticated communications software, and can easily be programmed to answer all incoming lines and offer callers a directory of options. Voice mailboxes, greetings and other interactive options are all controlled by the computer. How can these features work for your salon?

Automated answering and interactive directories

As much as many people prefer to hear a real human being answer the phone, automated answering is a standard in the business world. The reason is simple: It's efficient and cost-effective. Automated answering and interactive directories allow callers to access the information, departments or people they want without the added payroll expense of operators or receptionists.

Some of the ways automated answering and interactive directories can streamline your salon or spa:

■ A professionally recorded directory eliminates common inconsistencies in client greetings (e.g., miscues or rushed hellos). Many companies specialize in writing and recording automated phone greetings. Professionally recorded directories start at approximately $175; the final price depends on length and complexity. Local radio disc jockeys (with those wonderful voices) are finding this service a new source of revenue.

■ The salon's main greeting can offer callers an interactive directory of the business and its services. They may select from options including booking an appointment, canceling an existing appointment, purchasing gift certificates or retail products, receiving directions to the salon, hearing a list of services and hours of operation, or accessing the staff directory. With automated directories, callers get to what they want quickly. The directory must be well-designed and clearly communicated. Frequent callers can quickly bypass the main menu by directly dialing the department or extension they desire.

■ Callers equate automated phone systems and directories with sophisticated businesses. Given this, your phone system can be a valuable image-enhancing tool.

Salon and spa information

Use the salon's directory and sub-directories to provide clients, especially first-time callers, a comprehensive overview of its services, products and capabilities via a consistent and controlled medium. New service, product or equipment introductions are easily accomplished through simple directory updates.

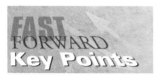

How many times has a client called on a busy Saturday for directions to the salon, when the front desk staff is working on the edge of chaos? "One moment please, I'll put you through to our directions extension. If you need further assistance, simply press 114." Directions will be accurate every time without human intervention or payroll cost.

BE CREATIVE: Showcase a different staff member each month, or dedicate an automated extension to special events or in-salon clinics for clients. Putting an automated phone system to work will build salon sales simply by informing clients of what the business has to offer.

Voice mail

Nothing interferes with staff productivity and the flow of business more than phone interruptions. Non-essential calls from family, friends, wives, husbands, significant others, kids, salespeople, telemarketers — you name it — can be distracting and a huge time-waster. And pulling staff away from paying clients for such calls is the biggest "no, no" of them all. Voice mail is the technological solution.

Imagine the simplicity and speed an automated phone system with voice mail could bring to a salon front desk, booking room or office: "I'm sorry, Matthew is with a client at this time. May I put you through to his voice mail?" The deluge of non-essential personal phone calls would be neatly and efficiently processed. To retrieve calls, a team member simply dials into the assigned voice mailbox.

An entry-level automated phone system with voice mail capabilities typically includes twenty-five voice mailboxes, and is upgradeable in increments of fifty mailboxes. (This is accomplished by upgrading the software which runs the system's automated programs.) Upgrades for many popular systems, such as those from COMDIAL, cost about $1,000.

Message-on-hold

One of the most logical features to add to your phone system is message-on-hold. For only a few hundred dollars, this feature can be added to most existing systems.

The *Bogen ProHold* is one of the more popular and easy-to-use units. The user simply inserts a standard audio cassette containing a pre-recorded "hold" message into the unit, which then creates a digitized copy. This copy is played back whenever a caller is placed on hold. To change the message, re-record and change the cassette.

The new marketing and image-building opportunities are as broad as your imagination. Professionals who specialize in message-on-hold recordings suggest 10- to 20-second messages separated by five seconds of music which complements the salon's image. Expect to pay $175 or more per recording. Again, it's worth contacting local disc jockeys to record your message.

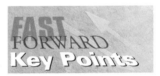

Marketing pros never miss an opportunity to sell. Message-on-hold is an efficient and highly flexible marketing tool that will pay for itself quickly.

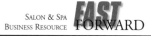
Internal paging systems

One result of the explosive growth of large salons and day spas is an increased need for efficient internal communications. Internal paging systems are a terrific solution.

Already in wide use at high-traffic restaurants which need to quickly contact customers waiting to be seated, internal paging systems offer salons a great way to communicate with staff. With the touch of a button, spa technicians can be advised that clients are checked in and ready to leave the reception area, or a stylist advised that a color client is ready for her haircut. Using a selection of alpha-numeric codes, or simple vibrations, these systems can eliminate the time and expense required to search out and communicate basic information one-to-one with staff.

Paging systems have become integral components of many salon and day spa operations. For example: With nearly sixty people on staff, Bob Steele of Bob Steele Hairdressers in Atlanta, GA, finds his paging system invaluable. The front desk staff can immediately notify a stylist located anywhere within a mile of the premises that her client has arrived. It's a simple and economical option for finding a needed technician, even though she may be anywhere within the 5,600 square-foot salon — or next door having a late lunch.

Bob Steele Hairdressers has also developed a code system to designate in which capacity a technician is needed. A stylist whose client has just arrived will receive code "0"; a stylist whose *new* client has just arrived will receive code "1." There are ten codes in all, including bang trim requests, schedule changes, and calls and messages waiting at the front desk. Every team member at the salon has his or her own voice mailbox, which clients, family and friends may access directly.

What do these goodies cost? It depends on the features. A basic pager can rent or lease for as little as $10 per month. Then there are the "top of the line" systems, such as Motorola's *Tracker,* which commands a considerable initial investment. The *Tracker's* base station costs about $3,500 and pagers start at around $220 each.

Though start-up costs can be intimidating, the advantage in buying outright is that the system will pay for itself in a few years, which may be better than the salon making perpetual payments.

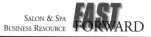
Computer systems and software

P erhaps the most universal fear, shared by people from all walks of life and at all levels of business, is the fear of things unknown. But the belief that a lack of knowledge on a subject equates to a lack of ability to acquire that knowledge is fallacious. Beyond the excuses offered by salon owners who feel that their artistic license trumps the need for technological and operational procedure, there is the need to relentlessly pursue every avenue that presents an opportunity for business growth. In today's business climate, it is impossible to grow without a computer. Clients' demand for prompt, uninterrupted service has set the service bar. How well your salon scores is up to you.

Computers are meant to do more than gather dust at a cluttered front desk. Their impact on salons will be enormous, measured not only in hours saved on routine paperwork and record-keeping matters, but also in the salon's overall efficiency rating, including productivity levels and inventory control. Benchmarks such as clients' service and retail histories, technicians' schedules, client appointments, inventory turns, retention and attrition numbers — and a host of other items — may be recalled with a few simple keystrokes. The introduction of the computer into the salon environment also signals the demise of paper appointment books and half-erased, illegible etchings of client names. Control of both client and staff schedules is centralized at the front desk, at the fingertips of the coordinator.

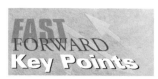

Key Points

A good computer system responds to every scenario, capturing information at the time events occur. Salons are complex by nature, and the time to capture information is at the time it occurs.

Taking your salon to "the next level" — introducing growth strategies solidly rooted in objective performance criteria — can only happen when management is organized and information is easily accessible. It's time to stop rummaging around in years' worth of paper piles, which only get thicker and more confusing as time passes. The technological future predicted decades ago by scientific visionaries is upon us. And though we may still be light years from the ability to "beam" employees and co-workers from the break room to the styling floor, we can certainly utilize computers to maximize the operational efficiency of a salon business.

Where computers are taking salons and spas

Computers have waited a long time to pass through the doors of the salon industry. Owners are often hesitant about wandering into uncharted territory, and are concerned about the impact computers will have on their businesses in the form of hardware and software investments, and the time and costs of training. Yet the benefits that technology offers a properly prepared salon far outweigh the initial trepidation it inspires.

The growing presence of technology in salons heralds an important realization, according to MIKAL'S Fred Dengler. Technology is no longer "on the way" into salons, says Fred. It's here. "The attitude of salon owners and managers is changing. They are now asking for technological help in their own businesses rather than viewing computers as belonging somewhere else. However, many owners still aren't maximizing their utilization of technology."

The most significant difference between automated and non-automated salons, according to Kent Crabtree of INNOVATIVE BUSINESS COMPUTER SOLUTIONS (The Salon/Spa Manager), is efficiency. He asserts, "Computers move salons away from the 'mom and pop' perception. Organizing mailings, and working with sales totals and projections is too time-consuming for most salon owners today, and it costs money to get someone else to do it." A good software system, however, offers options — and will engender what Kent calls a "remarkable transition."

"When utilized correctly," says Ross Neill of EXTENDED TECHNOLOGIES (SalonBiz and SpaBiz), "computers enable us to run our businesses more efficiently. Today, they are not so much an advantage as a necessity — for tighter margins, price competitiveness and the ability to provide a greater level of customer service at

Salon Industry Software Vendors

VENDOR	TELEPHONE	INTERNET WEB SITE
CLIENTRAK!	800.397.4582	www.clientrak.com
ELITE	800.662.ELITE	www.elite-usa.com
FINGERTIP ACCESS	800.382.5510 or 404.252.1519	www.ftaccess.com
HAIRMAX	800.HAIRMAX	www.imall.com/stores/hairmax
LEPRECHAUN	800.373.1684 or 412.766.0993	www.leprechaun-software.com
MIKAL	800.448.5420 or 513.528.5100	www.mikal.com
MILANO	800.667.1596 or 905.884.4888	www.milanosystems.com
THE SALON/SPA MANAGER (IBCS)	800.682.2998	www.spasalon.com
SALONBIZ	800.632.5527	www.salonbiz.com
SALON PRO	800.830.9992 or 847.584.9377	www.salonpro.com
SALON PROFESSIONAL	800.710.3879	www.prosalon.com
SALONSCAPE	800.995.0045	www.salonscape.com
SALON SOLUTIONS	888.813.2141	www.salon-solutions.com
SALONTEC	800.221.5236 or 727.360.8000	www.salontec.com
SALON TRANSCRIPTS	800.766.4778	salontranscripts.com

a lower price." But what price does the salon owner pay for the decision to automate?

"The appointment book is the greatest fear," states Steve Smith of HairMax. "It may be an unfounded fear, but many salon owners and managers wonder: What if it doesn't work?" Ron Mataya of Leprechaun refers to the process as crossing a chasm. "People in this industry tend to be very creative, and a computer is the antithesis of creativity," he says. "Crossing that chasm is the big hurdle. Most owners are so busy working that they have no time to make money; they are so consumed by the business that they don't see the need to step back."

"The sheer volume of work is the biggest problem for most salons making the move from paper to computer," says Kent Crabtree. "Plus, the keyboard and mouse still frighten a lot of people. However, a modern system minimizes the need for training. And the ability to decentralize the front desk by setting up separate booking rooms allows for better customer service."

New customer service tools

On the subject of booking rooms, Ross Neill states, "Consumers are becoming more demanding; they want value-added service. Salons need to be able to book electronically, and a big salon can take this traffic off the front desk altogether. This allows the desk staff to concentrate on retail and customer service, and cuts client wait time considerably. Salons with multiple locations utilizing a single call center will have better phone coverage. As for economic feasibility, a booking room can occupy less expensive space than the salon's retail area."

Steve Smith offers a similar opinion: "The quality of service at the front desk and over the phone is being shredded. You can't tend to client needs at the desk when it's swamped. If a salon can allocate a private area where someone can answer the phone and work on a networked computer, traffic flow will improve dramatically. Higher volume salons must address this issue."

"If the salon can support the overhead," says Ron Mataya, "a booking room is a great idea. The majority of salons today just

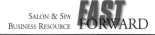
don't have that luxury. But we are in transition. Our industry likes to think of itself as avant-garde, on the leading edge of style. We are now on the leading edge of our own wave of technology."

Riding the wave

The greatest advantage technology offers salons, according to Fred Dengler, is that it "sharpens" every aspect of the business it is applied to: "The idea is to let the computer do tedious tasks such as tracking inventory and tabulating sales. Let the computer compute so that you don't have to!"

There are other advantages to automation — some of them further removed from the basic operation of the salon. As all business owners are aware, client perception is crucial to success. Steve Smith says, "Salon clients are exposed to computers in their own jobs and homes. They are happy to see that salons are 'keeping up with the times.' Clients are generally full of encouragement and willing to help salons through the implementation period."

Finally, there is perhaps the most important item of all: salon owner sanity. Ron Mataya offers this tip: "Technology can help owners and managers preserve their quality of life. Unless you're computerized, the salon will consume your life."

There is no doubt that salon owners are beginning to accept and capitalize upon the impact of modern technology on their businesses. Yet this acceptance requires a major shift in the way business has always been conducted and considered. "It is a change, and change is always difficult," says Ross Neill. But this one is definitely worth it.

Know your computer lingo

To many, computer lingo is difficult to comprehend, no matter how interesting it sounds. In the spirit of good sportsmanship, STRATEGIES' web architect, Jim Verrilli, compiled a list of common web-affiliated terms for our readers.

■ BOOKMARK: A placeholder which you ask your World Wide Web browser (a program that displays Web pages) to mark for you so that you can come back to the same spot later. AMERICA ONLINE (AOL) refers to a bookmark as a "Favorite Place."

■ BROWSER: A program that displays Web pages.

■ CACHE: A place on your hard drive that stores text and images from Web pages so they come up quickly when you visit them more than once.

■ COOKIE: A piece of information a Web page might store in your browser for use when you return. (For example: Storing information entered in forms, such as billing and shipping addresses, saves time because you don't have to reenter the same items each time you place an order.)

■ HOME PAGE: A page that an individual, club or company creates on the World Wide Web.

■ HTML (Hypertext Markup Language): The format of documents on the Web.

■ HTTP (Hypertext Transfer Protocol): The way computers exchange Web information. When you see an Internet address that begins with "http://", you know that address points to a Web page.

■ HYPERLINK: Text or images that take you to another place on the same page, another page, or another site entirely. Hyperlinks usually appear as underlined text.

■ HYPERTEXT: Text documents which are linked by hyperlinks.

■ INTERNET EXPLORER™: A popular Web browser developed by Microsoft (also called MSIE). Internet Explorer is the Web browser built into most versions of AOL software.

■ JAVA™: A programming language. It works the same for Macs,

PCs and other computers, and is popular on the Web because it works for all platforms (i.e., anyone can download the same piece of software and use it).

■ NETSCAPE/NETSCAPE NAVIGATOR™: A popular Web browser developed by NETSCAPE COMMUNICATIONS CORPORATION.

■ PLUG-IN: A small program your browser uses to do things it can't do by itself. For instance, the ShockWave plug-in lets your browser show small multimedia programs embedded in some Web pages.

■ SEARCH ENGINE: A program that looks through things for you. On the World Wide Web, this has come to mean a Web page from which you can search the entire Web. There are some search engines that do other things, like search news groups or phone books.

■ SSL (Secure Sockets Layer): A technology that encrypts information that travels from your browser to the Web server. While you send and receive information within a secure server, your credit card number and any other information you send and receive is much harder for anyone to steal. When you enter a secure server, the browser will prompt you with a message such as: "Encrypted data with valid server authentication."

■ SURF: To travel through cyberspace, usually by clicking a series of hyperlinks.

■ URL (Uniform Resource Locator): An "address" pointing to a site on the Internet.

■ WEBMASTER: A person who manages and maintains a Web site.

Jim Verrilli is director of 123THEWORLD, *a marketing and image development studio specializing in brand-building and promotion planning. With over 15 years' experience, four focusing specifically on web site development, Jim has effectively bridged the publicity-building gap between new and traditional media outlets.* 123THEWORLD *offers industry-specific services through its* DAYSPAMARKETING *division. You may reach Jim via telephone at 970.498.8975; e-mail at* jim@123theworld.com; *or the internet at* www.123theworld.com *or* www.dayspamarketing.com.

Computers: How to select the right system

We talked to Catherine Renaud at SOFTWARE CREATIONS, INC.

When thinking of automating or changing automation, consider the dynamics of your current operation. How does a client move through the salon and out the door? Analyze your paper flow. What changes would you make to improve the current system? Once you identify the ultimate process, the chance is good of finding a software solution that closely matches the salon's process. After all, there are about thirty vendors competing for your business.

Software requirements dictate hardware requirements. If your software vendor does not sell hardware:

- Ask for a list of requirements to provide to the network and hardware vendor.
- Ask for a list of qualified, recommended network engineers in your area. Make sure the hardware vendor has certified engineers in the specified network you plan to operate.

A *network* allows computers to share information. Hardware located on the premises constitutes a local area network (LAN). Multiple computers linked from remote locations comprise a wide area network (WAN).

Partnerships are vital

It is important to find a software vendor that takes an "arms around," rather than an "arm's length," approach. Automation is a difficult process, no matter how easy the software is to use. It takes time to adapt and to learn something that may be totally foreign to your nature. However, industry pioneers have paved the way for new computer users, and history indicates that salons are better off for having taken the automation plunge.

On average, salon teams need about thirty days to adapt to automation. Then it becomes like a part of the wallpaper — if it's good. If not, you will always be dealing with computer problems

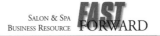

rather than serving clients. Selecting application software is the most important aspect of automation, and may be your most important business decision.

SOFTWARE CREATIONS, INC. (SCI), sells Finger Tip Access (FTA) application software products in two segments: Million-dollar-plus salons (which need sophisticated processes to keep track of 100–1000 or more clients per day), and "more intimate" salons which receive 75–100 clients per day. Since 1986, SCI has listened to the requirements of spas and salons, and written software to match. SCI's suites of products are designed to mold themselves to their environment instead of forcing the spa or salon into the requirements of the software.

Many salons start with a software product, only to find that after a year or so they outgrow the system. This is a natural result of growth, but may entail an expensive and time-consuming conversion unless you purchase upwardly compatible products. SCI replaces a lot of entry-level software because the spa or salon has reached a functionality saturation. To address this growing need, SCI introduced FTA for Windows, which is upwardly compatible with FTA Gold — ensuring a smooth transition as the spa or salon grows.

DOS versus Windows...

SCI introduced FTA for Windows in 1998. The focus of FingerTip Access Touch Screen for Windows is on spas and salons that maintain an intimate setting, with under seventy-five guests per day. FTA for Windows makes navigation as simple as possible by displaying large buttons with pictures on the touch screen.

Photos of clients and technicians can easily be scanned in to aid the operator in running the spa or salon. E-mail, warnings when products run low, PIN password protection, and internet updates are only a few of the features utilized by FTA for Windows.

Whether your software runs on Windows, DOS or both, make sure it's an on-line–real-time system. Access to information is the key to success, and anything but on-line–real-time will fall short of your ultimate goals for automation.

What's the scoop on DOS versus Windows? The only thing they have in common is that they are both operating systems. (The operating system is the traffic cop of the entire system.)

DOS is used effectively in large environments that require instant transaction processing with little or no interruption by the operating system. DOS is usually not visible to the end user and is rarely used or accessed once the application software is installed.

Windows interacts with the user in what has become a standard for this generation. Windows requires more knowledge of the operating system and takes more time to navigate but opens opportunities to use multiple software applications, such as word processing, spread sheets, accounting software and relational data bases.

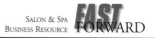
Guidelines for software vendor selection

We talked to Catherine Renaud at SOFTWARE CREATIONS, INC.

When searching for a system, consider application software which generally contains:

- Point of purchase
- Appointment booking
- Inventory
- Marketing
- Reports

As you come to understand and rely on these areas of functionality, the business will improve.

- When considering a software company, be sure to check at least six references and require the company to provide at least twenty from which you may randomly choose. (This will help prevent a sales set-up among friends of the vendor.)
- Software vendors are segmented by functionality. Ask the vendor for a list of functions the software provides and make sure your wish list is covered.
- Look for a software system with security built around information that is only accessible to authorized employees.

Salons that require only one computer may find a Windows environment more appealing and useful than salons that have many workstations on a network. Salons or spas with networks find DOS more useful on the front desk and appointment booking stations, while the office may prefer Windows, with the application software appearing as an icon. (Icons are the pictures you click to launch the software program.)

FTA Gold's enhanced gift certificate database was pioneered by DePasquale, who prints the certificate at the point of purchase on a HEWLETT-PACKARD laser printer. SCI offers customization to spas and salons that wish to automatically print gift certificates at the point of purchase. Regardless of format, FTA Gold can integrate your gift certificate into the process for on-demand printing.

The goal of every salon is to operate a hassle-free environment for the client. An efficient, paperless system provides that capability. Staff can check schedules, send notes to the front desk, and review client formulas — all at the touch of a button or two.

Catherine Renaud is president of SOFTWARE CREATIONS, INC., *located in Atlanta, GA.* SCI *offers FingerTip Access software for salons and spas. For more information on FTA for Windows and FTA Gold, call 800.382.5510.* SCI's *web site is* www.FTACCESS.com.

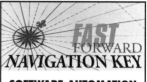

NAVIGATION KEY

SOFTWARE AUTOMATION

STEP 1: SHOP AROUND. No program is right for every salon, but chances are there's one that's right for yours.

STEP 2: COMPARE RESULTS. Which program holds the most promise for taking your salon to the next level?

STEP 3: SUPPORT IS CRUCIAL. Will your software vendor be there when you need them? Check their reputation for backing up their software with training and support.

STEP 4: MAKE A DECISION. When the results are in, it's time to lock into the company that will best serve your business.

STEP FIVE: BUY THE SERVICE CONTRACT. Data integrity and technological upgrades are critical. Questions and problems will arise. Buy it.

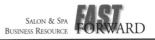
Going Paperless: Thinking outside the box

F TA Gold is the software around which the term "paperless" originated. Industry leaders such as Frederic Fekkai, Bumble & bumble, Charles Ifergan, DiPietro Todd and Jose Eber pioneered this concept using FTA. Paperless is not for everyone but, for anyone who operates a large and complex environment, paperless is best. For example: A paperless system is cost-justified when you operate a salon or spa with ten chairs or more. Consider:

- Time is money. The return on investment becomes evident when paper bills decrease, productivity improves, and clients are better served and return more often. Plus, paper is environmentally insensitive.
- Paper is cumbersome and not a convenient means of communication for a technician.
- Paper has a way of disappearing along with your money.
- Clients are suspicious of paper: *Is that my name on there? What are they saying?*
- Paperless improves communication among the team by passing information electronically and, therefore, immediately.
- Paperless improves the process of client service, allowing instant access to information.

An *evolving ticket* increases retail sales and can change the way merchandise is sold in a salon. With an evolving sales ticket, technical staff can add products to a client ticket while still on the floor. Just as product is positioned near or in the service area, so is a touch-screen computer workstation. Technicians easily adapt to seeing what they need and touching the screen.

A system that responds quickly and accurately is important to the life of the salon. Good computer software makes it simple to respond to daily requests from clients. (For example: When a client decides on a spur-of-the-moment purchase, the technician can walk to the workstation, touch the client's name and the name of the product, and the item is automatically added to the sales ticket.) Additionally, a printer in the retail area may produce a "picking ticket" and the front desk staff can have the items bagged and waiting for the exiting client.

A PAPERLESS COMPUTER SYSTEM HAS TO BE ON-LINE–REAL-TIME TO WORK. In a paperless environment, computer files are continuously updated. Therefore, when a staff member needs information about a client, it is there immediately. A batch system, on the other hand, collects information all day and updates at the end of the day. In such a system, paperless could not work because you have "yesterday's news" today.

PAPERLESS DOES NOT MEAN PAPER-FREE. Paper reports are run daily when balancing the drawer or analyzing salon productivity. *Paperless* involves access to information regarding the clients' welfare while in the salon. It means a smoother transition for clients as they move comfortably through relaxing treatments.

Convenience is our society's watchword. When salon clients arrive for services, they want to be pampered, and pampered they are. Technicians are trained to be accommodating, and that should extend to the check-in and check-out process. With a paperless environment, accommodating the client is easy because information is always accessible.

Salons do change, often becoming day spas. Think of the future when planning computerization. Make sure the software incorporates processes that can function efficiently in the spa regimen.

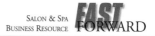
Using e-mail to meet business objectives

Depending on your salon's position and objectives, e-mail can be a profitable growth tool. Step one is to begin compiling addresses from clients and constructing a comprehensive database. An e-mail campaign can be considerably less expensive than traditional marketing techniques. For example: There are no postage, printing, design or web site costs involved. All that is needed is a little creativity in developing promotional offers, and some time devoted to maintaining the database.

With a steady client base, it's easy to "work" e-mail. Electronic messaging makes it simple to offer special service marketing to clients who receive particular services (e.g., tips for maintaining a permanent wave or making color last longer). Developing your salon's affinity for this technology can lead to improved public and client relations, a greater number of referrals, more successful promotions and higher retention rates. If marketing is really the name of the game, e-mail can do it for your salon.

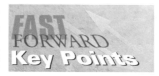

E-mail marketing to your client base is an opportunity too good to miss. It's lightning-fast and inexpensive. Consider doing a monthly e-mail update newsletter to clients. Keep it short and sell, sell, sell.

Should your salon be on the World Wide Web?

As the technological capacity for on-line ordering increases, so does the number of businesses taking advantage of this new source of revenue. While many lament the demise of "personal" attention, blaming it on the propagation of answering machines, voice mail and other automated systems, these devices are rapidly becoming indispensible to growing businesses. (To discover how much so, just call your health maintenance organization or credit card company.) Offering a menu of departments and persons for clients' consideration can save the business considerable time and expense.

But does your salon belong on the World Wide Web? The answer depends on your current market position and goals for the future. It depends on the amount of time and money allotted to the salon's technological and marketing agenda. It's far better to not have a web site than to have a poorly designed one, according to Jim Verrilli of 123THEWORLD.

It's also worth remembering that salons which depend on a mostly local clientele can reap the same benefits from print campaigns and radio spots. Day spas and destination spas, however, may generate additional interest through a web site because they can derive a greater portion of their business from tourists who may be scouting ahead. "No matter the nature of your business or the results you seek, it is crucial to remember that internet-savvy clients will evaluate the professionalism of the business based on the web site," says Jim.

Marketing is the name of the game. "There has to be an objective," says Jim. "If exposure is all you want, a single web page containing a logo can accomplish that. But in order to achieve the objectives of reaching new clients and growing the business, you must implement a full marketing program, or find someone who can do it for you."

What will a web site accomplish?

T he interactive format and visual appeal of a web site make it an even better marketing tool than e-mail. The main objective, according to Jim Verrilli, is to "work the 'net for business development." There are a number of conditions to consider concerning the web's relation to a salon business:

■ TIME: If clients have access to descriptions of services and service providers prior to contacting the salon or spa, phone time is reduced dramatically. This equals less time on hold for them, and less time devoted to non-productive service and product descriptions for the front desk or booking room staff. *(See chapter 5.)*

■ EASE OF ACCESS: A growing number of offices and homes are becoming equipped with internet access capability. Today, it's practically a given that a business has a web site. For example: An English language search on AltaVista (an internet search engine) using the key words "day spa" yields well over one million web pages, most developed for privately owned businesses. (NOTE: Some spas are listed more than once because they have more complex sites with multiple pages that have

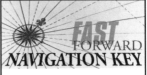

NAVIGATION KEY

WEB SITE WARNING

Set realistic expectations for your web site. Answer these questions before investing in one:

How can it help you better serve existing clients (e.g., e-mail, appointment scheduling, service offerings and descriptions, product purchasing)?

What interesting features will attract new clients (e.g., unique services/products, specialized skills, gift certificate purchases, questions and answers)?

Commit to keeping your site fresh and exciting — or don't do it.

either been submitted by the owners or robotically indexed by the search engine. This means more exposure for them.) The prevalence of internet service providers and the simplicity of getting on line has opened a new avenue of information exchange for salons and day spas.

■ ECONOMICALLY SPEAKING: The cost of developing and maintaining a web site will depend on the complexity of its content and presentation (i.e., the number of billable hours required). There are few benchmarks by which to estimate expenses. Many local internet service providers (ISP's) will design web sites for a nominal fee, but they may not accomplish the desired result. "Many aspects of a webmaster's service are esoteric and invisible," says Jim Verrilli. "To reflect your salon's style and market position, you will need to hire a professional firm with marketing and development skills. If your resources are limited, there is the option of only producing a single page, perhaps listing hours of operation and providing an e-mail link. This is the most basic application, simply telling clients what you do."

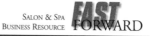

Hallmarks of a "great" web site

Logic is the largest player in deciding how to structure your salon's site. A web presence is an extension of the salon's newspaper, magazine and Yellow Page ads. It is an amalgamation of marketing materials including service and price menus, team profiles, the salon newsletter, promotional advertisements, updates on community projects and full-color images portraying the salon's best work. Every item that can be used to promote the salon can be displayed (and archived, if desired) on a web site.

Presentation

Without a friendly format — an invitation to visit, peruse and interact — your salon or day spa web site will not achieve its primary goal: attracting clients. Of course *friendly* is a relative term, but your web site should appeal to as many groups of people as possible. Just as the asymmetrical haircut which looks fashionable on a Paris runway may not "cut it" at the corner office, a web site could actually limit interest in the salon if it is perceived to cater too much or too little to certain groups. If this is a marketing objective, so be it, but do not unwittingly allow your salon to be typecast. Make the statement you wish to convey, but maintain control of the creative process.

Interactive

A salon web site must encourage client interaction. Brevity may be a virtue, but multiple pages will pique people's interest. A good web site will enable clients to navigate through several areas of interest.

- SERVICES: This is the perfect arena to thoroughly explain the team's skills and display color images.
- PRICING MENU, INCLUDING THE ABILITY TO CUSTOMIZE PACKAGES AND DAYS OF BEAUTY: In much the same way that customers pick and choose which compact discs to buy from COLUMBIA HOUSE, it is possible to allow clients to construct the perfect packages

for themselves and others, and e-mail their choices to the salon. Web access can complement a powerful software package at the front desk, preventing double bookings and services booked without the appropriate treatment rooms reserved. And the inconvenience of client callbacks for those who request complex packages is replaced by brief, simple confirmation calls to let them know their e-mails are not lost in cyberspace.

■ SERIOUS INTEGRATION: It is possible to organize the salon's technical systems into a single integrated array. This is known as "back-end integration." With this type of configuration, the salon's database, including the appointment book and other software applications, will seamlessly interact with the web site. The catch? According to Jim Verrilli, this type of technology can be costly, running into thousands of dollars. For the average salon, the return on investment would not justify initial costs. For most salons, a single- or multi-page site with an e-mail link will suffice.

Informative

The purpose of a web site is to distribute information about your salon business. In the flurry to explain the features and benefits of services and products, don't forsake the basics, such as:

■ HOURS OF OPERATION: Especially convenient if the salon maintains seasonal or irregular hours. This information can also be easily incorporated into your phone system's hold message.

■ DIRECTIONS: It's always a courtesy to offer verbal directions to clients, especially new ones. Posting them on the web site is an added convenience.

Enticing

■ BROWSING BUSINESS: Mention product lines and explain why the salon carries each one. It will attract new retail clients.

■ MOST WANTED: The salon story will help potential clients decide that yours is the salon they have been looking for. Team member profiles will build trust in the salon's ability to fulfill client needs and desires.

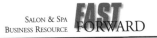
EVALUATION FORM

BUSINESS APPLICATION SOFTWARE FOR THE SPA & SALON

PRODUCT	VENDOR	CONTACT NAME & PHONE #

	(Y)ES OR (N)O	PRIORITY (1: low – 10: high)
Number of references		
3	____	____
4 – 8	____	____
9 – 15	____	____
16 – 20	____	____
20 +	____	____
Years in business		
1 – 3	____	____
3 – 5	____	____
5 – 10	____	____
10 – 20	____	____
20+	____	____
Software		
Reliability reference check	____	____
Speed reference check	____	____
Down time reference check (Provide %)	____	____
Lost data reference (Provide %)	____	____
Software user interface		
Keyboard	____	____
Touch screen	____	____
Touch screen & keyboard	____	____
Mouse driven	____	____
Mouse & keyboard	____	____
Platform		
MSDOS	____	____
Windows	____	____
NT/Windows Workstation	____	____
Novell Network	____	____
Linux	____	____
Citrix/Winwork	____	____
Citrix/Winframe	____	____

Customer service

7 Day / 24 hour	_____	_____
5 Day / 10 hour	_____	_____
5 Day / 8 hour	_____	_____
Hourly	_____	_____
Other	_____	_____
Reference check service	_____	_____

Client portfolio

Client look-up by name	_____	_____
Client look-up by phone number	_____	_____
Client look-up by room number	_____	_____
Retention factors (e.g., new, non-request)	_____	_____
Follow-up date	_____	_____
Client referral tracking	_____	_____
Client formulas	_____	_____
Client demographics (age, occupation, etc.)	_____	_____
Medical and allergy forms	_____	_____
Accumulated historical charges by client	_____	_____
User-defined flagged information	_____	_____
Maintains service and retail history	_____	_____
Selection of historical charges by client base	_____	_____
Credit card information	_____	_____
Special comments field (bounced check, etc.)	_____	_____
Preferred customer field	_____	_____
Total money spent on services/products	_____	_____
Discounts given	_____	_____
Outstanding accounts	_____	_____
Client clubs	_____	_____
Frequency of visits	_____	_____

Appointment booking

Real-time access to system	_____	_____
Prevention of duplicate booking	_____	_____
Books standing appointments	_____	_____
Book 1 month out	_____	_____
Book 1 – 3 months out	_____	_____
Book 3 – 6 months out	_____	_____
Ability to book as far out as necessary	_____	_____
Automatic multiple service booking	_____	_____
Package booking	_____	_____
Ability to book lunches	_____	_____
Book a room with a technician	_____	_____
Automatically books room with a service	_____	_____
Tracks room type	_____	_____
Automatic start times	_____	_____
Individual service time slots by technician	_____	_____
Individual service price by technician	_____	_____
Allows two technicians to a room	_____	_____
Preset packages (unlimited)	_____	_____
Modify packages on the fly	_____	_____

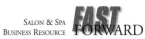
Search for openings   ____   ____
View technician's openings   ____   ____
Identify conflicting client appointments   ____   ____
Predefine technician groups & display on screen   ____   ____
Find opening by preset group   ____   ____
View technician's schedule eight days out   ____   ____
Color-coded client type in appointment book   ____   ____
When canceling, looks at all appointments for the same day   ____   ____
Captures who booked appointments   ____   ____

Client/appointment booking integration

Select the employee and time   ____   ____
Select the client   ____   ____
Select the services   ____   ____
Color booking with automatic processing time   ____   ____
Client arrival list   ____   ____
View and/or print the client's bookings   ____   ____
View client bookings for today and the future   ____   ____
Add new client data from the booking screen   ____   ____
Display note from client record when booking   ____   ____
Automatic wait list   ____   ____
Move appointment automatically without cancelation   ____   ____
Wait list with move capability   ____   ____
Technician start times visible in book   ____   ____
Standing appointments   ____   ____
Access purchase history from book   ____   ____
Access formulas from book   ____   ____
Automatic package booking   ____   ____
Alternate search sequences for packages   ____   ____
Insert technician request in predefined package   ____   ____
Add or delete service in predefined package   ____   ____
Restaurant reservations   ____   ____
Spa reservations   ____   ____
Booked value report   ____   ____
Book appointments into future (no limitations)   ____   ____

Confirmation

Lists all customers scheduled for next day,
    with phone numbers   ____   ____
Automatically dials client's number   ____   ____

Point of sale

Client receipts   ____   ____
Bar code scanning   ____   ____
Product look-up   ____   ____
No limit on total dollar amount in a day   ____   ____
Open register to give change without a ticket   ____   ____
Alternative menu mode instead of bar codes   ____   ____
Automatic price look-up   ____   ____
Un-tax by item   ____   ____
Displays options for form of payment   ____   ____

Discount tracking	____	____
Voids	____	____
Returns	____	____
Complimentary	____	____
Store credits	____	____
Outstanding store credits	____	____
User-definable tender types	____	____
House charges owed & paid	____	____
Petty cash control	____	____
Add product to open ticket & print remotely	____	____
Instantly calculates every sales transaction	____	____
Cash drawer reconciliation	____	____
Receipt transaction log by the day	____	____
Balance sheet recap	____	____
Cumulative balance sheet (any range of days)	____	____
Day end close out – multiple shifts	____	____
Multiple cash drawer balance recaps	____	____
Price override	____	____
Print or view ticket for today (traveler)	____	____
Tracks each technician's total	____	____
Escape to add a product or cancel a ticket	____	____
Change credit for sale at ring-up	____	____
Add tip to sale at ring-up	____	____
Service tax	____	____
Retail tax	____	____
Credit card & check authorization	____	____
Ability to receive change from credit card or check	____	____
Employee ID tracking at P.O.S.	____	____
Integrated settlement	____	____

Client/point of sale integration

Membership tracking	____	____
Series tracking	____	____
Returned product tracking by client	____	____
Client IOU's	____	____
Charge purchases to the room	____	____

Gift certificates

Track purchaser and receiver information	____	____
Track who sold	____	____
Capability to have blank receiver	____	____
Automatically number and print certificate	____	____
Capability to include tips	____	____
Automatic expiration date by gift certificate	____	____
Number and dates	____	____
Automatically appears in purchaser history	____	____
Fully auditable – appears in balance reports	____	____
Prints voided certificates and who voided	____	____
Prints outstanding certificates	____	____
Prints expired certificates	____	____
Text line for customer	____	____

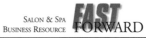
Today's client check-in

Color-coded client arrival and departure   ———   ———
Color-coded guest types   ———   ———
Client retention tracking   ———   ———

Today's client movement

Daily list of clients with appointments   ———   ———
Easily view client's ticket   ———   ———
Easily view client's purchase history   ———   ———
Easily view client's formulas   ———   ———
Easily view client notes & comments   ———   ———
Identify the location of the client in the facility   ———   ———

Today's client check-out

Add product or service before ring out   ———   ———
Cancel product or service before ring out   ———   ———
Change price on product or service before ring out   ———   ———
Change technician credit before ring out   ———   ———
Past purchased retail items are viewed on screen   ———   ———
Updates productivity, inventory, client retention   ———   ———
Book an additional service that adds to ticket today   ———   ———
Automatic selection of service provider and rate   ———   ———
Write and view special notes on client   ———   ———
Color-coded client status system   ———   ———
Suggests future appointment by displaying history   ———   ———
Automatic removal from list when checked out   ———   ———
Automatic no-show report   ———   ———

Staff participation today

View service provider's appointment schedule   ———   ———
View client formulas   ———   ———
Write and view client notes and comments   ———   ———
Add a product to the ticket before ringing   ———   ———
Change any price on ticket before ringing   ———   ———

Technicians

Productivity by sales totals   ———   ———
Productivity by classification   ———   ———
Client retention by technician   ———   ———
Technician daily transaction log   ———   ———
Goals & trends   ———   ———
Technician profile in booking module   ———   ———
Cannot book a service for wrong technician   ———   ———
Technician schedules (viewing & printing)   ———   ———

Inventory

Supports bar codes   ———   ———
Bar code printing   ———   ———

Price label printing	___	___
Reorder points with reorder capabilities	___	___
Suggested order based on sales history by product	___	___
Vendor capacity (provide number)	___	___
Brands capacity (provide number)	___	___
Backbar tracking	___	___
How often product turns over	___	___
Tracks returned product	___	___
Tracks shortages	___	___
Tracks profitability of all products sold	___	___
Value of current inventory report	___	___
Sales and on-hand report by classification	___	___
Shipping from central warehouse	___	___
Receiving at remote location	___	___
Hand-held inventory capture	___	___

Reports

View or print daily schedule for each employee	___	___
View or print customer flow tickets with technical cards needed	___	___
View and print appointment book by the day for specific technician	___	___

Marketing reports

By birthday	___	___
By new client	___	___
By clients who have not returned	___	___
By retail purchase history	___	___
By service purchase history	___	___
By clients seen in the last ten days	___	___
By clients spending over XX amount	___	___
By client referral	___	___

Payroll commissions

Individual pay plans	___	___
Leveled commissions (provide number)	___	___
Product deduction	___	___
Spa and/or salon deduction	___	___
Tracks services and retail commissions	___	___
Produces gross pay report	___	___
Produces gross pay report and provides accounting	___	___
Manage multiple shifts	___	___
Splits commission between two people	___	___
Track sick leave, holidays, etc.	___	___

Security

Track who made appointments	___	___
Track who rang sale	___	___
Password protection – reports	___	___
Restricted access to certain screens	___	___

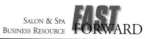
System features

Multiple appointment books using client DB	___	___
Technician capacity – up to 20	___	___
Technician capacity – 21 to 40	___	___
Technician capacity – 41 to 100	___	___
Technician capacity – 101 to 1,000	___	___
Technician capacity – 1,001 to 9,999	___	___
Separate services into different categories	___	___
Separate retail products into different categories	___	___
Set up different price levels for each employee	___	___
Set up default durations for appointments	___	___
Central booking	___	___
Open system to external software	___	___
Unattended dial-up (polling)	___	___
Speed of system	___	___
OBDC compliant	___	___
Password system	___	___
Customize features to suit environment	___	___
Modification requests accepted	___	___
Intuitive use of color	___	___
Paperless ability	___	___
Floor workstations viewing, and password access	___	___
Floor workstations viewing only	___	___
Multiple salons on-line to home office	___	___

Training

On site: 1 day	___	___
On site: 2 – 3 days	___	___
On site: 4 – 6 days	___	___
On site: 7 – 15 days	___	___
Other (provide number)	___	___
Study program for practice	___	___
Modem training	___	___
Pre-training consultation	___	___
Post-training consultation	___	___

Future direction

On DOS and moving to Windows95 or '98	___	___
On DOS and moving to HTML	___	___
On Windows95 or '98 and staying	___	___
On Windows95 or '98 and moving to HTML	___	___
Appointments accepted from internet	___	___
Data warehousing component	___	___
Automatic ordering from manufacturer	___	___

Things to do:

■ If you are not yet automated — it's time.
   Research the software companies and systems available to find one
   that best suits your salon's needs.
   Remember to look for these all-important applications:

   > POINT OF SALE
   > APPOINTMENT BOOKING
   > INVENTORY
   > MARKETING
   > REPORTS

■ Get to know your software, and what it can do. Learn to run
   reports to help your business grow, as well as what they mean:

   > RETENTION
   > AVERAGE TICKET
   > PRODUCTIVITY
   > SALES
   > GIFT CERTIFICATES

■ Explore World Wide Web options. What will an Internet presence
   do for your salon?

■ Evaluate your current phone system and consider upgrading to a
   more advanced, sophisticated one which may include:

   > VOICE MAIL
   > MESSAGE ON HOLD
   > INFORMATION BOXES (FOR DIRECTIONS, HOURS, ETC.)

■ For larger salons: Look into the benefits of an internal pager system, a terrific solution to internal communication challenges.

MAXIMIZING YOUR HUMAN RESOURCES

3

*Staff recruitment & review,
and career development*

A poll of salon and day spa owners would likely show that well over 50% have experienced walkouts. Staff turnover has always been an industry nemesis. It disrupts business, disappoints and confuses clients, and causes needless stress for all involved. Moreover, it's expensive. It drives up operating, recruitment and training costs. Turnover has placed salons in the high-risk/high-cost bracket with insurance providers. "Unstable" and "flighty" are terms regularly used to describe the salon workforce.

Success for employees in the salon and day spa industry *appears* straightforward: graduate from cosmetology school, get your license, find a busy salon, develop your skills, build a clientele. It's a mad dash to get booked solid, gridlocked and burned out. This is the evolution of a "successful" stylist. But problems often arise during this cycle...and they rest squarely on the shoulders of salon owners and managers.

Many salons restrict work to a one-dimensional path: Build your clientele, get your commission, get booked solid, raise your prices. But because so much responsibility for salon growth is casually passed off to the staff, the driving force that should inspire that growth simply doesn't materialize. Daily routines and complacent behaviors contaminate the salon's culture. The lack of leadership, direction and the challenge to achieve great things leads to unrest and dissension in the ranks. At this point, staff turnover is inevitable. For these salons, the want ads should read: "Stylist with following wanted — because we don't know where we're going and need to borrow your customers for a while."

Where is your salon going?

What's your vision? Is it exciting? Do you have a game plan to get there? What are your sales and profit goals? What is your breakeven point? Does the staff know the salon's sales goals, and their responsibilities in achieving them? What skills and behaviors does your vision require? Does your pay program encourage these skills and behaviors? Do staff play a key role in moving the salon forward? Is your staff challenged, inspired, motivated and driven by the salon environment? Do they know the salon's quality, performance and financial goals?

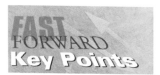

FAST FORWARD Key Points

Career-minded individuals gravitate to businesses that are exciting and growing. They look for salons driven by a strong and challenging vision, with high standards of quality and service.

Career-minded individuals gravitate to businesses that are exciting and growing. They look for salons driven by a strong and challenging vision, with high standards of quality and service. They look for leadership, openness, uncompromised trust, high ethical standards, fairness and the opportunity to participate in growing the salon. When one or more of these qualities is missing or compromised, a divide grows between the vision which drives the business and the personal agendas of employees.

Individual employee agendas *will* derail the forward momentum of your business. The salon industry can reverse its dismal staff turnover rate by looking beyond the confines of individual followings and commissioned sales, and focusing on unified vision, leadership, team performance and empowerment. *(We'll tackle leadership in chapter 4.)*

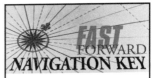

STAFFING ASSESSMENT

Before you embark on a recruitment campaign, step back and assess your real needs. For example: If you just lost a productive stylist, is it necessary to immediately replace the individual? Analyze the total productive hours of the remaining stylists. Perhaps a part-time stylist can satisfy your production needs, and save both payroll and benefit money.

When performing a staff assessment, analyze the technical skills needed by the salon. Will a color technician bolster color sales? Will a nailcare specialist attract more business? Will a haircutting expert raise the skill level of all stylists?

Establish hiring objectives before seeking new staff. This will keep payroll under control. But before you do anything, make sure you are optimizing the production capability you already have.

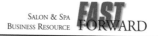
Sell "careers" – Not "jobs"

The cry, "I can't find employees," echoes throughout the industry. The labor shortage is real; competition for employees, both right out of school and experienced, is stiff. And by all indications, the shortage will get worse before it gets better. This simple bit of reality will force salons to rethink their staff recruitment and retention strategies and programs.

Staff recruiting is an ongoing process. Seeking employees only when you need them doesn't work today. By the time a recruiting effort is in place, the game is half over. Salons that treat recruiting as a process have the greatest success in quickly and efficiently securing staff.

Why do many salons have no trouble finding competent help? The answer is simple: THEY OFFER CAREERS, NOT JOBS. These salons entice the best workers by selling the salon's strategic vision, and the long-term advantages of being part of their team. This big-picture view focuses on a positive work environment, skill development, professional growth and advancement, and benefits and income. By focusing on career growth opportunities rather than job openings, you will increase the quantity and quality of applicants.

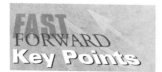

You'll never win today's competitive recruiting game if you're a part-time player.

What does turnover cost?

The issue of recruitment and retention takes on an entirely new perspective when you consider the true costs of employee turnover. And with a growing shortage of qualified staff, these costs will surely increase. Consider the costs a salon incurs from turnover by calculating the *actual* expense of each item on this list.

- …lost management time invested in training the former employee.
- …recruiting costs.
- …compensation paid to the former employee while he or she was in training.
- …lost sales while the position was vacant.
- …management time spent interviewing candidates to fill the position.
- …training a new employee.
- …compensation paid to a new employee before he or she becomes productive.
- …the extra time management and key staff must invest in the new employee.
- …the mistakes a new employee makes when first on the job.
- …disruption at the front desk, and paperwork expense caused by the departing employee.
- …impact of the person's loss of expertise on business and client satisfaction.
- …productive time lost due to the internal gossip that traditionally follows an employee's departure.

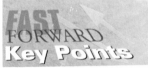

With a growing shortage of qualified staff, turnover costs will surely increase.

These are just some of the costs a salon experiences when an employee resigns or is fired. No matter the type of salon you own or manage, make sure you fully understand them. Your employees, clients and bottom line will all benefit from this understanding.

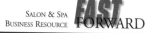
Getting ready to recruit

B efore diving head-first into the recruitment process, perform a personal assessment of your management style and recruitment capabilities. The objective is to identify hidden problems that could disrupt the recruitment process.

Excessive staff turnover, whether by resignation or termination, is a clear indication that problems exist at the managerial level. If not addressed, these problems will defeat any positive results produced by your recruitment efforts.

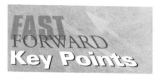

Excessive staff turnover, whether by resignation or termination, is a clear indication that problems exist at the managerial level.

Using a scale of 1–10, in which 1 is "no" and 10 is "yes," respond to the following questions. Be honest!

Am I really a good manager?

If you constantly battle employee turnover and repeated performance problems, your answer should be less than five; and the more turnover and performance problems you have, the closer you move towards one.

This question is meant to sensitize you to your management and leadership style. Are you *dominant,* focusing the troops on a vision and driving them toward it at all costs? Are you an *inducer,* managing by vision, consensus and diplomacy? Are you a free-wheeling *entrepreneurial* manager, always "shooting from the hip" and moving from one crisis to the next? Are you *steady:* not too aggressive, and most comfortable not rocking the boat? Or are you a *compliant* manager who avoids confrontation and is mostly passive when dealing with people…better known as the wimp?

The key to understanding your management style is understanding how you approach various situations. Consider:

There are times when a dominant manager can accomplish more by becoming an inducer. A dominant style may be just what the doctor ordered to turn around an ailing business, but may destroy an already efficient salon. If you're a compliant, passive manager, it's likely you chose the wrong career path — but you're not alone. Many very successful stylists have found management to be more of a curse than a step up the career ladder. *(We'll discuss shifting leadership styles in chapter 4.)*

AM I A VISIONARY LEADER WHO CAN MOTIVATE AND EMPOWER EMPLOYEES?

You can't lead without a vision to guide, motivate and empower your team. When Patton wanted to lead the first army into Berlin, he used his vision to motivate and empower his troops. Where do you want to take your salon business, and how will you use that vision to motivate and empower your staff to get there?

DO I HAVE THE DISCIPLINE AND SENSE OF PURPOSE TO LEAD BY EXAMPLE?

"Do as I say and not as I do" doesn't work in the world of management. The only rule that works is "if you talk the talk, you'd better walk the walk." People learn best by emulating role models and leaders. Likewise, employees will interpret every deviation as a sign that management no longer supports certain behaviors.

Performance and turnover problems can often be traced back to management. Many good employees either are fired or resign due to poor indoctrination and lack of appropriate role models.

DO I TRULY FIND MANAGEMENT A REWARDING PROCESS?

You're not doing anyone any favors if you are in management, but don't like managing. Moreover, you cannot efficiently recruit, select, train and lead new employees if you don't enjoy creating sparkling gems out of diamonds in the rough. Evaluate your management style and objectives; then make the necessary adjustments. *(Motivational techniques are discussed in chapter 15.)*

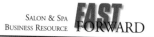
Recruiting guide: Create a hiring profile

A hiring profile is an essential recruiting tool. It forces you to clearly define the type of people who are "right" for your salon. One wise business executive said it best: "If you want a company full of eagles, hire eagles. No matter how much you train them…no matter how much you pay them…no matter how hard you work to motivate them…a turkey will never soar like an eagle. Rather than soaring, all you'll get is lots of wings flapping, frenetic running around and gobble gobbles."

Create your hiring profile by carefully assessing and listing the characteristics of people who have succeeded in your salon or day spa. Include the attitudes and skills each position requires, and the attitudes your salon's vision demands. Aggressively pursue these characteristics in all applicants.

The staff can help form a hiring profile. IDEA: Make it a topic of your next staff meeting or meet privately with key people to gather opinions on the subject. When the hiring profile is complete, share it with the staff. Inform them that their behavior characteristics helped form the profile. This will provide positive reinforcement, as well as "give notice" to individuals lacking certain behaviors.

ONCE THE PROFILE IS COMPLETE, STICK TO IT. During interviews, ask probing questions to reveal applicants' past behavior in situations dur-

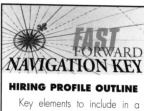

NAVIGATION KEY

HIRING PROFILE OUTLINE

Key elements to include in a comprehensive hiring profile:

APPEARANCE
PROFESSIONAL DEMEANOR
COMMUNICATION SKILLS
OPENNESS
TEAMWORK
RELIABILITY
ETHICAL STANDARDS
FOLLOW-THOUGH
TECHNICAL SKILL SETS
SPECIALTY SKILL(S)
POISE
CONSULTATION/SELLING SKILLS
YEARS OF EXPERIENCE
WORK HISTORY
ADVANCED EDUCATION
ABILITY TO WORK UNDER PRESSURE
ORGANIZATIONAL SKILLS
TIME MANAGEMENT

ing which they may have exercised the behaviors you're seeking.

CHECK REFERENCES CAREFULLY. Research state laws concerning informational queries on an applicant's work history. Have applicants sign a release allowing you to contact references regarding their work history.

When checking references, go back at least three jobs or five years. References must be filtered because recent employers may be concerned with the legal risks of honest answers.

(See also "Creating a leadership team," chapter 4.)

Money as a motivator

Money is not the all-powerful motivator most owners and managers think it is. In fact, it and other forms of compensation get more attention than they deserve. Studies show that money ranks fifth or sixth on most employees' priority list. People work for many reasons…money is just one of them.

To maintain proper perspective, commit your compensation package to paper. The objective is to offer new employees a program that rewards "team" performance, the ability to retain clients in the salon, superior customer service and their support of the salon's vision.

Rewards in the form of recognition, promotion and compensation are among the strongest statements you make to your team about their work. If you don't thoroughly communicate your compensation program, or if it doesn't deliver strong customer-service standards, you're missing a powerful opportunity to link staff behavior to your customer-driven vision. Creating monthly group and individual goals can dramatically improve overall staff performance and service quality.

You can recognize good performance without paying a great deal of money. Too many salon owners focus solely on the monetary aspects of employment, and pay out more in compensation and bonuses than necessary. An internal survey by METROPOLITAN LIFE shows that their employees, given a choice, preferred management recognition for good service over cash rewards. Most employees simply don't know they are truly appreciated.

Your compensation package must be affordable, performance- and behavior-driven, and fair to all parties. With a little creativity and a lot of vision, you can develop a package that, combined with other growth incentives, attracts qualified people who fit your mold. *(Compensation systems are discussed in chapter 13.)*

How to recruit in a shrinking labor market

When your salon must replace an employee…is recruiting, interviewing, hiring and training a struggle? Finding the right individuals can be frustrating. But there are strategies which can streamline the process, even though there is a shortage of qualified salon professionals.

The ability to recruit qualified employees is crucial to business success. Progressive businesses are *always* looking for new talent or individuals with specialized skills that could benefit the company. Salons must do the same.

Where to begin

Many salons and spas regard recruiting as nothing more than placing an advertisement in the classifieds and interviewing applicants. But in reality, this is only one small piece of the recruitment puzzle. Determining the kind of salon and/or spa you wish to own, and the kind of team you wish to build, are the all-important first steps. Your recruitment program must reflect this vision.

Just as your salon's advertising program consists of media advertising, direct-mail campaigns, newsletters and other promotions, your recruitment program will contain a variety of elements… each designed to communicate a specific message to prospective employees. This message will reflect your salon's vision and intention to attract candidates who share similar goals and values.

RECRUITING MUST BE AN ONGOING PROCESS. The day an employee leaves is not the time to hit the ignition switch on your recruitment program. *It's already too late.* Salons that continuously recruit are better prepared for unexpected staffing needs because they're always prospecting and interviewing candidates. Every growing company, regardless of size, must have qualified people to call upon when the need arises. Well-organized recruitment efforts can deliver big dividends by reducing potentially damaging situations to nothing more than bumps in the road — not to mention providing the peace of mind of knowing you are prepared.

Building your "red file"

Maintain a "red file" of employment candidates whom you can call when a real need emerges…after a resignation or termination, or when salon growth dictates a need for additional staff.

Constant recruiting efforts are much more important than an occasional ad in the classifieds. Get into the beauty schools, and offer presentations that define your competitive advantage in the marketplace. Send letters to every person in your immediate area who holds a cosmetology license. (You may order the list, organized by zip code, from your state cosmetology board.) Hold an open house for those who want to discuss employment opportunities at your salon.

If you place classifieds ads, read the competition's ads as well. Does yours stand out? You only get about *one second* to catch someone's attention, especially someone who is not actively seeking a new opportunity but likes to see what's available. Many salon employees occasionally peruse the classifieds. Many stylists aren't "looking" for a job, but are always "listening."

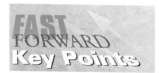

FAST FORWARD Key Points

Every growing company, regardless of size, must have qualified people to call upon when the need arises.

Some salon owners have tried a different approach with classifieds, placing a different ad every week to create ongoing interest. Each focuses on a different aspect of the salon, making potential applicants wonder what will be divulged next.

For some applicants, nothing takes the place of discretion. If you use classified ads to attract stylists, make the process as easy as possible for the applicant. One STRATEGIES reader asked stylists to send resumés and work histories to a post office box — a recruiting practice proven to work in the corporate world.

Open houses and career days provide an excellent platform to showcase your salon. These events are easily promoted through classified ads and local cosmetology schools. If you put together a good public relations campaign, you may receive valuable free press coverage.

If you belong to a local salon owners' association or know other owners who would like to pool resources, a career day can become an exciting event. But it can be even more exciting when your distributor gets involved. A large meeting room at a local facility will provide ample space for interviewing attendees. Distributors may charge a nominal fee to offset costs, but it's a great way for distributors and salons to work together.

Through your recruiting program, maintain contact with as many people as possible who can refer qualified individuals to your salon. This networking strategy is one of the most effective ways to secure employees. The application and interview process should be strong enough to weed out applicants who do not meet your requirements.

What can you offer local beauty schools in return for their cooperation? Your objective is to gain access to students. Schedule a presentation targeting resumé preparation, how to dress for an interview, the realities of salon life, working with the public or other topics that will benefit students. Most schools welcome the opportunity to present these types of programs. Consider a presentation (slides, video, or Microsoft PowerPoint) that takes students on a virtual tour of your salon. Leave information about the salon, including its vision statement, indoctrination and training programs, employee packages, growth opportunities and an employment application. The school may even provide a private room to conduct on-site interviews.

Vision and the glass slipper

When candidates do apply to your salon, what will you offer them? Because the supply of qualified stylists is far short of the demand, you must be able to answer the question: "Why would a stylist want to work at my salon instead of the competition?"

There are many factors that attract applicants to a salon. The ambiance, clientele and compensation package are all key ingredients. But most powerful of all is the salon *vision*.

It is imperative to communicate your salon's vision to every prospective employee. Just as your vision guides the behavior and performance of the staff, it will help quickly weed out individuals who don't fit the teamwork mold. When you have a salon vision statement, you are prepared to explain precisely *where* the salon is going and *how* it plans to get there. Often, this is a key criterion as candidates decide whether to join a company.

Encourage candidates to talk with existing staff and leadership team members. Observe and evaluate: Do they "fit" in terms of skill, attitude and personality? The best working relationships occur when the fit is right for both the stylist and the salon.

After making a selection, don't forget the applicants you *didn't* hire. Ask them back; don't just send a form letter. Let them know your salon is growing, and there will be job openings in the future. Make them feel "plugged in" to your salon. Keep the process positive and upbeat. You never know when your paths will cross again or how many other prospects they will be in contact with. Add them to your red file.

MENTAL TICKLE: Qualified applicants not chosen today may be your best employees tomorrow. Treat all candidates, whether you plan to hire them or not, as future employees of the salon.

A STRATEGIES WANT AD
WITH A PROVEN RESPONSE RECORD

Stylists and expert colorists: Your search for the perfect salon is over. Imagine the perfect balance of upscale ambiance, impeccable quality service and business sophistication. Imagine attractive starting salaries, income growth potential, performance bonuses and excellent benefits. Stop imagining! We have openings for a few very special, highly professional stylists and colorists at our salon/day spa. Clientele not required — talent and enthusiasm are. For a confidential interview, call our salon manager at XXX.XXX.XXXX.

Salon 218…Recruiting according to plan

**Recruiting staff doesn't have to be a nightmare —
creativity can go a long way to completing your team**

Just when you think things are finally going your way, a new roadblock lands right in your path. Client retention rates are up, you've fine-tuned your management systems and created a working environment in which the entire team is motivated to grow the salon. Your salon is pulling in so much business that it can't keep up with the number of clients walking through the door. Productivity is through the roof and staff is burning out. Worst of all, clients are having trouble getting into the salon, which is counterproductive to the customer service standards you've striven so hard to attain.

Are you doing something wrong? Did you make a mistake somewhere? No — these are all signs of salon growth. All indicators are telling you that, to realize the true potential of your salon, your next step is (gasps and moans from around the industry) to recruit more staff take on the extra workload. But how do you recruit staff that will adapt to your finely tuned salon structure?

One owner's experience

Angela Adams, owner of Salon 218 in Huntington Beach, CA, was confronted with this challenge. Her staff was completely gridlocked, but she realized after attending a Strategies Incubator that the salon still had more potential. It was obvious that she must expand her staff for the salon to operate at a higher level.

The first step was to communicate her intentions to the existing team. Salon 218 utilizes a salary/team-bonus compensation system, so she communicated in great detail that more stylists on the floor equals more revenue-producing hours to sell. With more hours sold, the salon brings in more money, which allows the team to hit their bonus more easily. Everyone was excited. Additionally,

Angela called upon her team to help develop a recruitment process to ensure each new recruit would be compatible with SALON 218'S culture and management. "During weekly huddles, my staff always comes up with ways to cut costs and grow the salon," says Angela. "That involvement should extend into the recruitment process."

Options and considerations

The SALON 218 team has worked hard to develop a clientele devoted to the salon rather than to individual stylists, so Angela wasn't forced to search for "star" stylists with existing followings. Clients were already waiting to get into the salon, so she was more concerned with finding new staff motivated to contribute to the team. Angela began her search at the one place she knew she could find young, motivated individuals: her old beauty school. "I volunteered to instruct two classes at the school," says Angela, who is also one of seventeen salon owners who comprise the school's advisory board. "My sole intention was to give the students an escape from technical education and give them a chance to see the creative work others are doing in the industry."

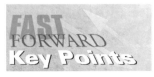

SALON 218 had thirty-one stylists respond to their invitation.

The two classes were entitled *Building Your Career Through Legendary Customer Service* and *Goal-Setting Your Way To Success.* "The school encourages its advisory board members to instruct classes," Angela says. "But I'm the only one of seventeen who has taken them up on it. Frankly, it amazes me how many salon owners ignore the incredible recruiting opportunity of getting in front of a classroom full of students and promoting the culture and techniques that make their salon a special place to work."

Angela's "first cut" effort

In addition to providing students with a much-neglected element of beauty school curriculum, Angela's classes also acted as a "first cut" for her recruitment efforts. "Only those truly interested in my message and the working environment we promote in our salon responded," Angela says. This ensures a beneficial and productive recruitment process for both the salon and potential recruits. She and her team designed very simple invitations to a "recruitment night" to be held at her salon. Prior to each class, each student received an invitation.

So, do alternative recruitment methods really attract more interest than the trusty old newspaper ad? You'd better believe it. *SALON 218 had thirty-one stylists respond to their invitation.* Angela's class showcased her commitment to stylist education and industry awareness. For inexperienced stylists just out of beauty school, a nurturing team environment is an inspiring place to start.

Recruits get the client treatment

Recognizing the importance of finding team members to fit SALON 218's philosophy, Angela and her team wanted to structure their recruitment night so that it accurately represented the salon's culture and philosophies. Most importantly, it had to be a team event. Responsibilities were delegated according to what the team refers to as SALON 218's *four guarantees.* Angela explains, "These are four mandatory guarantees that every client must experience when visiting SALON 218. What better way for new recruits to learn these criteria than to experience them?"

■ WARM GREETING WITH TOUCH AND OFFER OF A STYLE CHANGE. "This makes the client feel comfortable and lets her know the stylist is willing to try a new look," says Angela. For recruitment night a *hello* team was assembled to greet attendees and offer either a handshake or a warm touch to the shoulder. The sign-in team handed out name tags and short questionnaires, as well as complimentary gifts for attending. Because no services were being performed, the style change concept was discussed, though not offered.

■ MASSAGE THERAPY WITH EVERY SERVICE. "A complimentary shoulder or hand massage is a very rewarding three-minute service," explains Angela. "Clients are relaxed, and we can cross-promote services." During recruitment night, this guarantee was met by the *tour* team, who incorporated massages as a stop on their tour through the salon. New recruits experienced the SALON 218 tour as if they were clients, learning about the retail center and massage and nail areas, as well as receiving introductions to the entire staff.

■ A WRITTEN LIST OF ALL PRODUCTS NEEDED to maintain the new style at home. The most powerful tool for selling product is the professional recommendation. SALON 218 has grown a lucrative retail business supported by an enthusiastic staff — a point well made by the tour team. A professional recommendation requires product knowledge, and the gifts ensured the beginning of the applicants' research.

■ MAKE-UP TOUCH-UP, PRE-BOOKING OF APPOINTMENTS and a guaranteed confirmation call 24–48 hours prior to appointments. "Again, the make-up touch-up lets us cross-promote services," says Angela. "Pre-booking and confirmation calls enable us to keep client retention rates up. We tried to stress the importance of these efforts during recruitment night."

Final selection

Throughout the recruitment night, an evaluation team recorded remarks on the new talent and took Polaroid pictures of each individual to make it easier to remember whom they were talking about later. They kept all remarks concealed and, more importantly, stressed only positive attributes. Those who did not fit SALON 218'S culture were easy to pick out. The final selection of five new team members was made in a staff meeting after the event. The most promising candidates made positive

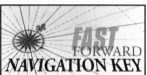

FAST FORWARD NAVIGATION KEY

Heartfelt communication made SALON 218's recruitment effort a success. Angela and her team knew the type of individuals they were looking for. With a little creativity and planning, they made those individuals come to them. In an industry that constantly hears the cry for good help, SALON 218 is breaking new ground with their resourcefulness and strict focus on the final goal.

TT965
.D83
2000
3196700068
261506

Ducoff, Neil.
   Fast forward salon & spa business
resource : -- Centerbrook, CT : Strategies
Pub. Group, c2000.
   482 p. : ill. ; 19 cm. -- (Fast forward
platinum business series)

   ISBN: 0970102801

   1. Health resorts--Management.
2. Beauty shops--Management. I. Cross,
Matthew. II. Flinn, Nancy A.
III. Slater, Heather. IV. Title.

TT965 .D83 2000   646.7/2/068   00-711107
                                                     MARC

$59.95

4~/2

impressions throughout the evening. Careful preparation and thorough planning greatly facilitated the final choice of the new team members. Everyone left the event with feelings of assurance and inspiration. SALON 218's team was evolving, and will continue to do so because of ever-increasing interest generated by the event.

During the recruitment night, Angela shared some observations on the beauty industry. "I was honest with them," she recalls. "I told them I believe the industry is broken, but as a team we have an incredible opportunity to mend it. People are much more inspired when they can impress their own voices on the vision."

In the words of business guru Tom Peters, "No longer is it the big eat the small — now the fast eat the slow." And in today's game of recruiting new staff, the tried-and-true help-wanted ad isn't exactly breaking any sound barriers.

Perfect your interviewing skills

R ecruiting new staff this year? Getting people through the door will be tougher and more expensive than ever because the base of quality talent is shrinking. Now is the time to perfect your interviewing skills and hire people who are right for your salon.

The human resource specialist

Imagine yourself as the director of human resources for a major corporation. Your job is to interview and hire the very best people to work for the company. Success in your job, and the future of the company, rests on your decision. Would you simply hire the first person to come through the door? Probably not. Chances are, you would find a way to match the perfect candidate to the perfect job. In most cases, you would also find it better to not hire at all than to hire the wrong person.

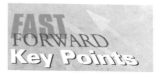

During interviews, many entrepreneurs get too wrapped up in telling their own story. They forget the prime objective: to ask leading questions that will reveal the true qualities and potential behaviors of the applicant.

In an interview, the owner or manager should do more listening than talking.

PROBING FOR CLUES: Your first challenge is to uncover why a candidate may or may not fit salon standards. Thoroughly peruse the resumé, ask insightful interview questions and check references.

The resumé

A well-written resumé tells the story of a job candidate's career up to a certain point. It should include an objective (the candidate's goal), the names of previous employers (including dates of employment and duties performed) and educational experience (including dates of attendance).

Always look over a candidate's resumé carefully. Take note of long gaps in employment, frequent job changes, scope of education, and other things about which you may like to ask.

Revealing questions

Asking probing questions during an interview increases the odds of hiring the right person. The answers may shatter your initial impressions, but the time together will show how well the two of you interact.

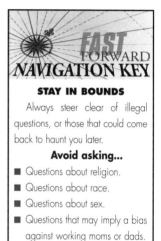

STAY IN BOUNDS

Always steer clear of illegal questions, or those that could come back to haunt you later.

Avoid asking...

- Questions about religion.
- Questions about race.
- Questions about sex.
- Questions that may imply a bias against working moms or dads.

- PROBING FOR MOTIVATION: Why did you apply for this position? What are your long-term goals? How do you plan to reach these goals? Where would you like to be in five years? What do you want from your next job that you are not getting now?

- PROBING FOR STABILITY: What were the reasons for leaving your last job? How have your goals changed over the years? What's your greatest disappointment so far in your career?

- PROBING FOR RESOURCEFULNESS: What was a difficult problem you faced in your last job? How did you solve it? If you started working here today, what expertise would you bring to the job immediately? Describe a time when you were treated rudely by an employee of another business. How did the person act? How did you react?

- PROBING FOR COMPATIBILITY: For what characteristics or actions has your last manager complimented you? Describe a time when he or she criticized you. How did you react?

The reference check

Request employment references if they are not included with a candidate's resumé. Then, after the first interview, call to verify.

Finally — if a candidate matches your requirements, has an admirable personality and seems like a true overachiever — go for it.

Listen to previous employers' responses to inquiries on their former employee. Sometimes you can pick up clues regarding the applicant's performance, personality, ethics and other behavior patterns.

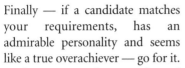

NAVIGATION KEY

VERIFY REFERENCES

Hiring by guesswork can teach expensive lessons. Every candidate's resumé must be put to the test by calling previous employers and checking the following:

- Dates of employment
- Reason for termination of employment
- Salary history
- Ask: "Is he/she rehirable?"

When checking references, note whether character references are supplied by the applicant. Also, previous employers can be easily omitted from an application. Look for time gaps in employment histories and ask for explanations. Listen carefully to what's not said. Body language can often identify sensitive issues.

Indoctrinating and training new staff

Poor behavior and work habits can develop quickly during the first days and months of employment, but they take a long time to correct. When it comes to servicing clients, maintaining quality standards and supporting your vision, *nothing* can be left to chance.

Educate thoroughly and continuously

To get the most from your team, you must educate them continuously. You can't afford *not* to, for the following three reasons:

- It provides an opportunity to communicate and emphasize the salon's vision.
- It provides concrete skills staff need to succeed at your salon.
- It offers alternatives to old ways and allows employees to create their own new ways of serving clients better.

Good training enables people to develop the "right" skills and behaviors quickly. In a salon environment, *new* employees must live up to *established* customer expectations. There's no room for "Sorry about that. I'm new here," when clients expect the best from your salon on every visit.

- How do new employees behave before training?
- Define how you want them to behave after training.

Demonstrate the behavior expected at the salon. Teach the technical and service skills they will need. Lastly, teach them about your salon vision. HINT: One thing you *can't* teach is attitude. People simply don't respond to lectures or courses telling them to smile at customers. But if your salon demonstrates in other ways that it really cares about customers, if the indoctrination and training program teaches the vision and skills to help them grow, you *will* change attitudes in the process.

Developing your training program

Once you hire eagles (avoiding the turkeys), do everything you can to keep the eagle mentality alive. During the first days on the job, newly hired employees are still highly impressionable. Those first few days may be your only chance to mold and shape a new employee. This is where your training program begins.

No matter how much experience new employees have, everyone must complete the same indoctrination program. During the program, all new staff members learn firsthand the details of the salon's vision, performance expectations and operating systems... including client handling procedures, client retention programs, quality standards and other specifics that will directly impact their ability to succeed.

Mandatory training for all new employees should last at least five days, each one packed with training and role-playing projects supervised by key staff members. The goal of this *behavioral* training is to quickly indoctrinate new people into the behavior patterns that support your vision. Many behavior problems could be avoided if owners instituted a formal, rigorous indoctrination process.

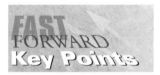

No matter how much experience new employees have, everyone must complete the same indoctrination program.

Each day should focus on a specific aspect of behavior, such as customer-handling procedures. Begin by describing the procedure's objectives, and why they are integral to the salon's service quality program. Next, demonstrate the behaviors the salon expects in all customer contact situations: telephone calls, front desk greetings, client check-in and check-out, shampoo procedures, styling, color, etc. Leave nothing to chance.

The DISNEY CORPORATION teaches this process at Disney University. Even the groundskeepers go through four days of training to learn the company's vision, procedures and other key aspects vital to maintaining superior service standards. If a visitor asks a groundskeeper the location of a particular ride, he'll have the right answer. Salons can and must do the same.

A few key points to boost your indoctrination program are:

- Teach part of the program yourself. Demonstrate your commitment to the principles and behaviors your salon expects of employees.
- Drive home your salon's vision, and give new team members an opportunity to use it. Have them answer the phone, book appointments and greet new clients. Remember, this goes for everyone — including the "star" you just hired with twelve years of salon experience. Your salon is different. The indoctrination program will show them why and how.
- Involve key staff. Ask new staff members to work with the receptionist or coordinator on one day, and a senior stylist the next. Be certain to present a key part of the program yourself.
- Work them hard. Each day of indoctrination should be packed with information, demonstrations, role-playing and hands-on work. It's boot camp salon-style, and every new recruit should experience a feeling of accomplishment, teamwork and camaraderie at the program's conclusion.
- Commit your program and schedule to paper, detailing each day. Prepare a three-ring binder, with extra paper for notes. The program should be as structured as possible.

Don't miss this opportunity to instill and reinforce your vision with all new staff members. The benefits are extraordinary.

Teach: Expect and expected

Candidates and new employees need to know how they fit into your vision. Tell them what to expect.

- What should they anticipate, good and bad, in their daily work? The simple act of telling people what to expect can save a great deal of future pain. Don't push the "ups" and hold back the "downs." If new employees must sweep floors, shampoo clients and rinse color for the first six months, tell them.
- How will you measure their performance? Nothing is more important to new employees than knowing how their performance will be evaluated. Offer a detailed explanation of your performance and evaluation program.
- How will you recognize and reward them for good work?

Raises, bonuses, prizes, promotions and other types of recognition show employees that you value them and their work.

■ HOW VITAL IS CUSTOMER SERVICE TO EVERY SALON ACTIVITY AND RULE? Tell staff members what to expect daily, and how you will monitor, reward, recognize and promote them. It will encourage them to pursue maximum levels of excellence and customer satisfaction.

Problem employees

Problem employees can make life miserable for everyone in the salon, including clients. Their behavior must be addressed before it disrupts the rest of the business or impacts client service. Your management style will be important.

Will you be a dominant boss, attacking the employee? Will you attempt to consult and counsel? Will you be the steady manager who explains that "rules are rules, and must be followed"? Or will you wimp out and hope the problem goes away?

Management experts agree that problem employees must be handled quickly and efficiently, in much the same manner as a problem client. Most employee behavior problems are brought on by a lack of training, poor understanding of the salon's vision, or a personal problem the employee is unable to keep from interfering with work. You must get to the root of the problem, discuss corrective measures and develop a verbal and/or written contract through which the behavior will be corrected.

Customer service champions

Your salon team has been painstakingly recruited using your hiring profile, rigorously indoctrinated into your vision, and empowered to use the vision to move the salon and themselves forward. The product of your recruitment efforts is a well-oiled team of professionals capable of achieving a level of success only a select group of salons ever experience. It's business at its best.

Why build a skill certification program?

I n-salon skill certification is a long-overdue quality assurance process. Today, salon success depends upon consistent technical and customer service quality. To achieve this, salons need a formal skill program to train and indoctrinate new staff members, and to monitor and update the skills and services of long-standing staff.

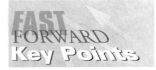

The program's objective is to ensure the quality and integrity of your salon, by allowing staff members to perform only those services for which they have been certified. Isn't that what clients expect from a True Quality salon or day spa?

What exactly is it?

A SKILL CERTIFICATION PROGRAM IS A FORMAL, ORGANIZED APPROACH TO EVALUATING STAFF SKILL AND ABILITY IN A VARIETY OF TECHNICAL AND CUSTOMER SERVICE AREAS. The program's objective is to ensure the quality and integrity of your salon, by allowing staff members to perform only those services for which they have been certified. (For example: Coordinators will know whom to assign clients requesting certain services; and if technicians sell services they are not yet certified to perform, procedure will require that the coordinator assign a certified team member.)

But a skill certification program must go well beyond technical skills. It must also include customer service, communication and other non-technical skills. Designing a certification program requires the same attention to detail as designing a salon. Begin with clearly defined objectives that reflect your vision for the salon. When fully designed and implemented, your skill certification program becomes "what you sell": quality technical service, superior customer service, and all the intangibles that will separate your salon from the competition.

Let's examine some key aspects of skill certification:

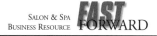
DON'T EVEN THINK ABOUT TRUE QUALITY WITHOUT IT.

Service is your product. To deliver a quality service, you must have established processes, quality objectives and standards of performance. True Quality will *not* happen without a skill certification program. The tenets of True Quality demand that no one provides a service of any form (technical or interpersonal) unless he or she can perform to established standards. Given this, most salons will never meet the most basic True Quality requirements.

SALON SIZE DOESN'T MATTER.

If you're already thinking your salon is too small to justify a formal skill certification program, you're wrong. Size is not the issue; customer satisfaction is. How good do you want your salon to be? Are you willing to accept mediocre technical and customer service? Are you willing to accept the costs of otherwise avoidable redo's? Are you willing to accept low client retention rates? Are you willing to fund the costs of inefficiency and poor productivity? Even the most basic certification program pays major dividends and gives most salons a competitive advantage.

ITS ABSENCE IS MEASURABLE.

At most salons, clients are assigned to staff based on availability first, and competency second. This practice, combined with a lack of quality assurance mechanisms, has produced a dismal industry-wide first-time client retention rate that barely exceeds 30%. In other words, almost 70% of all first-time clients are not sufficiently impressed with their salon experience to return for a second visit. A 30% retention rate is unacceptable. The only sure way to improve your salon's client retention rate is to implement a skill certification program.

IT PROVIDES PATHWAYS FOR GROWTH.

What does it take to succeed in your salon? What are the skill requirements? What's expected of new staff? How can they move into the higher pay levels? Your skill certification program will provide the answers, while showing staff the salon's path for growth.

In recent years, the business world has shifted to skill-based pay systems that encourage employees to develop and perfect new skills. These programs benefit the company, employee and consumer. Yet salons are still stuck in, and limited by, "percentage of sales" pay methods. The promise is: Sell more, earn more.

Sales are clearly important, but where do quality assurance and customer service fit in? When pay is based solely on individual sales, everything else takes a back seat. High sales have nothing to do with quality service; they simply show that an employee can sell in spite of skill and customer service deficiencies. In salons and spas, quality-driven pathways for growth are critical.

IT BUILDS CLIENT LOYALTY TO YOUR SALON TEAM.

Stylist followings are a relic of the past, with no place in today's salon. Every day, more forward-thinking salons are proving they can service clients as a team of professionals, and that client loyalty can shift from individual stylists to the team. Skill certification will be your most powerful tool in this shift. It will build client trust in your team-service approach. Trust is all clients need to become a team client.

IT'S A POWERFUL MARKETING TOOL.

Don't keep your skill certification program a secret. It's a powerful marketing tool. Aggressively promote it through advertising, consultations and all potential and existing client contacts.

Designing your skill certification program

D ue to the the residual problems of years gone by, salon owners today are faced with the choice of whether to even train staff. First, high turnover (plus a poor industry image) leaves ever-fewer working stylists in an already lean job pool, creating a human resources nightmare. Second, the emergence of career-minded stylists means salon owners must prove they can offer career development pathways. And third, the abandonment of the art gallery image in favor of corporate structure means stiff competition looms ahead. But perhaps the choice has already been made. If a little time and money up front results in a burgeoning future, secure staff and profitability, then *ante up* and start training.

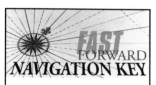

NAVIGATION KEY

Too many salon owners rush to complete an in-salon skill certification program, only to get frustrated.

Plan on three or four months to complete entry-level technical and non-technical portions. Intermediate and advanced certification programs could take up to six or eight months to complete.

WHERE DO YOU START? Commit to developing a customer-driven, high-quality, consistent salon. Add solid leadership and a clear vision. Then delve into the following program blueprint. It contains everything you'll need to build a basic skill certification program.

The elements of the plan

Nearly all salon skills which require certification fall into one of three major training areas: *technical, professional/organizational,* or *personal/cultural.*

■ TECHNICAL TRAINING encompasses the skills which generate revenue for the salon. They include retailing; performing hair, nail, skin and spa services; and telephone and consultation skills.

■ PROFESSIONAL/ORGANIZATIONAL behavior strongly supports an understanding of the salon's vision and goals. Although not critical to everyday operation, it is vital for long-term success. Associated skills include the ability to understand retail goals, etiquette, client indoctrination, decision-making, profiling, profit and loss, client treatment and retention rates, and how to handle complaints.

■ PERSONAL/CULTURAL skills relate to working relationships: staff to staff, staff to client, and staff to leadership team. They include upholding cultural requirements which contribute to the over-all salon environment: participation in salon meetings, relating to co-workers, maintaining and enforcing salon culture, partic-ipating in projects, contributing ideas, supporting the salon mission and vision, and leading projects.

These are only partial skill listings. Detail your salon to find oth-ers that should be included in the training program. You may not discover them all the first time, but keep searching. If you find a few that seem to fit into more than one category, try to find which they best fit into.

The heart of your program

The *written, practical* and *benchmark* sections of the program will include the bulk of training information, and can be used for any skill in any of the above categories, from a technical training program for haircolor to the personal/cultural skill of complaint handling. The plan can be used for any skill needing certification. To gain a better understanding, let's use the technical skill "perming."

The written portion

Writing down all aspects of a skill solidifies teaching methods and makes it tangible to you and the staff. Preparing each part of the written section will help you methodically list the skills to be learned. Once it's written, continually refer to it. Skill training should not become a guessing game later.

To create a comprehensive written analysis for a particular skill, gather as much support material as possible: magazine articles, notes from other training sessions, anything to enhance the learn-

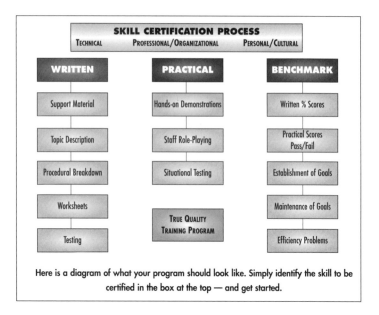

Here is a diagram of what your program should look like. Simply identify the skill to be certified in the box at the top — and get started.

ing process. After gathering the materials, create a topic description explaining how to master the skill. Make bullet point notes. For our perming example, topic descriptions would include hair analysis and consultation, and perm selection, wrap and processing.

A PROCEDURAL BREAKDOWN consists of all bullet points from the topic description. Precisely outline the steps for performing that particular skill. This will give the staff an agenda to follow, and ensure the skill is performed correctly and without confusion. A perming example:

- STEP ONE: Perform consultation.
- STEP TWO: Shampoo hair with deep-cleansing shampoo.
- STEP THREE: Begin perm wrap using technique outlined by perm consultation.

Use your procedural breakdown to develop worksheets. (Use key points to form review questions.) Utilize these worksheets as quizzes to reinforce the learning process.

The practical portion

The major thrust of the practical portion of a skill certification program is visual learning — learning by showing.

HANDS-ON DEMONSTRATIONS reinforce the written material already covered, by allowing staff to see a particular skill applied in a real-life situation. When showing the steps for perming, actually wrap a model. Show all aspects, including section size, rod placement and wrap technique. Show the entire process if desired.

Role-playing encourages staff to repeat new skills, and allows them to try new techniques and methods in a controlled environment. For example: Staff can work on models, repeating what they have seen. Video taping is effective in critiquing some skills.

Situational testing, much like written testing, allows staff to be evaluated on their newly acquired practical skills. Testing can range from role-playing to basic observations about the hands-on demonstrations.

The benchmarks

When written and practical training are completed, it's time to establish benchmarks: parameters which measure how well the staff retains new skills. Some benchmarks must be achieved before certification is granted; others must be achieved afterward, to ensure consistency.

PRE-CERTIFICATION BENCHMARKS INCLUDE:

- WRITTEN TEST SCORES…should range from 85%–100%.
- PRACTICAL TEST SCORES…rated pass/fail. They should be scored by a certification trainer.
- ESTABLISHMENT OF GOALS…Set attainable, realistic objectives to help your staff master new skills and become certified. An example: Perm wraps must consistently be completed within twenty-five minutes.

POST-CERTIFICATION BENCHMARKS INCLUDE:

- GOAL MAINTENANCE…ensures skill levels remain consistent and comply with certification requirements; encourages staff to master new skills. For perming, staff may be required to perform a minimum of ten perms per month to remain certified.

■ EFFICIENCY PROBLEMS…isolate aspects of new skills that trouble staff. For example: Excessive re-perms may indicate the need to isolate and analyze a problem, and retrain staff if necessary.

Conclusion

When implementing a skill certification program in an existing salon, it must grow with the business. It needs adequate time to incubate. Staff, especially new members, must be certified before performing services. This will keep quality high and decrease mistakes. Stylists already performing services should continue, but also be trained and formally certified within a specified time period.

Get help developing your training program if necessary. Consider your staff when looking for qualified trainers, or ask your distributor. The benefits of a certification program will far outweigh the time spent building and maintaining it. A training and skill certification program is a cost-effective way to secure the future of your salon and staff. It can improve quality, consistency and efficiency.

Skill certification case study:
One salon's practical certification experience

Salon owner Albert Tromblay talks about how he focused all of his salon's energies on consistent, quality work that can be performed by each team member

A big part of our salon's problem was the lack of confidence in each other's skills. Techniques varied between staff, and we were feeding the new clients to the least experienced stylists and expecting them to exceed expectations. We faced low client retention and high stress levels. We worked hard for our good reputation, but our inability to address performance inconsistencies was jeopardizing our future.

Realizing the inevitable

We felt a comprehensive skill program was needed. All technical, professional and cultural skills had to be defined, but how? We took a leap of faith and shared our burdens and vision for TROMBLAY SALON with the staff. We explained why we thought a skill certification program would be the answer to our problems. Overwhelmed by the magnitude of this task, we asked for help. Our two senior stylists came to our aid and formed our leadership team. Their biggest fear was that the program would eliminate creativity; therefore, we designed our standards to allow room for individual interpretation.

We began with weekly two-hour meetings to identify and categorize skills, which were divided into four levels of difficulty. We watched each other perform the service, agreed to one set of standards, then practiced it again and again. Then we presented it to the staff with a hands-on demonstration. Stylists honed their skill until they were ready to be certified, under the observation of a senior staff member.

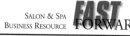
Looking back

We have been adjusting, and adding new and more advanced skills as we go. Documenting and identifying what we do has given more meaning to our work. It's getting easier to recognize accomplishments and strengths instead of weaknesses and faults. We have even tied our compensation plan into the skill program.

Ultimately, we would like to say that no service is booked with a stylist who is not certified in that skill, but that is easier said than done. It's not always known at the time of booking what the result of the consultation will be. So, now all new clients get a consultation with at least two stylists. This creates a win-win situation. The client has better access to our salon, receives a more consistent service and has the input of more than one stylist. The staff has more confidence in each other, has a better understanding of what is expected and receives skills and knowledge that are of value in today's market.

We now believe that anything can be solved with good communication. The skills program is making our business healthier. The consistency and service of our salon is definitely making us stand out in a community fueled by 90% booth rental. *It's working in Kalamazoo, Michigan.*

Things to do:

■ Design a compensation package that rewards team members for overall performance, including:

> SKILL LEVEL
> TEAMWORK
> RETENTION
> PRODUCTIVITY
> ATTENDANCE
> ATTITUDE
> APPEARANCE

■ Design a hiring profile that clearly defines the type of employee who is right for your salon.

■ Develop an ongoing recruiting plan which reflects your salon's vision.

■ Perfect your interviewing skills in order to hire the right people for your salon.

> MAKE A LIST OF INTERVIEWING "DO'S AND DON'TS."

■ Develop a training program for new employees. Put it in writing. Describe what each training day will consist of.

■ Build a skill certification program to monitor and update the skill of all employees.

■ Design a detailed performance evaluation form to measure the progress and performance of new hires, as well as long-standing employees.

LEADERSHIP

Staff coaching and performance

L eadership encompasses the very essence of what it takes to move a business forward by moving its people forward. It is a call to action in the quest for vision, values, strategic objectives, communication, standards of performance, motivation, inspiration, steadfastness, flexibility, compassion, good judgement and opportunity.

LEADERSHIP IS A STATE OF MIND. It's the innate understanding and acceptance that "the buck stops with you." You can delegate, collaborate and seek consensus but, ultimately, decisions regarding the future of your business are in your hands. In this regard, leadership may be either a burden or a privilege of the highest order. True leaders rise to the challenge, and stand above the crowd. They relentlessly pursue the top rungs of the success ladder. Their nature is to create and lead, not to follow. Their reward is progress and accomplishment. Their nemesis is stagnation.

LEADERSHIP IS ABOUT CHANGE. *Caretakers* keep things neat and tidy. Their vision is of maintaining a standard. *Leaders,* on the other hand, thrive on change because they understand it is a relentless force in business. Trends come and go. Markets shift. Without

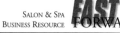
change, there is stagnation. Especially in the salon industry, change is the energy that drives the leadership spirit and keeps it fresh.

Barber shops became an endangered species because their leaders functioned only as caretakers, and failed to respond to shifts in the market. Wash-and-set salons met a similar fate in the early '70s when owners failed to recognize the haircutting boom as more than a passing trend. The day spa concept represents yet another shift in the marketplace, as consumers, both men and women, look to salons for services and products that focus on beauty and wellness from head to toe.

FAST FORWARD
Key Points

Change is relentless.
It's the energy that drives the leadership spirit and keeps it fresh.

LEADERSHIP IS EARNED. Too many salon owners cling to the fatal assumption that "leadership" is somehow a preordained fact of ownership. It isn't. Whether you are an owner, stylist, colorist, nail technician or spa therapist, leadership is earned through deeds and actions. Employees don't follow a *title*. They follow the individual behind the title, one who can take them to a better place, who offers opportunities and prosperity. A leader gains respect and authority by earning it. Likewise, leaders lose respect and authority by being dictatorial, egotistical or abusive — or by simply failing to lead.

IN THE ABSENCE OF LEADERSHIP THERE IS CHAOS. If you abdicate leadership responsibilities, the culture of the business will free-float into unfocused chaos. "Hostage management" is nothing more than a by-product of neglecting one's leadership responsibilities. Perhaps some owners lack sufficient leadership skills, or perceive certain aspects of leadership to be disturbingly confrontational… but without leadership, the salon's culture can be irreparably damaged as anarchy takes over.

Leadership and salon culture

LEADERSHIP CREATES STRUCTURE AND FOCUS…AND CULTURE. It's the beacon that guides a salon to fulfill its vision and strategic objective. *Don't confuse leadership with management.*

At the moment you conceived your salon business, its culture began to form. As new staff join, their personalities, behaviors and beliefs will further shape its culture.

Carefully maintained and nurtured, this culture will quickly evolve into a collection of governing values, beliefs and standards of performance which will make the salon strong and fill it with vitality. Left unchecked, it will become contaminated, and forward motion will stop.

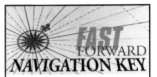

You can "see" the culture your leadership creates

Culture is more pertinent to salon success than many people realize. Perhaps it's because they perceive "culture" as an abstract which they can't see or touch. But the fact is, you *can* see, touch and experience culture…especially in a personal service business. Much of what is done in the salon and provided through services is behavior-driven. *Culture defines behavior.* You can observe, experience and, especially in a salon, feel behaviors in the form of applied technical and interpersonal skills.

To MANAGE is "to direct or control the use of; to exert control over; to make submissive to one's authority, discipline or persuasion; to direct or administer; to direct, supervise or carry on business or other affairs."

To LEAD is "to show the way by going in advance; to serve as a route for; to guide the action or opinion of; to direct the performance or activities of."

Are you a leader or a misguided manager? To rally the forces and effectively work with staff every day, you must know the difference.

Thanks to Webster's Dictionary

THE STATE OF SALON CULTURE TODAY: Let's suppose you introduce a new promotion to your staff. You explain it thoroughly and ask for feedback. What kind of culture exists if the responses include, "I don't want lose my commission; let the newbies do it," or, "We've tried that before; it won't work here"? Suppose you want to implement a True Quality team-driven program through which clients are encouraged to utilize the skills of the entire staff. The objective is to balance productivity and improve performance by reducing

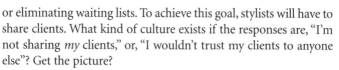

or eliminating waiting lists. To achieve this goal, stylists will have to share clients. What kind of culture exists if the responses are, "I'm not sharing *my* clients," or, "I wouldn't trust my clients to anyone else"? Get the picture?

LEADERSHIP SKILLS PLAY A PIVOTAL ROLE IN SHAPING AND NURTURING A SALON'S CULTURE. Without constant attention, coaching and support, a culture can become contaminated. Sometimes a staff member doesn't fit your culture, and must be removed before the balance of the salon is disturbed. A strong positive culture can weed out those staff members who do not fit in.

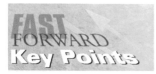

A positive culture defines what is right and acceptable behavior in your salon.

A positive culture is a powerful force. It defines appropriate and acceptable behavior, and sets standards of performance that team members strive for and protect at all costs. A positive culture gives the salon the stamina to overcome adversities faced by all growing businesses.

Are you a manager or a leader?

D o you proudly bear the title "manager"? If so, you are indeed an authority figure…though others may not necessarily do as you tell them. "Managers" manage resources, *things* (e.g., schedules, supplies, bills).

When you're in front of people, you're more likely a leader — unless no one is following. By definition, a leader needs one or more followers. But you can't become a leader simply by adopting the title. You earn the title when you are recognized as a leader by your followers. And don't forget: Followers can always fire a leader.

Leaders put themselves on the line. They take personal risks — emotional, physical or both. They commit. They develop and empower their followers by stepping back to let others gain experience. They are not intimidated by the skills of others, but encourage excellence. Great leaders strive for team success, and ascribe these successes to the team's efforts, not their own. Leaders come in all shapes, sizes, colors and ages, and from both sexes. And, contrary to popular belief (although some people do appear to be born with them), it is possible to develop leadership skills at any point.

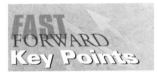

Always remember, you manage things…and lead people.

What it takes to be a leader

People become leaders when they demonstrate a strength, or combination of strengths, that attracts followers. One may be physically strong, or knowledgeable or charismatic. Strength may emanate from an inner conviction or set of values. Whether viewed by history as good or bad, *true* leaders have two things in common:

1. They know and understand the needs of the people they lead — and their goal is to fulfill those needs.
2. They may not be the most-liked person, but they have earned the respect of their followers.

Hannibal was a strong leader, but someone had to feed the elephants and clothe the troops. History says little about the supporting roles of his managers and staff, yet we know he didn't achieve his victories without well-fed elephants. It is possible to be both a leader and a manager. The *way you manage* either supports your leadership role or keeps you from it. What is an effective leader?

An effective leader

- …is flexible rather than rigid, choosing from a wide range of behaviors and tactics.
- …is aware of the forces within him- or herself, among the staff and in any given situation.
- …chooses a leadership style *after* assessing these forces; is honest with followers.
- …lets the followers know their influence on a given issue and how leadership authority will be exercised.
- …does not "duck" responsibility by involving others in the decision-making process.
- …ensures necessary decisions are made by the followers whenever feasible, or by him- or herself if the situation requires.

Five typical leadership styles

1. TELLING: The leader identifies the problem, considers alternative solutions, chooses one and tells the followers what to do.
2. PERSUADING: As before, the leader makes the decision but, instead of simply announcing it, tries to persuade the followers to accept it.
3. CONSULTING: The leader allows the followers the opportunity to influence the decision from the beginning by suggesting alternative solutions. The leader then selects the most promising.
4. JOINING: The leader participates as any other member, and agrees to abide by the group's decision.
5. DELEGATING: The leader defines a problem and the boundaries within which it must be solved, then turns it over to the team and agrees to support their decision if it is within the stated boundaries.

Before choosing a leadership style, assess...

WITHIN THE LEADER: values; confidence in the followers; feelings of security; personal inclination toward a given leadership style.

WITHIN THE FOLLOWERS: knowledge and experience; need for independence; readiness for responsibility; interest level; understanding of company values, vision and mission; expectations of the leader; personality variables.

WITHIN THE SITUATION ITSELF: type of organization; demonstrated effectiveness of followers; nature of the problem; constraints (e.g., resources, rules and regulations).

Leaders exhibit the following qualities:

- The *vision* to spell out clearly what they will do for those who depend on them.
- The *drive* to share that vision with those who have the largest stake in the business' success.
- The *courage* to challenge status quo, stimulate change and make decisions to move the salon forward, even in difficult times.
- The *ability* to inspire people to action, individually and in teams, to achieve goals.
- The *foresight* to empower people to learn new skills and stretch their capabilities.
- The *wisdom* to listen and learn, and translate that knowledge into valuable performance.
- The *integrity* to serve as a good example through actions that consistently reinforce basic values.
- The *willingness* to recognize accomplishments, and celebrate individual and team successes and contributions.

THE DOWNSIDE: A leader must take responsibility for the work of others, and learn to guide and coach rather than issue orders. This means accepting a lesser degree of control. Even people you trust will stumble from time to time. You must pick them up, assuage their fears and be supportive.

A leader needs to be:

- *Objective*...no prejudice or bias concerning people or projects. Insist on the truth.

- *Sensitive*…able to understand followers' needs and frailties; welfare of the organization is a top priority.
- *Competent*…knowledge, skill, experience, inspiring attitude.
- *Fair without being soft*…tough-minded without being tough; willingness to do unpopular or unpleasant things.
- *Consistent*…"rules of the game" apply to everyone; messages communicated convey a common thread or vision.
- *Humble*…not arrogant; able to laugh at him- or herself.
- *Steady under fire*…calm and composed; can be counted on.
- *Confidently supportive*…believes in followers; unswerving support; ready to accept unconditional responsibility for followers' mistakes.
- *Guiding light*…able to cope, sometimes with seemingly insurmountable odds.
- *A winner.*

Understanding your leadership style

Many businesses today are shifting their cultures through employee-participative, team-based and empowered styles of leadership. Each is a "democratic" leadership style. The driving force behind this widespread shift is the realization that top-down, autocratic management no longer works. Why? It's impossible to instill quality, consistent behavior (i.e., to encourage employee involvement and teamwork) within a "command-and-control" environment. You cannot *dictate* employees into taking responsibility for quality and growth, but your leadership style can create a culture that encourages team performance through a whole-systems view of business growth.

Workforce trends clearly show employees' concern with the quality of their work life. Simply put, they are interested in "more say, not more pay." Given this, your leadership style will determine your success. Can you be the kind of leader you want to be, achieve the results you desire, *and* stay true to your values and beliefs?

The Lippitt Model of Leadership

The Lippitt Model of Leadership was created to help leaders better assess their own style and, if necessary, shift to another. Leadership styles and resulting cultures are represented graphically on the following model.

- The AUTHORITARIAN leader creates the business, its management structure, and its goals and vision. Command-and-control is the way things are done. Authoritarian leaders hold their cards close to their chest. Hidden management agendas abound.
- The DEMOCRATIC leader actively coaches, mentors and supports team members. Teamwork is the mandate; employees behave as stakeholders who co-create strategic objectives, programs, performance goals and organizational structures. Individual and leadership team agendas are more open. Communication, information exchange and cooperation are highly valued. Growth is steady, and easily accelerated.

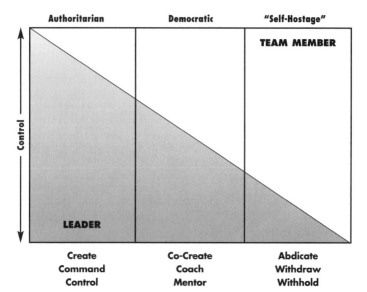

THE LIPPITT MODEL OF LEADERSHIP
As published in Preferred Futuring
Created by Ron Lippitt and Ralph White

- The "SELF-HOSTAGE" leader withdraws from involvement, typically abdicating responsibility for the business. Little structure, coaching or mentoring is provided. Key information is withheld, largely because no formal communication system exists between leaders and team members. The business culture has no direction, so counterproductive behavior is normal. In the absence of leadership and structure, team members create and settle into their own unfocused culture, which seldom reflects the leader's vision. *In short, there is no leadership.*

Shifting your leadership style — Can you do it?

The Lippett Model is an excellent visual tool to help salon owners and managers identify their leadership styles. But identifying your style is the easy part; shifting to a new one is the true challenge, especially if the desired style clashes with your personality and temperament. Discerning the type of leadership your business demands is the first step — heavily authoritarian and self-hostage styles can both discourage teamwork.

The driving force behind today's cutting-edge leadership thinking is a *whole-systems view*. Identified on the Lippett Model as the democratic leadership style, it focuses the energy of every team member on growing the business. It engenders a trusting, open and systems-driven culture that thrives on the power of the team. Everyone contributes to the design and improvement of business systems. HINT: Remember, you manage *systems,* not *people.*

When every team member has a whole-systems view of the business, everyone is responsible for success. All members understand their roles in and contribution to the growth process. Even the busiest stylists or technicians take responsibility for the success of young rookies. Leadership's role is to nurture and strengthen the salon's culture by keeping it focused, and responsive to change.

Whenever leaders attempt to shift between styles, they create an organizational craziness which is often costly to productivity and stability. Here are two common traps:

TRAP #1: GOOD INTENTIONS, NO FOLLOW-THROUGH. An authoritarian leader will likely confuse team members with a new "let's co-create our future…I want you to take responsibility" style. The knee-jerk response is usually fear and distrust; it isn't easy to let go years of distrust created by a lack of input in the business.

A common assumption of business owners is that if *they* undergo a transformation of consciousness, the rest of the team will also make the shift. In reality, people and cultures don't change easily. Sometimes, resistance to a new democratic culture can frustrate leaders so much that they revert to

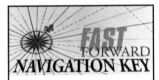

FAST FORWARD NAVIGATION KEY

No matter how much talk there is of teamwork, most salon and day spa employees have a "tunnel-vision" view of their individual roles in the overall business.

But the business world is rapidly shifting to a whole-systems view, with evolving cultures and leadership styles to drive it forward.

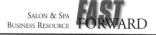

their old authoritarian styles. Consequently, team members become frustrated, and the attempt to shift leadership styles fails.

TRAP #2: A "SELF-HOSTAGE" TAKES CHARGE. When self-hostage leaders attempt to shift to a democratic style, resistance can be considerable. The culture has free-floated for so long that attempts to instill structure and focus may be construed as an invasion of personal space.

Resistance is a natural and expected response to change — no matter how great or small. A self-hostage leader must work diligently to communicate a vision of the future, and the benefits to the entire team. He or she must exercise patience; instilling structure and focus in a structureless culture takes time and communication. Even the most battle-hardened change leaders know that it is wiser to move forward in manageable stages than to sink the ship and force your team to swim the remainder of the voyage.

Perhaps the most significant quality a self-hostage leader must exert is *tenacity* in staying the new course. The challenge is greatest when individual staff members boast large clienteles. Self-hostage leaders who cannot dispel the belief that employees are in control will be held hostage indefinitely because they tend to back down at the first hint of resistance. Doing so encourages employees to say, "I knew this wouldn't last. Things will never change here."

The "bookmark in time" strategy

To successfully shift your management style and, in turn, the salon's business culture, try the *bookmark in time* strategy. (A bookmark simply indicates a key point of reference.) When initiating sweeping change in salon culture and leadership, a bookmark in time identifies the precise point of transition from what *was* to what *will be*. It can also be used to measure progress, such as a cultural or leadership shift, along a pre-determined path.

Shifting leadership styles and changing a salon culture requires powerful communication. Imagine calling a staff meeting to announce that "today, we're changing everything," and that, "from now on, I will be a different, more democratic leader." Employee responses would likely range from confusion to boredom.

Now imagine the same meeting, with the same change objectives, but this time including the bookmark in time strategy. Explain the frustrations of management and of team members. Detail the ways in which your leadership style and the resulting business culture contributed to everyone's frustrations. Then announce, "Today represents a bookmark in time for our salon. We cannot change the past, but together we can co-create an exciting and rewarding future." Paint a picture of the future; detail a fresher, more exciting work environment. Paint this picture with large brush strokes, touching on personal and professional growth, income opportunities, training and education.

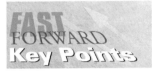

Self-hostage leaders who cannot break free from the belief that employees are in control will be held hostage indefinitely.

Share a *realistic* image of the salon's future, but one that dramatically differentiates yesterday from tomorrow. The future begins this very moment, at the bookmark in time. All progress should be measured against the condition of the salon at the time the bookmark is set, and communicated to staff through updates, meetings and huddles (fast, concise performance updates, with a heavy dose of motivation).

THE FIRST NINETY DAYS OF THE BOOKMARK STRATEGY ARE CRITICAL. Measuring progress, even small gains, is a powerful tool that will pay big dividends.

Confidence to change requires a plan

The best way to describe the Japanese approach to change and progress is: "Ready, ready, ready…ready, aim, fire, bull's-eye." The typical American entrepreneurial approach is: "Aim, fire, miss. Aim, fire, miss. Aim, fire, bull's-eye."

The temptation to charge ahead in reengineering is hard to resist, but doing so without a well-conceived plan can stir up toxic waste from the bottom the business pot. This toxic waste equals resistance, fear and, sometimes, even sabotage of new programs.

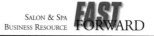
HINT: Dictating change is much different from inspiring and nurturing it. Change needs a plan to give it direction.

Change strategy

In *The E-Myth Manager* (HarperBusiness), Michael Gerber outlines specific steps to ensure a *complete* change strategy.

1. WHAT IS *YOUR* PRIMARY AIM? What do you want? This is about you, *not* the salon or your position in it. But the answer has global implications because it concerns your vision for your life, and can take you in surprising new directions.

2. WHAT IS YOUR STRATEGIC OBJECTIVE FOR THE BUSINESS? What type of salon or day spa do you want? What are your sales objectives for the next one to five years? How many locations? How many employees? Be specific.

3. WHAT IS YOUR FINANCIAL STRATEGY? First, you must know where you are; this requires a financial evaluation. *(See chapter 12.)* There is no better way plan a short- and long-term financial strategy than to complete a twelve-month cash-flow plan. (You can download a free Microsoft Excel cash-flow template from the STRATEGIES web site at WWW.STRATEGIESPUB.COM. Click on "Freebies.") The cash flow determines your revenue goals and spending budgets; it is a detailed guess of how your salon or day spa will perform financially. Without a monthly cash-flow plan, your business is flying financially blind.

4. WHAT'S YOUR ORGANIZATIONAL STRATEGY? For the moment, disregard your salon's current organizational *structure*. Instead, picture the structure that will best achieve your stated strategic *objective*. Which leadership and management positions will you need? What will the front desk and/or booking room require? What about training and education? Who will be responsible for planning, managing and organizing sales? The organizational strategy needn't be perfect; it will evolve as necessary.

5. WHAT IS YOUR MANAGEMENT STRATEGY? What management systems do you need to achieve your strategic objective? If you are shifting to a more democratic *whole-systems view,* team members must co-create the systems, and participate in their devel-

opment and application. For example: Open-book management has taken on a life of its own in the business world. By design, it brings team members into the entrepreneurial process. Team-based pay and team bonus are two more forward-thinking systems. Which systems will take you where you want to go?

6. WHAT IS YOUR PEOPLE STRATEGY? How will you help the team master the systems that drive the business? How will you teach them to play, and win, the salon business game? Communicating, training, evaluating, mentoring, coaching and focusing are integral parts of a "people strategy."

7. WHAT IS YOUR MARKETING STRATEGY? Everything about your salon or day spa business exists to attract customers. Do you have internal and external strategies to ensure success?

If you follow this very condensed overview of Michael Gerber's *E-Myth* system, you will be prepared to shift your leadership style and redesign your salon's culture, to delve into the process of reinventing and/or reengineering your business. Just the exercise of answering these questions can jump-start your entrepreneurial engine…and the change process.

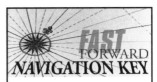

FAST FORWARD
NAVIGATION KEY

THE E-MYTH MANAGER

Michael Gerber is a master of entrepreneurial success strategy. His best-selling book *The E-Myth Manager* (HarperBusiness), presents a step-by-step game plan for building a dynamic, systems-driven, self-sustaining business. Read it.

Also of interest: *The E-Myth* and *The E-Myth Revisited*.

Anatomy of a leadership team

Even the largest salons and day spas are small businesses. And small business owners and managers wear many different hats to accomplish the myriad of tasks necessary to maintain and grow the business.

But shouldering the responsibilities of management by oneself breeds business inefficiency and stagnation…and high personal stress. That's why forward-thinking owners distribute management tasks to leadership teams. Creating an organized, vision-driven team improves salon efficiency and long-term success.

Contemplating a change in leadership structure? Consider three indicators of need: *overwork, poor performance* and *lack of clarity.*

1. The overworked and overburdened

At many salons, one or two people bear management responsibilities, but the owner is ultimately responsible for everything. Others may assume certain tasks, but the owner must assure that marketing, human resource, operational and financial functions are adequately discharged.

In other salons, there is a "manager," laden with all the responsibility he or she can handle. When something happens (or doesn't happen), it's the manager's fault. This results in more negative reactivity than positive proactivity.

Whether owner or manager…one person *can* be overworked and overburdened by the responsibilities of business. Managing and growing a salon requires a lot of thought and planning.

The days of an owner wearing all the hats and being the sole problem solver are gone. Today's economic climate dictates the proactive use of shared responsibility. True Quality and empowered work teams are more than business fads — they have become entrenched in the management structure of nearly every industry.

There's more to do in most salons than one person can handle. *Delegation* is the key to making any organization work properly.

2. Inefficiency and poor performance

Poor performance is a result of poor leadership design. If you are frustrated, the staff is unmotivated and the salon is stalled, it's time to restructure your management and leadership strategy. If the salon is not growing…is anyone responsible for growth? If it is not profitable…is anyone responsible for productivity? If it is disharmonious…is anyone responsible for morale and culture?

If the salon is not meeting expectations and moving forward, it needs leadership. Assess the roles of each department leader and team member in bringing together all the salon's resources (e.g., time, money, people). Is the existing environment predisposed to failure because the staff doesn't have the support (e.g., mentors, information) they need? Open communication is imperative.

3. Lack of clarity, purpose and direction

If no one on the leadership team knows what anyone else is doing, your team-building efforts must change. Salons often duplicate management efforts (i.e., two or more people work on the same kind of project). This makes for chaos, especially in human relations, if staff don't know to whom they should turn with specific problems. The solution?

TAKE A TEAM POLL: Do staff feel that communication with the salon leadership team is adequate? Find out if they know to whom they should go with specific queries. If there are gaps in the flow of information, now is the time to bridge them.

As the owner, do you know who bears ultimate responsibility for each of the salon's functional areas? If you are constantly searching for the person with just the right piece of information to complete whatever puzzle you're working on, it's time for a new structure. If key people cannot contribute comprehensive information on a specific functional area (providing you with all the data necessary for decision-making), your plan of employee empowerment may have gone awry.

Can your salon's structure deliver the success you want? If not, it's time to create one that can.

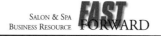
Creating a leadership team

A salon business needs an *effective* management structure comprised of specific duties and responsibilities for team leaders. Short-changing any of them will compromise the integrity, efficiency and vitality of the salon business.

Study the salon/day spa leadership chart below. We broke with tradition, using a wheel chart and placing the title of president/salon owner in the hub. The vision, values and culture of the business are nurtured at the hub. If the hub is weak (self-hostage mode), the entire organizational structure is compromised. If it is strong and

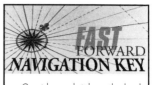

NAVIGATION KEY

Consider each job on the leadership chart and, on separate pieces of paper, list the results needed from each to achieve your strategic objective.

Targeting "results" rather than specific tasks adds clarity to each position's responsibilities.

SALON/DAY SPA LEADERSHIP TEAM

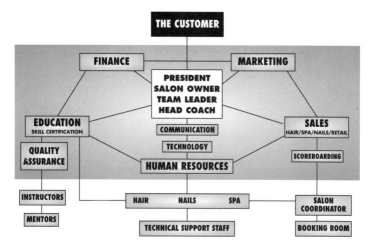

driven by a whole-systems view (democratic mode), the structure is dynamic and all team members are working toward a common goal. If it is on life support (authoritarian mode), the structure is weak because everything is created and controlled by one person.

Since "the customer" is the ultimate boss, this title sits symbolically atop the leadership chart. Too often, the needs and demands of the customer get lost in the fog of daily activity.

Study every position on chart. Complete the project described in the accompanying Navigation Key by compiling the *results* required from each position. Listing the results first simplifies the process of defining and prioritizing the *systems* needed to produce those results. Mental tickle: You manage systems, not people.

Staffing your leadership team

Most important in this process is ensuring key responsibilities are assigned and addressed. It can be frustrating for salons with limited staff and resources, but a position's function and responsibilities cannot be allowed to flounder due to lack of attention. This may require an owner to wear all the hats for a while. The objective is to create a

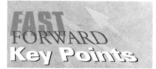

A major stumbling block at salons is the assumption that successful, high-revenue technicians will thrive in a leadership role. Technical success is not a leadership qualifier.

leadership team structure that will achieve the salon's strategic objective. The team will take shape as the business grows and resources become more readily available. Hint: Patience is key. Adding leadership personnel too fast can strain precious resources.

Building a leadership team is akin to recruiting a championship sports team. There is even a salary cap, defined by the payroll line on your cash-flow projection. The challenge is to find the best talent possible *and* stay within the boundaries of the payroll budget.

Begin your search internally, among existing staff. Are there *natural leaders* with the skills necessary to fill key positions? If the leaders are present but the skills are not, can the skills be developed? What will this require in time, money and other resources?

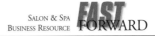
A major stumbling block at salons is the assumption that successful, high-revenue technicians will thrive in a leadership role. Technical success is not a leadership qualifier. In fact, thrusting a talented technician into a leadership role could be detrimental to the individual, no matter how strongly he or she believes it to be a positive career move. Very often, the true attraction is the glamour of the *title* — not the responsibilities, duties and accountabilities of the *position*. Defining and communicating the results expected from the position will assist all parties in the selection process, and ensure a proper fit.

FAST FORWARD Key Points

Maintaining focus at every level of the organization is the leadership team's primary challenge.

If you must recruit outside the business, use each position's results list (as defined by the NAVIGATION KEY exercise) to create a *hiring profile*. A hiring profile determines the type of individual who will best fill the position; from outward appearance and personality to experience and skill, applicants must complement and enhance the salon's existing culture. (This applies to all new hires, not just the leadership team.) For example: If you need an individual who shares your whole-systems view to manage the day spa department, the last person you want is an authoritarian leader.

BUILD YOUR LEADERSHIP TEAM WITH CARE. Have team members wear multiple hats when necessary, or until the best candidates are secured. Larger salon and day spa operations may have greater personnel and financial resources, but size also adds complexity. Communication must be systematized throughout the leadership team in order to maintain a strict focus on the strategic objective and key performance data such as client retention, productivity rate, average ticket and current sales performance versus goals. Maintaining focus at every level of the organization is the leadership team's primary challenge.

Knowledge is power: Meetings and huddles

Shared knowledge within an organization keeps it competitive, creative and amazingly flexible and adaptive to change. Shared knowledge creates energy and focus. Investment in knowledge is powerful, because it makes organizations fast.

Information accumulates quickly in business. To function efficiently and remain focused on the strategic objective, every member of the leadership team needs to be in sync and well-informed. Only then can information cascade outward to the entire team. But many salons and day spas rely solely on monthly meetings, and share only bits and pieces of information. Some have no formal meeting schedule at all.

How often should you meet? The answer depends on your organizational structure and the aggressiveness of your strategic objective. Monthly meetings may hit on the big picture, but are not sufficient to maintain momentum. If you want to shift your salon into fast forward, you must hold formal meetings supported by frequent, rapid-fire team huddles. (The prime objective of team huddles is to maintain focus on strategic objectives. Huddles are weekly, or even daily, events.)

Avoiding mental barriers: What would be your salon's potential if every team member focused on specific revenue and performance

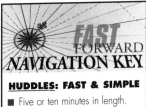

HUDDLES: FAST & SIMPLE

- Five or ten minutes in length.
- Huddle in teams: leadership teams, department leaders, front desk, hair, spa, etc.
- Same time every day, or same time and day every week.
- Stick to a fixed agenda; focus on performance data. *It's not a gripe session.*
- Update the scoreboard.
- Address timely opportunities and areas needing improvement.

goals? What would happen if everyone knew the daily and weekly score? Aside from some individual performance objectives, most salon employees operate from week to week and month to month with no knowledge of what the business must produce to sustain itself and grow. In these instances, individual agendas take precedence over the strategic objectives of the business.

Some salon owners are reluctant to share key performance information, and many actually *withhold* it. On the Lippett Model of Leadership, this denotes an authoritarian style which is not dynamic, and inhibits the development of a whole-systems view of the organization.

Withholding information slows forward momentum. Sharing information — and teaching employees how to use it — will shift your salon business into fast forward.

Scoreboards: The power of focus

T here is much more to a scoreboard than the random collection of numbers it first appears to be. There is a theory behind the idea of keeping score — that staff should have the knowledge they need to grow the businesses they work in; that it is not unthinkable to treat employees like rational and intelligent people; that people will respond enthusiastically when given the chance to ensure their own success. But in order to reach beyond the theory and help stylists and technicians truly understand the importance of scorekeeping, salon owners must confront the numbers. They must be able to use numbers to explain the theory.

PUTTING THE BUSINESS FIRST: The truth is, most stylists and technicians need to be taught why the security of the business' future is more important than their immediate gratification. Bringing in a new client is wonderful, but *keeping* her will make the salon profitable. Continuing one's education is wonderful, but sharing new knowledge with others is essential for team growth. It may seem to many salon employees that "the thing to do" is to fill individual chairs and pursue personal growth. But salon owners cannot allow this to happen at the expense of the salon. If the needs of the business are not attended, the business cannot survive. The livelihoods of owners and stylists alike depend upon the health of the salon.

RESERVE PLAYERS HAVE PASSION TOO: Given a choice, people will most often decide to get involved, to find ways to make the changes necessary for growth and success. Too few salon employees have that choice. The only way to get the staff to feel the same passion for the salon that you feel is to impart to them a sense of what it is to be a business owner. This means divulging certain information and delegating responsibility and accountability to everyone on the team. It means keeping score and posting regular progress reports.

PEOPLE NOT ONLY WANT TO BE PART OF SOMETHING SUCCESSFUL; they also want to be part of the reason for that success. Get your salon's reserve players off the bench and into the field. They have too much to contribute to be sidelined.

Why should I scoreboard?

What if you could get your employees to think and act as if they owned the salon? What if you could get them to think the way you do? Interestingly, many companies in various industries throughout the United States are learning to do just that. They use an idea called open-book management. In open-book companies, employees do interesting things:

- They stop thinking of themselves as "hired hands" and start thinking of themselves as "business people."
- They stop doing as little as they think they can get away with and start doing whatever needs to be done.
- They try to do their best work all the time because they know it influences the success of the business.
- They care about the success of the business because they know that's what puts money in their pockets.

Scoreboards bring about change

One powerful technique for information sharing is scoreboards: charts on the dispensary or break room wall which show how many customers the salon is serving, how the sales figures look this month, how much money the business is making. Once people understand the importance of those numbers and how they can affect them, they start paying *close* attention to them.

A good method of getting people involved is to ask them to help set goals for weekly customer totals, revenues, product sales, etc. Then, track the salon's progress toward these goals on the scoreboard. It's human nature: When people set their own goals, they take pride in hitting them. They want to hit them. Suddenly coming to work is a little more fun than it was before.

These steps are the basic elements of open-book management and scoreboarding. Implement them and you'll find that you are indeed keeping your best people, that they are indeed doing their best work — and that your business is succeeding to an extent you had only dreamed possible.

Scoreboards: Getting visual

On the following page is a standard scoreboard which many salon owners use successfully. It is basic and to-the-point…a great advantage when first introducing the concept of open (or semi-open) books to salon staff. But there are ways to dress up a scoreboard and make it more interesting and creative.

Scoreboards can be designed in any manner your imagination can conjure. Imagine laying a brick in the foundation of your "new salon" every time a goal is met. How about skipping along the yellow brick road or racing around the track in Indianapolis? *Scoreboards become more effective when they are less clinical.*

A salon owner attempting to implement a scoreboarding system must keep it interesting. Each employee's participation is important; it is crucial that their interest not wane after a few weeks or months. Like any new system, scoreboarding can be exciting for a while, but then quickly become mundane, or even boring. So, how does one sustain the staff's interest? It is up to the person who carries the salon's fiscal responsibility to maintain timely updates. The quickest way to kill staff interest in any salon procedure is to give the impression that management isn't interested.

- Be original with scoreboards.
- Involve the staff in every step. Let them flex their creative muscles. Designing a scoreboard is a great team meeting project.
- Choose a method of conveying the salon's progress that is pertinent to your particular area or marketplace. The scoreboard must make the numbers real for the staff; everyone must understand their significance. Each goal accomplished may signify a step along a trail with an oasis at the end, or a step on the path to a mountainous summit.

THERE IS NO WRONG WAY TO DESIGN A SCOREBOARD. Most important is to prevent it from falling into neglect. A scoreboard is a visual record of salon performance; without regular updates, your team is once again working in the dark. You must keep the light burning.

Developed by SALON BUSINESS STRATEGIES – 800.417.4848   Copyright ©1999   www.strategiespub.com

MONTH: November '98

REVENUE LEGS	GOALS	Week 1 DATES: 2 to 7	Week 2 DATES: 9 to 14	Week 3 DATES: 16 to 21	Week 4 DATES: 23 to 28	Week 5 DATES: 30 to -	TOTALS	% OF GOAL
Hair	25,000.00	5,400.00	5,400.00	5,000.00	4,876.00	345.00	21,021.00	84.1%
Nails	3,400.00	500.00	500.00	485.00	511.00	59.00	2,055.00	60.4%
Spa	2,000.00	398.00	398.00	450.00	465.00	265.00	1,976.00	98.8%
Retail	7,200.00	1,800.00	1,800.00	2,184.00	2,210.00	187.00	8,181.00	113.6%
Gift Certificates	2,600.00	475.00	475.00	675.00	695.00	110.00	2,430.00	97.2%
Total Sales	$40,100.00	$8,573.00	$8,573.00	$8,794.00	$8,757.00	$966.00	35,663.00	88.9%

PERFORMANCE GOALS							Average	% OF GOAL
Productivity	80.0%	75.0%	85.0%	90.0%	68.0%	75.0%	79%	98.3%
Ave. Svc. Ticket	$30.00	$28.00	$31.00	$32.00	$29.00	$28.00	$29.60	98.7%
Ave. Retail Tkt.	$15.00	$13.00	$13.00	$13.00	$13.00	$10.00	$12.40	82.7%
Client Visits	500	55	108	132	118	114	527	105%
% Pre-Book	40.0%	45.0%	47.0%	50.0%	45.0%	45.0%	46%	116%

THE STRATEGIES SALON SCOREBOARD

This scoreboard was created in Microsoft Excel; it is available *free* at the STRATEGIES web site. Go to WWW.STRATEGIESPUB.COM and click on "freebies." The scoreboard contains preset formulas to calculate your progress toward monthly revenue and performance objectives. The scoreboard can easily be adapted to meet your salon's performance tracking needs. NOTE: You must have Microsoft Excel installed in your computer in order to work with the scoreboard file. *It is not a stand-alone program.*

Getting started

The salon industry lends itself incredibly well to the implementation of scoreboarding systems. By its very nature, it is comprised of elements which are easily tracked and measured for improvement or decline, such as sales of hours and retail product. What steps are necessary to implement a scoring system in your salon?

- MAKE THE DECISION. Consider the salon as it is. Is it profitable? Could it be more so? If you see great potential for the future — do you know the steps to take to realize that potential? If these thoughts plague you every day (or night), then it's time to explore the scoreboarding option.

- DETERMINE YOUR TEAM'S THRESHOLD FOR CHANGE. How will they respond to a new level of responsibility and trust? Will they be excited about keeping score and about seeing information that was always before deemed "inappropriate" or "unnecessary"? Chances are, they'll rise to the occasion.

- MARSHAL THE RESOURCES. Gather all the business information you can. Most salon owners intuitively feel whether the business is doing well. Developing a scoreboard will quantify your opinions. Consult the bookkeeper, accountant or whoever maintains the financial records and monitors the cash flow. You will need to see sales figures, overhead and payroll costs, retail and backbar product costs — each and every number which pertains to the salon's overall performance and profitability. Then, decide which of these you will share with the team.

- GIVE THE STAFF THE BUSINESS' NUMBERS. Post them on the break room wall. Let everyone see the financial condition of the business and involve everyone in creating ways to put the salon on a path of constant improvement. It's time to involve everyone in the game, but first you have to give them the rules and regulations. This is where the scoreboard is vital. You don't need to reveal everything, but one can't expect to see dramatic improvements in sales and productivity until the entire team is aware of what needs to be done.

KEEPING SCORE IS NOT THE SAME AS KEEPING TABS. Posting a scoreboard allows the entire team access to information; it can never

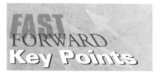

Key Points

Posting a scoreboard is a method of empowering every employee to make a difference in the salon's bottom line through individual and team contributions.

hide it or misrepresent it in any way. Posting a scoreboard is a method of empowering every employee to make a difference in the salon's bottom line through individual and team contributions. The best thing you can do for your salon is get the team involved in its continued growth and stability.

Mentoring is part of leadership

A mentor is a trusted counselor or guide, an experienced individual who knows the ropes and is charged with the responsibility of transferring that knowledge to another. In business, mentoring is an integral part of the human resource development process, especially in bringing new team members up to performance standards. Mentoring offers unique opportunities in four important areas:

1. THE MANAGEMENT TEAM: A mentoring program gives management a reliable and methodical system to indoctrinate new staff into the salon's culture.

2. THE MENTOR: What better way to utilize and reward the salon's tried-and-true performers than to bestow the mantle of "mentorship" upon them? A key benefit for long-standing high performers is that mentoring provides a meaningful diversion from their day-to-day responsibilities. Many mentors openly regard their work and contributions in this area as the highest form of job enrichment.

3. THE TRAINEE: A mentoring program is the perfect vehicle to quickly move new team members through the awkwardness of becoming acclimated to a new business environment and culture. And what more could a new hire ask than to work under the coaching wings of the best in the organization? From a benchmarking standpoint, mentoring provides new hires with a clear picture of how their performance measures up to the top performers.

4. BEYOND NEW HIRES: The benefits of mentoring are not confined to new hires. Mentoring can help existing team members develop new skills and accelerate the learning curve when promoted to positions that require new skills.

Qualifying for mentorship

Individuals must meet specific performance standards to qualify for mentor status. The biggest mistake many owners make is to assign high producers to a mentor program without prequalification. The last thing you want is an ego-driven mentor. *Respect is the cornerstone of any mentor program.*

Qualifications should include technical and non-technical criteria such as:

- years of service.
- advanced education and training courses attended.
- hands-on experience as an educator or trainer.
- skill level in specific technical disciplines.
- personal performance accomplishments.
- professional appearance, welcoming personality.
- patience and positive demeanor.
- leadership skill, ability and experience.
- appropriate personal communication skills.
- client retention rates.
- productivity rates.
- average ticket.
- retail sales.
- consultation skills.
- ability to follow through on tasks and projects.
- time management skills.
- organization skills.
- respect of peers.
- willingness and desire to help others.

A series of mentor relationships

A mentorship program should consist of a series of progressive learning experiences. Advancement must be built around the salon's internal *skill certification program.* Trainees should be tested through both written and practical exams. In salons with performance-based pay programs (whether salary, hourly or commission), pay increases should be tied to successful completion of each mentoring level. It is

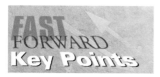

amazing how eagerly salon employees learn new skills when pay increases are tied to skill development. If your current pay program does not tie raises to skill development, it may be time to reevaluate and upgrade.

Leadership team, mentors and quality assurance

Leadership team members and mentors work in tandem to develop human resources. Specifically, the leadership team looks to mentors as a means to achieve the highest levels of consistency and quality. Given this, the mentor program can be the salon's best *quality assurance* mechanism.

Values and evaluations

B ehind every evaluation, there must be a purpose. What do you expect an employee evaluation system to accomplish? Have you set guidelines for staff to follow in the time between evaluations? HINT: Behaviors that are reinforced will be repeated. There are many areas on which salon or spa managers may focus, and therefore reinforce, through evaluations. You can:

- emphasize client satisfaction and retention.
- create a unique salon image based on appearance, ambiance, ability, etc.
- foster business growth and build profits.
- build strong, cross-functional teams.
- enhance the skills of every staff member.
- provide a way to compare actual performance to established standards.
- increase staff's individual productivity and quality of service.
- provide legally recognized documentation to support personnel policies and actions (e.g., hiring, firing, affirmative action, cultural diversity, promotions, compensation).

Be careful when flying without a net

With no evaluation system in place, you may have little basis for comparing actual performance (based on individual objectives, work standards, skill certification and job descriptions) to the salon's stated goals. In the absence of baseline data, an "evaluation" is little more than an opinion. You can't implement an evaluation system based on quality of work without a way to measure it.

- Develop a baseline for evaluating each position.
- Ask each team member for a list of achievements during the last evaluation period, the areas in which they could improve, and their personal goals. Then *you* do the same for each employee, and compare the lists. Discuss and clarify the differences, and agree on improvement goals. Record the actions you agree to take in support of an employee's goals. You should both sign the

paper. Give the original to the employee, and retain a copy as a basis for periodic review.

- Call a staff meeting to brainstorm potential evaluation criteria. Maintain a list of suggestions. Clarify ideas, but do not judge them. Evaluation comes later. Simply get as many ideas on the table as the staff can generate.

Formal evaluation and appraisal — Issues to consider

Does your formal evaluation system yield the desired results? Is it too productivity-oriented to maintain quality? Is it more focused on keeping employees than clients? Will it withstand a legal test? (A completed evaluation form is usually treated as a legal document. Choose content and language carefully.) Do evaluations result in improvements, or are they an exercise on paper only?

FAST FORWARD Key Points

You can't implement an evaluation system based on quality of work without a way to measure quality.

BLINKING RED LIGHTS: Does your evaluation system rely on subjective ratings of subjective data? Is appraisal based on personality traits which bear little relation to work behavior? Will the rating process stand up to a consistency test? Is your compensation system based on evaluation outcomes? Does your appraisal system recognize star qualities over team qualities?

If the evaluation is in any way based on *quantitative* data:

- Is there a clearly defined and communicated standard, objective or expectation?
- Is the method of collecting and measuring data clear?
- During the evaluation period, can each person learn how he or she is doing?
- Is evaluation data above suspicion in accuracy, consistency, completeness, and in how and by whom it is collected and reported?
- Is the evaluation approach and the data used sensitive to areas and situations over which individuals may have no control?

Do evaluations help?

Some believe evaluations are useless because there is no single way to evaluate staff…but people *want* to know the score. They want to know where they stand in relationship to owner and team expectations. Much of the problem with evaluations is that many employees don't have a clue what's expected of them, or how they are performing against those expectations. Often, performance feedback is restricted to "screw-ups." Resolving this situation is the first step in instituting an effective evaluation process, and understanding the team-based systems which have all but eliminated adversarial boss-to-subordinate evaluations.

Form and formulation

The design of an evaluation form is much less important than the way you and your team perceive the intent and outcome of an evaluation. Designs and length range from *none* to six- and eight-page formal reports. HINT: Form should follow function. Decide the salon's purpose, collaborate with staff on the criteria to include, and design a simple form to meet your needs.

The form's primary purpose is to summarize items discussed, agreements reached, actions to be taken (and by whom), and on what criteria future evaluations will be based.

Because each salon has its own staffing and skill-level demands, a cookie-cutter salon evaluation is of limited use. But instead of viewing this as a roadblock, consider it an opportunity to fine-tune your own programs. The effort will be well worth it in the long run.

The perfect staff evaluation form is one you and your staff create together to reflect the needs of the salon. No one can build a better evaluation for you than you.

A values exercise

Employees' suggested evaluation criteria are founded in their individual value codes, and personal values are reflected in professional performance. So, it's worth the time to devote a team meeting, or series of meetings, to developing an overall salon values code. Here's how:

- Compile a comprehensive list (50–75) of values you see or would like to see in the salon or day spa (e.g., truth, efficiency, teamwork, honesty, originality, integrity, artistry, collaboration, support).
- Put the list aside. When you can be objective, choose the three values most important to you.
- Share the list, *not your choices,* with each team member. Ask each to select three values from the list, or write in their own.
- Create a new list using everyone's choices. Values chosen by more than one person do not receive "favored" status. All are equal on the new list.
- Repeat the selection process until only a handful of values — a number small enough to discuss at a team meeting — is left. Large day spas and salons may require more iterations than those with fewer staff.
- Discuss the remaining values as a group, deciding on the three most important.
- Post these three values throughout the business. They will guide all management and staff decisions.

Evaluation guidelines

The elements of an effective salon employee evaluation should include:

- performance criteria relating directly to True Quality and client satisfaction goals.
- clear standards and measurements.
- procedures and descriptions that promote a positive, forward-thinking view rather than a negative focus on past deficiencies. Focus on what the salon can learn from past performance, even in areas not up to current standards.
- a formal process to inform staff of what they must do to improve performance before the next evaluation.
- employee opportunities to receive (or provide their own) feedback to help them keep track of their progress. Don't let too much time elapse between staff feedback sessions; the channels of communication should be constantly open.
- an understanding of the support *you* will provide to help the employee improve performance and enhance skills.
- a clear-cut understanding of the link between salon performance, pay and career growth.

Because staff members are the core of the evaluation program, a superior system will include provisions for them to:

- determine criteria for evaluations.
- collect and analyze their own data, enabling self-evaluation. Staff should also be able to evaluate you as their leader.
- receive peer evaluations.
- receive client evaluations.
- renegotiate standards, objectives or expectations as business conditions change.
- work within a compensation system that does not limit the number of high-performance employees.
- work within a system that equitably shares profits.
- receive rewards based on team recommendations.

Survey your leadership and culture

To help identify and measure those elusive things called "leadership" and "culture," we developed the following staff survey. Its purposes are to:

- offer a sense of the breadth and depth of salon culture.
- provide a device for collecting key data about that culture.
- enable you to pinpoint some aspects of salon culture you may desire to improve.
- develop a way to measure progress within a changing culture.

Begin with a staff letter

To the staff member:

There are no correct answers to this survey. Answers should represent your honest opinion, not what you feel the answer "should" be.

Unless all staff members elect to openly share their responses, individual responses will remain confidential. The leadership team will compile responses and communicate a summary to the team.

The survey is meant to provide data which can be used to identify and clarify critical assumptions, beliefs, values, perceptions and behaviors in the salon. Your opinion is vital to this effort.

Write in the number (1–7) which most clearly represents your opinion at this time. Select from the following list:

7	Totally agree, without reservation
6	Strongly agree
5	Partly agree
4	Can neither agree nor disagree
3	Partly disagree
2	Strongly disagree
1	Totally disagree, without reservation

The survey

___ 1. Communications are informal throughout the salon.

___ 2. There is a clear picture of where the owner or manager is leading the salon.

___ 3. The salon's vision and mission have been shared with all team members.

___ 4. Team members are rewarded fairly for their performance.

___ 5. All staff members participate in creating action plans to specify what needs to be done, how it will be done, who will do it and by when it must be done.

___ 6. Team members receive all the information they need to complete quality work.

___ 7. Team members are excited about their work.

___ 8. Staff are recognized and praised when they do a good job.

___ 9. Performance standards are clearly defined and communicated to everyone.

___ 10. Staff have the opportunity and support to develop and grow within the salon.

___ 11. Mediocrity is unacceptable.

___ 12. The business' decor is changed every few years to create a more pleasing environment.

___ 13. Staff have sufficient time to perform quality work.

___ 14. The team receives frequent, useful training.

___ 15. A certification process is in place and working.

___ 16. The salon is a fun place to work.

___ 17. There is no differentiation between staff when scheduling appointments, unless a client requests a specific person.

___ 18. Staff meetings are held regularly.

___ 19. The leadership team truly cares about the physical health and safety of the staff.

___ 20. Salon management supports decisions made by staff, provided members are acting in the best interests of the salon.

___ 21. The chain of command and organizational structure are clear.

___ 22. Staff have the authority to make decisions to get their job done.

___ 23. The salon treats employee training as a long-term investment, not an expense.

__ 24. Staff know and understand how their performance is measured.

__ 25. Every team member receives honest answers from the leadership team on issues of concern to them.

__ 26. Usually, clients are assigned to staff in order to make the best use of team members' skills.

__ 27. Compensation is fair, and administered consistently throughout the salon.

__ 28. Staff generally has a strong desire to complete high quality work.

__ 29. The team receives a variety of informal rewards for work done well (e.g., praise, memos, time off).

__ 30. The salon's furnishings and equipment are up to par.

__ 31. Client satisfaction and loyalty is the salon's primary concern.

__ 32. New hires are carefully selected, based on salon requirements and standards.

__ 33. Salon policies and procedures are clearly communicated to all team members.

__ 34. On average, staff enjoy working at the salon.

__ 35. Staff members are able to assess various pressures and demands, and identify which ones are really important.

__ 36. The salon is ideally located for both attracting and retaining clients and staff.

__ 37. Team members feel their jobs are secure (i.e., no worries about being laid off or the salon going out of business).

__ 38. When staff members are faced with personal situations that interfere with their ability to work effectively, the leadership team is supportive — but it is clear that work must be performed according to established standards.

__ 39. A dress and grooming policy enables the salon to present a unified and professional image to clients.

__ 40. The client booking system is fair to all staff members.

__ 41. Leadership treats each team member fairly and consistently.

__ 42. The owner or manager is a strong leader, seeks the counsel of staff, coaches and supports staff, delegates responsibility and authority, and praises the staff to clients.

__ 43. Client retention is high (above 50%).

__ 44. People in the salon help one another.

__ 45. Mistakes are seen as an opportunity to learn and improve and, unless repeated or clearly in violation of known rules , are not usually subject to disciplinary action.

__ 46. Products sell well and appeal to clients.

__ 47. Staff members are not stressed by excessive job pressures.

__ 48. The leadership team is openly receptive to new information, suggestions for improvement, and constructive criticism.

__ 49. In-house skill training is well-done and immediately useful on the job.

__ 50. To get the job done, staff members have the freedom to act as they need to.

__ 51. The owner or manager is more of a coach than a boss.

__ 52. Salon performance standards are challenging, yet achievable.

__ 53. When there is a business crisis, the team pulls together to help relieve the situation.

__ 54. Casual personal conversation between staff is discouraged while serving clients.

__ 55. The salon has the best possible range of staff talent for the clients served and the services offered.

__ 56. Co-workers put the good of the client, other staff and the salon ahead of their personal desires.

__ 57. Practices subject to disciplinary action are made clear to all staff in advance.

__ 58. Distributors are courteous, knowledgeable and helpful.

__ 59. The leadership team is ethical and moral in business dealings.

__ 60. The leadership team discusses the financial aspects of the business with each staff member in a way everyone understands.

__ 61. The salon has the best possible mix of clients.

__ 62. Staff are highly skilled and quality-conscious.

__ 63. Any behavior which is potentially distasteful to either clients or staff is frowned upon.

__ 64. Staff have the tools and supplies needed to deliver quality work.

__ 65. The leadership team would not begrudge staff pursuing a better job opportunity (assuming they leave on good terms).

__ 66. New hires always receive training on salon performance standards and practices.

__ 67. The current salon hours are best for the clients.

__ 68. The leadership team and staff trust one another.

__ 69. Staff are encouraged to take risks in getting their job done if they think the risk makes good business or ethical sense.

__ 70. The safety of clients and staff always concerns management.

__ 71. The team knows and understands the salon's long-term growth strategy.

__ 72. The leadership team takes appropriate steps to help any staff member not meeting expectations, even if termination results.

__ 73. Adequate time and preparation is allowed when a major change, such as introducing new management systems, is planned.

__ 74. All staff know where they stand in relation to the leadership team's expectations of them.

__ 75. Decisions relating to staff's work are made without unnecessary delay.

__ 76. Team members are treated as adults.

__ 77. The salon understands the needs and requirements of its clients.

__ 78. Staff are accountable for the results of work assigned to them.

__ 79. Work schedules and hours are fair.

__ 80. Any questions or complaints with policies and practices can be openly discussed, and an equitable (or at least understandable) conclusion reached.

__ 81. Staff receive training that prepares them to assume decision-making responsibility, clearly states the boundaries within which they may make a decision, and communicates the potential consequences of their decisions.

__ 82. Clientele are fairly assigned among service providers, regardless of the staff member's length of time on the job.

__ 83. The owner or manager is committed to True Quality Management, as shown by a personal involvement in making it work.

__ 84. Highly independent staff attitudes are considered counterproductive to the balanced best interest of the salon.

__ 85. Staff members are proud to be a part of this salon.

How to score the survey

1. Tally each team member's score. The highest possible individual total is 595 (85 x 7). The average total is 340. If most of your staff's totals are above 510, your salon's culture is in great shape. If you notice clusters of high and low totals, there are significant differences in the way the team perceives the salon's culture. Don't try to figure out who said what. Instead, discuss the findings with the entire staff.

2. Some statements may have received low-number responses on a significant number of surveys. Total the responses for these statements on all the surveys and divide by the number of respondents to determine the average. This will pinpoint areas for improvement. HINT: Be aware of patterns; some questions are directly related to others.

3. Repeat step two for statements which received high-number responses. Discuss these positive areas during team and individual meetings. Accentuating the positive aspects of the salon is a great way to reinforce behaviors and provide praise.

This survey should be sufficient in scope to help small- to medium-sized salons find "the keys to their culture." The primary value comes from the insights you will gain through staff discussions, and the actions that result.

Things to do:

■ Understand your leadership style and, if necessary, the shifts you must make to become a better leader and create a culture that encourages team performance.

■ To prepare to shift your leadership style and redesign the salon's culture, answer the following questions from *The E-Myth:*

WHAT IS YOUR PRIMARY AIM?

WHAT IS YOUR STRATEGIC OBJECTIVE FOR THE BUSINESS?

WHAT IS YOUR FINANCIAL STRATEGY?

WHAT IS YOUR ORGANIZATIONAL STRATEGY?

WHAT IS YOUR MANAGEMENT STRATEGY?

WHAT IS YOUR PEOPLE STRATEGY?

WHAT IS YOUR MARKETING STRATEGY?

■ Create a leadership team to improve salon efficiency and ensure long-term success.

■ Start using scoreboards to keep your team updated on performance and goals. Make them visual and exciting.

■ Schedule regular meetings and huddles to keep your team focused. Keep them brief and to-the-point.

■ Develop a mentoring program to offer experienced individuals the responsibility of sharing knowledge with new team members and bring them up to salon performance standards.

■ Develop an employee evaluation system which measures each employee's progress and performance based on salon standards and individual goals and objectives.

FRONT DESK STRATEGIES

Anatomy of the efficient salon/day spa front desk

F
IRST IMPRESSIONS: By definition, you only get one chance. And if a client's first impression is not a good one, the odds of a return visit to your salon are severely curtailed. This is why the front desk must act as a transitional station, drawing the client from the unrelenting demands of a hectic life into the serenity and calmness which are the hallmarks of so many successful salon and day spa operations. For the transition to be successful, the desk must be staffed by competent, enthusiastic, service-savvy employees who maintain an efficient and productive work structure.

In most day spas, it's nearly impossible to function without a full-time desk team, though many hair salons are still trying to do so. The lack of a receptionist, manager or coordinator to command and systematize the salon's communication hub leaves the business open to customer service inconsistencies, questionable bookings and other time-consuming productivity thieves. The front desk fulfills too many important functions and is too integral to the salon's overall profitability and smooth operation to be haphazardly manned.

The salon's front desk culture must be founded upon and always revolve around a single objective: total client satisfaction. But there is more to client comfort than smiling when extending a greeting or answering the phone on the second ring; it requires an overall efficiency which permeates every aspect of the client's salon visit. To achieve this, responsibility must be assigned. There must be someone to say, "This is my job."

And as your salon or day spa continues to grow and become busier, it is important to clarify roles at the front desk. Whose primary responsibility are the phones, appointment bookings, client greetings and salon tours, monetary transactions and balancing the cash drawer, inventory handling, payroll? Is there one person who can do everything? Probably not, especially if the business is large. Chances are, to achieve the efficiency level at which the salon must operate, it's time to divide and delegate.

Efficiency is the measure of your salon's customer service aptitude. It is a function of how long clients must wait on hold while attempting to book an appointment by telephone, the length of the check-in and check-out lines, the organization of the retail display — even the manner in which clients are guided through the building and their ease of access to stations and treatment rooms.

The goal of the front desk staff is complex and multi-faceted. Ensuring the level of service required to build and sustain the kind of reputation your salon or day spa deserves requires strong leadership principles and managerial skill. Every staff member at every position has a role to play.

Establishing responsibilities

W hichever title you prefer, the manager/coordinator position bears tremendous responsibility for salon operations, especially if the owner chooses to work as a technician in the business. A manager or coordinator is largely responsible for the fundamental day-to-day operations of the salon: payroll, inventory ordering and maintenance, and interviewing new employees. Fulfilling the requirements of the position requires an objective, analytical approach.

WHAT IS THE PRIMARY ROLE OF THE SALON COORDINATOR? Certainly, there is a long list of tasks to perform and accountabilities to answer for, but what is the position all about? If the front desk is the hub of the business, then the coordinator's function is to ensure that the hub stays stable and supports the other departments. Yet maintaining the hub's equilibrium by assembling and training a capable front desk team, resolving "personality incompatibility issues" and retaining one's own sense of balance *is but one step* in the intricate dance that is the coordinator's job. Just a few more of the steps:

■ INTERVIEWING, HIRING AND DISMISSING: Often, the coordinator will engage applicants in an initial interview and offer feedback to the owner. This requires not only a strong sense of intuition, but also a wide range of interpersonal skills. Protecting and growing the company is the highest priority. If additional staff is required, a salon owner must trust the coordinator's judgement. Likewise, when negative issues arise, the coordinator must possess the diplomacy and loyalty to the salon to reach resolution, even if it means releasing an employee.

■ INVENTORY MAINTENANCE AND ORDERING: How much inventory to carry? Which lines? How often to reorder? What's selling? How frequently does inventory turn? Depending on the retail presence the salon wishes to establish, answers to these questions will vary widely. And unless you employ a retail specialist, the coordinator may the only person with those answers.

- ACCOUNTING AND FINANCE, INCLUDING PAYROLL: There are many facets to maintaining a salon's fiscal security: accurate and prompt bank deposits and credit card authorizations; evaluation and budgeting of overhead costs; efficient and timely tax reporting and deposits; and a myriad of other tasks. Maintaining the finance department takes many long hours.
- CLIENT INTERACTION: Customer service can easily go unrecognized and unappreciated until a chink in the armor surfaces. It's up to the coordinator to make sure the chinks are few in number and non-recurring.

As anyone who has held the position will attest, a salon coordinator wears many hats and must fulfill different needs for different people. He or she must understand the inner workings of every aspect of the salon, including service processes, the time required for services, how to match new clients to appropriate technicians and which employees are most productive on which shifts. The coordinator's job is anything but simple. It requires tenacity, diligence and an almost supernatural ability to make the pieces fit.

Receptionist

Often underrated and undervalued, the receptionist position is critical to the salon's customer service capabilities. Along with the coordinator and manager, the receptionist is on the front lines, and is frequently the first voice heard or face seen by clients. Whether the responsibility is adequately acknowledged, the person chosen to fill this position commands a lot of power. It is true that the receptionist position does not usually require the same level of experience and professional expertise as does the manager or coordinator position. It does, however, require a gregarious and spirited personality; a professional demeanor and presentation; excellent communication skills and the ability to "wing it" when unexpected situations arise.

Especially in large salon day spa operations, schedules must be fitted together in much the same way as a five-thousand-piece, black-and-white, two-sided jigsaw puzzle. There will always be clients with inflexible or uncertain schedules, as well as inexplicable occurrences which conspire to prevent a normal day's operation at the salon: a staff member or client oversleeps, becomes ill or gets stuck in traffic; the weather turns inclement; the department of transportation decides to begin construction on your street. This single aspect of the receptionist position is so complex in many salons and day spas that owners are setting up special areas, completely isolated from the desk, devoted exclusively to answering clients' telephone queries.

The booker: New kid on the block

Whether the salon receives fifty or 500 calls per day, each must be handled as smoothly and quickly as possible. When clients wish to book or reschedule an appointment; inquire about a price, service or product; get directions or purchase a gift certificate, the salon response must be courteous and accurate.

If a client receives the level of service she expects, has your salon truly succeeded in its mission? Or is the goal to *exceed* expectations? Too often, it is impossible for an overwhelmed front desk staff to offer each client the attention she deserves. From this barely controlled chaos, the booker's position evolved.

Today's booker works exclusively on the telephone, often with a hands-free headset to make computer access easier. The sole purpose of the booker and the booking room is to remove the telephones from the front desk and allow a little more tranquility in the reception area. Though some salons retain one or two phone units at the desk which may receive rollover calls during times of high volume and can be used to dial out, others have removed them completely.

Booking room considerations

A s the complexity of salons and day spas increases, and requires more moving parts than ever before, many owners and managers are recognizing a need for departmentalization to keep the machine moving forward. This need to decentralize extends to the front desk. How many hoops can an overworked team jump through? Does the chaos at the desk signify a need for additional staff, or is it a symptom of inefficient operations? Is it time to consider a booking room?

CAUTION: The addition of a booking room does not automatically create a need for additional staff. A serious problem for many salon and day spa front desks is lack of organization. If neither hand is aware of what the other is doing, there is no way to effectively manage operations. There is no team. Organization, in whatever form it takes, is the first step to discovering whether your salon's front desk is truly understaffed, or if the existing team is simply overworked.

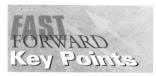

GETTING ORGANIZED

If neither hand is aware of what the other is doing, there is no way to effectively manage operations. There is no team. Organization, in whatever form it takes, is the first step to discovering whether your salon's front desk is truly understaffed, or if the team is simply overworked. Redirecting workflow and streamlining operations is often all that is necessary to regain control of the desk.

Create specific, detailed job descriptions for each team member who works at the salon front desk. Everyone must know his or her responsibilities, and accountabilities must be written into each position. If, with everyone working within well-defined parameters, the workload is still too great, *check the cash flow* and add new staff if feasible. However, redirecting workflow and streamlining existing operations is often all that is necessary to regain control of the front desk.

On-site or off-site?

SMALLER SALON DAY SPA OPERATIONS may find that practicality writes the rules concerning booking rooms (i.e., such operations are simply more convenient kept in-house, if they are necessary at all). Some booking rooms require only a single team member equipped with a computer, desk and headset; others are more elaborate. Most salons and day spas, however, do have the necessary space (an unoccupied or infrequently used treatment room, for example), and the cost is not as prohibitive as one may think.

Consider the investment in retail product that normally sits on the salon's shelves. Consider how much of it goes unsold because clients either cannot get into the salon for appointments or don't receive an adequate explanation of *why* they should purchase product. Chances are, for an investment smaller than the value of the retail product now sitting on the shelves, your salon can operate a booking room — which will free the desk staff to sell that retail, as well as additional services and gift certificates.

HIGHER VOLUME SALONS AND DAY SPAS are under more pressure. Consumers are more demanding than ever before, expecting value-added service. Cutting client wait times and improving traffic flow are no longer options. Yet neither is a hurried phone demeanor. Covering calls quickly but politely is crucial, as is the continued patronage of those very clients whose calls so often swamp the desk. Salons with multiple locations can utilize a single off-site *call center* to ensure better overall phone coverage. The call center can be located anywhere with working phone service, as long as it can be linked to the computers at each salon location.

Start-up requirements for a booking room include a computer connected to a local area network (LAN) for on-site rooms, or a wide area network (WAN) for off-site. Many salons already have LAN capability if they operate with multiple computers at the front desk or have units with access to scheduling information (though not necessarily the ability to make adjustments) elsewhere on the premises, such as in the dispensary or break room. In this case, the owner has several options, including buying a new unit or simply relocating a secondary computer to the new booking room.

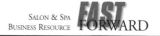
When utilizing an off-site call center, communication between locations must be instantaneous. This is called *real-time. (See chapter 2.)* Real-time automation prevents double-bookings in the event that an on-site receptionist or second booker at the call center attempts to place a client appointment in an already-occupied time slot.

Advantages of booking rooms

- ANNOYING, DISTRACTING RINGS DISAPPEAR: For the salon or day spa in which the reception area is near the service floor, or perhaps inconveniently adjacent to a treatment room, the isolation of a booking room can add a measure of serenity and peace for clients. The sound of a constantly ringing phone is often reminiscent of home or the office, preventing total relaxation.

- IMPROVED TRAFFIC FLOW: How many traffic jams are clients willing to navigate? The benefits of moving the phones away from the desk can be enormous. Daunting check-in and check-out lines can be virtually eliminated when the desk team has the freedom to move about the area discussing retail items, or to spring to the computer when needed.

- CLIENT CARE CAN SHIFT INTO HIGH GEAR: Booking rooms can relieve receptionists and coordinators of often cumbersome phone responsibilities — and free up more one-on-one time for responding to client needs in the salon. Questions about service and product benefits can be more thoroughly and

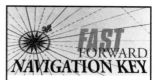

NAVIGATION KEY

A lot of salon owners would need little convincing to jump onto the booking room bandwagon. After all, there are some significant benefits:

- ANNOYING, DISTRACTING RINGS DISAPPEAR.
- IMPROVED TRAFFIC FLOW.
- CLIENT CARE CAN SHIFT INTO HIGH GEAR.
- INCREASED SALES OPPORTUNITIES.

patiently answered, billing issues resolved, compliments on new styles offered. All of the etiquette issues that need to be covered but are too often brushed aside at the overwhelmed front desk can be addressed properly.

■ INCREASED SALES OPPORTUNITIES: The front desk is a sales and customer service department. Adding a booking room provides the desk team a greater opportunity to flex their collective muscle and create new opportunities for overall salon growth. Up-selling, cross-selling, offering gift certificates, explaining promotions and encouraging the teamwork ethic can all receive more of the time they deserve and need.

When to consider adding a booking room

Just as the decision to expand or add a new product line depends on the market in which a salon operates and the best interests of its clients, so does the decision to add a booking room. But there are other considerations as well. If adding a booking room means hiring an additional staff member, will the return on the salon's investment offset the new payroll costs? Will clients truly be better served by the addition? Considerations include:

■ A high volume of calls that routinely interferes with the desk staff's ability to offer maximum client service.

■ Bottlenecks at the desk revolving around which team member will eventually have the time to check out an otherwise satisfied client.

■ Client comments or complaints about an inability to get through when trying to make an appointment by phone.

Finding just the right person

Hiring to fill a position at the front desk requires more than a dawning awareness of an ill-defined need. Once the need is intuitively felt, specific guidelines for its resolution must be developed. For example: If your desk is suddenly "more hectic" than usual, might it be due to a higher number of new clients and walk-ins, or increased retail traffic due to the introduction of a new product line? Many front desk problems have geographic solutions: the register can be moved to the other side of the desk, a retail display can be shifted a few feet, chairs can be added or removed. But…what if the issue is the sheer volume of business flowing through the salon doors every day?

Crafting a comprehensive job description is critical to a successful search for staff. What duties and opportunities will a position in your salon offer? What accountabilities will be attached to these duties and opportunities? What benefits of employment will a new team member enjoy?

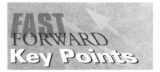

BEGINNING THE SEARCH: Where and how to find your perfect employee will depend largely on your market and resources. Cooperative partnerships, outreach programs, community and charity involvement, and referrals from current clients and staff are all valuable resources. It is important to make the salon or day spa's name known in every way possible. The more potential employees know about the salon, the more applications you will receive for available positions and, as some owners contend, the less "convincing" you will have to undertake during interviews when it's time to make a hiring decision.

BEGINNING THE SEARCH
Where and how you find your perfect employee will depend largely on your market and resources. Cooperative partnerships, outreach programs, community and charity involvement, and client and staff referrals are valuable resources.

Perhaps the most important qualification for desk staff is that they fit into the salon's culture and exhibit the promise of positive contribution. Whether you're looking for someone to assume the leadership mantle, to be sure the phones are answered consistently or to help turn the desk into a powerful sales position, the person chosen must display a conscientious desire to see the business grow to its full potential.

- SCHOOL PARTNERSHIPS: Many salons and day spas find that students from cosmetology school, high school or local colleges make excellent receptionists — especially those attending cosmetology school, for whom the practical experience could prove invaluable. Students are commonly willing to work flexible hours for a rate of pay that can easily be absorbed into the salon's budget. Salon owners that form continuing relationships with cosmetology schools through class instruction and open houses often encounter fewer problems recruiting because their names are already known to students.

- FASHION SHOWS AND OTHER SOCIAL CONTEXTS: No matter how it's done — a fashion show to showcase the staff's work, a wine and cheese reception or other event planned to generate some strategic exposure — opening the salon to the public, clients, and their families and friends will generate a lot of interest from many quarters. There is no way to anticipate from where future staff members will come, but displaying what the salon has to offer can attract interesting prospects. The answer to your business needs may already be observing the salon, but waiting for an invitation in.

- CHARITABLE EVENTS: Valuable public relations can be generated through contributions to raffles, club fundraisers and other events. In addition to staying in step with the community and doing a good turn for some worthwhile causes, the salon can get its name in front of a wide variety of people. There is a largely untapped pool of workers "on hiatus" who want to return to work after starting a family, traveling or just taking a break from the rigors of nine-to-five.

Training to ensure a perfect fit

B usinesses, whether it is consciously acknowledged or understood by their owners, are systems-driven. Every salon possesses inherent systems which dictate policy; whether they are controlled by, or in control of, the management team makes the difference between success and failure. For example: Most important to a salon employee's training is the owner's ability to outline the skills necessary to fill the position. Training a new employee is simply the synthesis of this knowledge.

Etiquette is essential

For many salon owners, the rules of the road are simple: Clients should be treated the same way one would treat a guest in one's home. They should not be allowed to enter without a proper greeting, or to sit unattended in the reception area without the offer of a beverage and other amenities. Every new client receives a salon tour, introductions to staff members and an overview of services. But such client care is possible only through a combination of systems and personality.

IT TAKES PEOPLE SKILLS OF THE HIGHEST ORDER. No matter how loudly one screams on the inside, the hectic atmosphere of the front desk cannot interfere with client service. Each deserves to experience the care and serenity promised by the salon's public relations and customer service creed. *Presentation matters.*

- THE GREETING: Clients are comforted by the sight of a well-groomed, smiling receptionist or coordinator who comes forward to greet them as they enter a salon. Formal greetings, firm handshakes and eye contact, and concern for their comfort appeal to clients' sense of professionalism and will engender confidence in the abilities of the entire team.

- WATCH THE TONE: Telephone and in-salon client contact must be efficient and time-conscious, but never rushed. Each client requires personalized attention to fulfill her individual needs.

- CLIENTS CANNOT BE WRONG: Well, perhaps they can, but they

should never be told so. It is the responsibility of the front desk team to ensure that client conflicts are resolved without pointing any fingers. Finger-pointing only gets one's fingers broken, and is injurious to staff morale and client retention numbers.

■ CONCLUDING THE APPOINTMENT AND CLOSING THE SALE: The opportunity to purchase product, pre-book future appointments and offer feedback on their salon experience is expected by many clients. The front desk staff must provide and encourage this interaction.

Customer service

IT'S ALL ABOUT CONTROL. It is impossible to provide the kind of service demanded by clients if one succumbs to the chaos of the front desk environment. The only way to maintain your sanity, and the sanity of your colleagues, is to maintain control — of yourself, your surroundings and those unexpected situations which arise throughout the day.

Salon clients are best served through honesty and a genuine effort toward resolving their problems and acknowledging their comments. Even if the news is not good for the salon — a client cannot control her new cut, is disappointed with a change of color or is not satisfied with a product purchase — experience truly is the best teacher. This is why some of the best salon coordinators and receptionists come from service-intensive industries such as restaurant and hotel management. Every team member at the front desk occupies a customer care position imbued with the power to make or break the salon's service record.

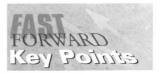

IT'S ALL ABOUT CONTROL

It is impossible to provide the kind of service demanded by clients if one succumbs to the chaos of the front desk environment. The only way to maintain your sanity, and the sanity of your colleagues, is to maintain control.

Procedure matters. Consistency is not an option. There is no area of customer relations too small for scripted responses, especially when a client is making an initial contact with the salon. Frequently asked questions (FAQ's) should be posted at the front desk. These are but a few:

- Why does a certain technician no longer work at the salon?
- Why do prices differ from stylist to stylist?
- May I return a product purchase?
- Why should I see another stylist?

In particularly challenging situations, as with a confrontational and highly vocal client in the salon, front desk staff must know how absolutely they are bound to protocol, as well as the freedoms they may exercise in resolving the situation.

Making contact: If technicians require varying lengths of time to complete services, post these requirements at the desk. Educate each member of the desk team about the personalities of each technician; good client matches will make for more pleasant experiences and higher retention. A strong software package can relieve many scheduling headaches.

COMPREHENSIVE TRAINING REQUIRES PRACTICAL EXPERIENCE IN ALL AREAS IN WHICH A NEW TEAM MEMBER MUST FUNCTION. In your salon or spa, this may mean that a new receptionist shadows a coordinator for a few days or answers telephone calls monitored by a manager. It may mean a crash course in the services offered and technology utilized at the desk.

There will always be a learning curve. Make sure that as much of it as possible is traversed before a new team member assumes his or her position.

A non-productive department?

A common fallacy of salon management philosophy is the belief that the front desk is a non-productive department, existing only to assist the technical staff. *Think again.* While it is true that a primary function of the desk is the efficient and productive booking of stylists and technicians, this responsibility is but the tip of the iceberg. This team does much more than assign clients to stylists and spa technicians. They control the salon's most precious resources: the appointment book and revenue-producing hours. But their responsibility is evolving.

Yesterday it was simply booking appointments. Today it's managing salon productivity and efficiency. For the savvy coordinator, an empty hour on the book or a client on a waiting list is a signal to shift into high gear. They know the capabilities of every team member. They know the clients. They solve problems, run reports, manage cash receipts, maintain inventory and order supplies. They turn chaos into calm. They protect the salon with special loyalty. The desk is their domain…they protect it.

Responsibilities and objectives

The goal of the salon coordinator is to lead, to carry the salon's "flag" onto the front lines and plant it firmly in the minds of clients, vendors, business relations and the public. It is to lead the other desk and technical staff to a new level of

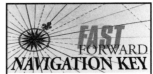

NAVIGATION KEY

The goal of the salon coordinator is to lead, to carry the salon's "flag" onto the front lines and plant it firmly. But these team members must be trained to become more than task-masters. Their responsibilities also include:

■ MONITORING revenue-producing hours and increasing productivity ratings.

■ CREATING efficient traffic and work flow.

■ BUILDING the salon's average ticket.

The reception area is a promotional, public relations and sales center.

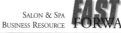
excellence, to lead *by example.* A salon in pursuit of excellence needs a commander-in-chief. When the owner chooses to work behind the chair, or decides the time has come to delegate some of the cumbersome responsibilities of management, the commander-in-chief position often falls to the manager or coordinator. But while it is easy to craft a competent job description of the technical skills required to ably fill front desk positions, these team members must be trained to become more than task-masters.

Revenue-producing hours and productivity ratings

Catering to the clients' needs is quite enough to keep the desk a busy place, and should be the top priority of the desk staff. But if salon owners are careful not to over-burden front desk staff with a lot of unnecessary hoops to jump through, their time will generate a lot more revenue for the business.

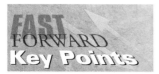

WHO'S FUELING WHOM?
Catering to the clients' needs is enough to keep the desk busy, and should be the top priority of the staff. But if salon owners are careful not to over-burden front desk staff with a lot of unnecessary hoops, their time will generate a lot more revenue for the business.

SALON AND SPA PRODUCTIVITY IS THE RATIO OF WORK ACTUALLY DONE TO THE TOTAL TIME AVAILABLE. But raw numbers can be deceiving; the front desk staff's job is to streamline them. For example: A stylist who is available for eight hours per day and likes to book out a full hour for a cut and style may claim 100% productivity (and burnout) if she sees eight clients. However, if she actually finishes the service in forty-five minutes, a more accurate productivity rating would be 80%, which is actually a highly desirable level. (CAUTION: Most salon staff realize that 100% productivity can quickly lead to burnout, as well as poor retention numbers for first-time clients. *Do not target 100% productivity.* The above example is meant to show that a salon's numbers must be examined closely for "time stealers" which can disguise low productivity rates.)

Every hour on the salon's books which is tagged for sale has the potential to be a revenue-producing hour. Hours which are not considered revenue-producing hours are those reserved for lunch, team meetings, in-salon training, etc. Only revenue-producing hours should be considered when calculating productivity. But alert receptionists and coordinators should be trained to see productivity "black holes" and turn them into viable salon time.

Efficient traffic and workflow

SERVICE BUSINESSES DO NOT HAVE ANY TIME TO WASTE. Keeping a finger on all the activities that swirl around the front desk requires the ability to put one's fingers to a computer keyboard. Many salons still rely on paper appointment books and information files, but the automation move is on. Computer knowledge is a prerequisite of employment in most businesses today. The salon can be no different. If it requires a ten-minute phone call for a single client to schedule an appointment, how many others won't get through? If a client must wait twenty minutes to pay for services, will she come back? Good customer service requires an appropriate length of time be spent with clients, but not more than necessary.

Every area of service in the salon will be positively impacted by increased organization and speed at the front desk. When desk staff are less harried and technicians less rushed, all are more efficient. Though initial automation expenses will depend on the equipment needed and the program chosen to run on that equipment, the resulting increase in accessible revenue-producing hours will create an influx of dollars — from retained clients able to schedule more convenient appointments and from new clients who are suddenly able to get in — which will easily and rapidly recoup the expense. You, your team and the salon's clients can then enjoy the business' new ability to work around the clients' needs.

There are several occurrences that salon coordinators and receptionists should look for and weed out of the business' traditional operating procedure:

- LONG LUNCHES: Whatever the assigned lunch break, everyone must abide by it.

- ARRIVING WITH THE CLIENT: What happens with a walk-in if the only staff members present are the ones who are booked? Absent stylists and technicians hurt the salon's earning potential as well as their own. If working hours are scheduled, the technicians must be on the premises.

- PERSONAL CALLS AND CONGREGATIONS AT THE DESK: Impromptu gatherings can seriously impair the desk staff's ability to function effectively. Make it a ground rule that the only ones allowed behind the desk are those required to be there.

- ACCESS DENIED: Similarly, the desk staff must be the only ones in the salon with access to the appointment book. Their job is to impartially assign clients to available staff members and encourage teamwork through their booking practices.

Building average ticket

IT'S ALL ABOUT SALES AS SERVICE. Many methods of boosting a salon's average ticket are centered at the front desk. The power of the desk staff resides in their ability to push sales through the roof by promoting the salon's culture to every client who calls or walks through the door. The reception area is the salon's promotional and public relations center. It *is* a sales center.

- GIVE CLIENTS A VISUAL through detailed, descriptive explanations of services on inquiry calls. Would you rather receive a "really good manicure" or a "luxurious hand treatment"? Front desk team members must be able to explain each step of each service in a way that entices clients to book an appointment.

- EFFECTIVE RETAIL DISPLAYS WILL SELL PRODUCT. With the sleek packaging manufacturers are now producing, many lines will sell themselves if they are within easy reach of the consumer.

- OFFER CLIENTS A RETAIL PURCHASE OR CONFIRMATION OF TECHNICIAN'S OFFER. The opportunity to purchase home maintenance products is a component of the complete salon experience. Do not deny clients the chance to look good between appointments. They are the salon's best advertisement.

- OFFER VALUE-ADDED SERVICES DURING WAIT TIMES. If a client is already in the salon, but a technician is running late, is the desk staff authorized to offer an impromptu manicure or conditioning treatment at a reduced price? Doing so may just get clients "hooked" on future bookings.

- PROMOTING PROMOTIONS ON THE PHONE AND AT THE COUNTER must be written into the job description of each desk team member. Since they are clients' first and last contact with the salon, these encounters should be productive.

- PROMOTING TEAM SERVICE AND CLIENT SHARING will help clients feel comfortable with many different technicians. Consequently, they will be less nervous about trying new services and trusting product advice — and that will send the salon's average ticket up.

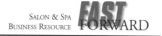
Team huddles: Your goals are our goals

Keeping everyone on the same page is no easy task without clear and constant communication — among the *entire* team. The most effective facilitation method is team huddles. Huddles provide an open forum for each staff member to share opinions and ideas, reflections on past performance and goals for the future. They also help bridge the chasms that often exist between salon owners and employees, and between different departments which may not be as familiar with each other's services as they need to be.

The front desk must be intimately acquainted with all salon service procedures. Otherwise, selling them is problematic. One method of familiarizing the entire staff with the full range of services the salon offers is to hold staff meetings in which the information is communicated in word and practice. If the receptionist or coordinator needs to know what a facial does for the skin or a massage for the circulation, have him or her *experience* it.

Huddles also enable the technical staff to comprehend the integral role of the desk in salon growth. To foster a mutual respect between the styling floor and the front desk, everyone must understand the pressures and responsibilities the desk team operates under each day, and the impact they have on individual technicians' productivity and earning potential. A strong focus on interactive team meetings will quickly produce measurable communications results.

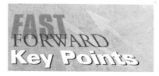

THE HUDDLE FACTOR

Huddles provide an open forum for each staff member to share opinions and ideas, reflections on past performance and goals for the future. They help bridge the chasms that often exist between salon owners and employees, and between departments which may not be as familiar with each other's services as they need to be.

The front desk team needs to participate in two kinds of huddles: those which involve the rest of the salon, and those devoted to issues specific to their goals and position. Huddles should be scheduled and conducted regularly. Consistent follow-through is imperative in emphasizing the importance of the topics discussed at these meetings.

Well, they're usually our goals...

The level of interaction and interdependence between the front desk and other salon departments determines how many of their goals are complementary. In certain situations, the desk works hand-in-hand with the technical staff.

- RETAIL PRODUCT SOLD: It is up to the receptionist who operates the cash register to ensure that each client has the opportunity to purchase product recommended by technicians. Stylists and technicians open the door and the desk team closes the deal. (Or, the desk team opens the door *and* closes the deal.) It's also important that retail displays be kept organized and dust-free to maximize their appeal to clients.

- GIFT CERTIFICATES SOLD: There are several ways to go about this. Many salons devote an unused station or construct original, free-standing displays to promote gift certificates — especially around holidays such as Valentine's Day and Mother's Day. Bookers and other team members who respond to client calls should mention these promotions to each caller. Receptionists and coordinators should not let clients leave without inquiring whether they are in need of a "perfect gift" for family, friends or co-workers.

...But not always

To ensure the level of productivity your salon's desk team is capable of, they must have their own goals, revolving around their position in the business. And, through regular huddles, each member of the desk team must remain up-to-date on *what* the goals are, *why* they are important and *how* to meet them. It's the only way they can support the rest of the business.

- PERCENT OF APPOINTMENTS PRE-BOOKED: All clients must have the opportunity to book their next appointment in advance. A client's prerogative to change her mind notwithstanding (the point is to make the offer), tracking pre-booked appointments has several advantages: managers can provide immediate feedback to the desk team; it's an area that's easy to improve quickly; and the gratification of seeing a goal quickly met can inspire team members to work toward other goals. Pre-booking is easy to track manually. It simply requires notations on client tickets or the daily master client list, which can then be tallied at closing. These numbers can be calculated for individuals and the desk team as a whole.

- CLIENTS STRANDED ON WAITING LISTS: A greater number of salon owners and managers than ever before believe that waiting lists can be detrimental to client retention. Therefore, they consider the number of clients on "hold" a measure of their business' front desk efficiency — or the lack of it. Can a client see an alternate technician? When was she last contacted to determine if circumstances have changed and she will accept a currently open appointment?

- HOURS FILLED ON APPOINTMENT BOOK: Are there a lot of fifteen-minute gaps in technicians' schedules which, if strung continuously, would allow time to see more clients? Do lunch hours run long? Do technicians' schedules begin late or end early? The appointment book is the possession of the front desk. The coordinator controls it, and must have the support of the owner in exerting the power to tighten schedules. Salon and spa productivity will soar as a result.

- CLIENT ISSUES RESOLVED: Receptionists and coordinators are sounding boards for clients and staff alike. How much authority does the team have to take measures — such as offering complimentary redo's or other services, or issuing certificates redeemable for product — to the occasional disgruntled client? A crucial component of salons (in addition to outstanding service) that hear very few client complaints is a business- and service-savvy desk team which insulates the styling floor and treatment rooms. Rather than scoring the team on how many negatives surface, score them on how many *do not*.

■ NUMBER OF TICKETS PROCESSED: Your salon needs to be automated to consider scoring this productivity measure. Some software packages will track the number of transactions processed by the front desk over the course of a day, week or month. This capability allows owners and managers to zero in on specific times of day and evaluate the desk's performance. How many tickets are actually processed (e.g., clients serviced) during the busiest hours? How many are processed at slower times? Perhaps the desk team's efforts can be better coordinated during hectic times or redirected to other areas in need of attention during down time. The people who work the desk know client flow and traffic patterns better than anyone. Get them to share what they know at regular meetings, and track their improvement in streamlining desk operations.

■ UP-SELLING AND CROSS-PROMOTION: This performance statistic is also easier to measure through a computer, especially when transactions are processed under operator codes. This way, service and retail purchases that were not included on the original ticket can be attributed to the receptionist or coordinator who completes the sale and rings the transaction; these numbers will clearly indicate the degree of emphasis the desk team places on sales goals.

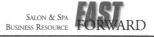
The value of efficiency

Competent, dependable management and desk personnel are crucial to the success of a salon or day spa venture, especially if the owner works in the business as a stylist or technician. And the competence and dependability of these positions must be adequately rewarded. Compensation strategies for the desk team are often planned blindly by salon and spa owners who have yet to decipher the many ways in which these players support the rest of the team.

Compensation for a job well done

The method and amount of compensation allotted to the front desk team depends upon the level of responsibility. A receptionist whose primary job requirement is answering the phone may be paid an hourly rate — rewarding his or her actual time spent in the salon performing required duties. But for the receptionist, manager or coordinator who devotes time to a variety of responsibilities and goes "above and beyond" the call of duty so often that non-routine activities soon become routine, a different strategy is required.

WHEN IT COMES TO HIRING SKILL AND TALENT, YOU GET WHAT YOU PAY FOR. Too many owners view the front desk as a void in the salon, and the staff's sole purpose for being to retrieve phone calls and book appointments. The irony is that treating the desk this way will prevent competent, effective people with the right skills and experience from even applying. Front desk positions now require a more professional employee who in turn expects to earn more. You do not want high turnover at this position.

Paying a little more for a professional administrator or someone with customer service experience pays off for many salons, and owners routinely go outside the salon industry when hiring front desk staff. Hotel concierges, restaurant hostesses and *maître d's*, retail associates and customer service representatives with phone skills are excellent candidates. While the additional training may initially seem to be a drawback, it ultimately forces the salon to improve the most important part of the business: the front desk, the customer service headquarters.

To determine starting pay, research what is being paid for comparable positions in your salon's marketplace. Local chambers of commerce and libraries often store this information. It is also critically important to consult the salon or spa's cash flow. Can the business support the additional payroll? If so, at what rate of pay? The wage offered by your salon must be fair both to the new employee and the business.

Determining the front desk's salary expense is as simple as dividing the number of dollars devoted to desk payroll by the salon or spa's total revenue figures. In the spirit of controlling payroll costs, the owner's goal is to decrease this percentage by motivating the team to increase sales — not by hiring unskilled labor at a lower hourly wage.

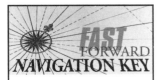

FAST FORWARD

NAVIGATION KEY

What is the objective of the front desk? Once a team is in place that can tighten schedules, push retail and pre-book appointments, they must be compensated for their efforts. *Look for results.*

- SALES TARGETS
- RETENTION
- PRODUCTIVITY
- AVERAGE TICKET
- FREQUENCY OF VISIT
- CROSS-SELLING & UP-SELLING
- MAINTAINING CONTROL

These accomplishments, though often rhetorically referred to as invaluable, can in fact be measured and evaluated.

Rating front desk performance

"WHAT IS THE OBJECTIVE OF THE FRONT DESK?" Once a team is in place that can tighten schedules, push retail and pre-book appointments, they must be compensated for their efforts. *Look for results.*

Does the salon have projected targets for sales, retention, productivity, average ticket, frequency of visit? If so, these are the numbers to watch. How effective is the front desk team at filling vacant hours on the book, no matter which technician's column they occupy? How good are they at cross-selling product and services?

Negotiating client difficulties? Maintaining control of the reception area, even during stressful hours, and making clients feel comfortable? These accomplishments, often rhetorically referred to as "invaluable," can in fact be measured and evaluated.

Efficiency records of front desk activity *can* be kept, and the results tabulated. Most of today's salon software programs can sort front desk transaction data, giving management and owners access to information such as the time of day the salon receives the most incoming calls and rings up the most tickets. This information makes some interesting calculations possible:

- USING THE COMPUTER, TRACK THE AVERAGE TOTAL OF DAILY TRANSACTIONS for the entire month. Divide this number by the number of team members working the desk at any given hour. This calculation yields the number of transactions per hour per employee, and will tell you when the salon is under- or overstaffed.

- IT'S A JUDGEMENT CALL: If the desk is handling a lot of transactions per hour, the team may not be able to provide great customer service. If the number of transactions for any given hour is low, the team may need other work to occupy their time — such as tracking and contacting "lost" clients, developing targeted marketing plans and instituting client reward systems.

There are methods of rewarding the desk team for performance beyond the call.

- SET QUARTERLY GOALS BASED ON (SEASONAL) PROJECTIONS. When these goals are met, it's bonus time. Let the team decide how to disburse their hard-earned bonus dollars. Make certain that the bonus amount is comparable to a substantial increase over their base pay.

- PERCENTAGE OF SALES OVER BREAKEVEN. Does the salon front desk team know what they have to do in service and retail tickets to break even for the week, month and quarter? (If not, how can they formulate effective goals?) If the dollars generated at the desk push salon sales past the break-even point, set some of this money aside for a bonus pool.

The Front Desk Acid Test

Employees add value or they add cost

"Does my salon's front desk…"

	NEVER				ALWAYS
1…operate with clearly defined performance goals?	1	2	3	4	5
2…keep <u>salon productivity</u> as its number one priority?	1	2	3	4	5
3…take total responsibility for client satisfaction?	1	2	3	4	5
4…put the needs and concerns of clients first?	1	2	3	4	5
5…recommend the skills of the entire salon?	1	2	3	4	5
6…regularly participate in leadership team meetings?	1	2	3	4	5
7…know the salon's weekly/monthly sales objectives?	1	2	3	4	5
8…assist in planning work schedules to avoid gridlock?	1	2	3	4	5
9…contribute to increasing average ticket?	1	2	3	4	5
10…operate with well-conceived systems?	1	2	3	4	5
11…have goals tied to a team-based incentive program?	1	2	3	4	5
12…present a professional personal appearance?	1	2	3	4	5
13…use good judgement when addressing problems?	1	2	3	4	5
14…maintain high levels of respect for clients and staff?	1	2	3	4	5
15…deliver value-added service?	1	2	3	4	5

TOTAL SCORE: _____

Total your responses. The highest possible score is 75; the lowest 15. Compare your score with the chart below to see how your front desk contributes to salon growth. If the salon scored less than 4 on any question, target that area for improvement. A 3 or less indicates an area that must receive immediate attention.

15 – 25
LITTLE OR NO CONTRIBUTION TO SALON GROWTH

26 – 45
MINIMAL CONTRIBUTION
Your front desk needs lots of work.

46 – 60
AVERAGE CONTRIBUTION
Your front desk needs systems, structure and training.

61 – 70
GOOD CONTRIBUTION
Your front desk is on the right track, but needs focus, organization and clearly defined goals/incentives.

71 – 75
FIRST-RATE CONTRIBUTION
Your front desk is well-structured, with high performance standards. Explore more advanced goals and incentive programs.

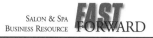
A priorities checklist

THE TOP TEN ASPECTS OF CUSTOMER SERVICE...
AS SEEN BY THE COORDINATOR

1. Clients should feel "at home"
2. A friendly voice on the phone
3. A smiling face at the desk
4. Place client with appropriate stylist
5. Maintain efficient scheduling
6. Clean salon environment
7. Total client focus; client comes first
8. Good first and last impression
9. Birthday and miss-you cards
10. Know retail and service preferences

THE TOP TEN WISHES OF OWNERS AND DESK STAFF
FOR IMPROVED CLIENT SERVICE

1. Product education
2. Technical "stylist" information
3. More room to move around desk
4. Move phones away from desk
5. Separate check-in and check-out
6. External motivational seminars
7. Training: How to be "professional"
8. Modern computer systems
9. Training: How to close the sale
10. Communication among staff

FRONT DESK STRATEGIES

Things to do:

- EVALUATE YOUR FRONT DESK: Take the front desk acid test on page 199. How does your front desk score?

- Define the primary role of front desk staff. Enlist the staff's help in creating specific, detailed job descriptions for each team member who works at the desk.

- Consider a booking room. It can take an enormous amount of pressure off the front desk and free the team to focus more clearly on client satisfaction.

- Develop specific guidelines for hiring for the front desk position. Know the qualities you need *before* beginning your search.

- Develop a training program which is geared toward customer service, and includes practical experience in all areas in which a new team member must function.

- Make productivity the top priority of the front desk staff.

- Give your front desk staff product knowledge classes. Teach them the importance of up-selling and closing sales.

- Set goals for your front desk staff. Use scoreboards and huddles to track progress and keep them informed on:
    PRODUCTIVITY
    RETAIL SALES
    GIFT CERTIFICATES
    PRE-BOOKING

MOVING TOWARD "TRUE QUALITY"

Today, *True Quality* is a necessity... not an option

INTRODUCTION BY:

> Matthew Cross, President
> LEADERSHIP ALLIANCE

A ccording to the legendary "Einstein of Quality and Business," Dr. W. Edwards Deming (1900–1993), all businesses are really in one business only.

Regardless of the business you are in — service, manufacturing, education, non-profit, etc. — there is one primary aim of which you must be acutely aware, and continuously strive to master, if you wish to grow and prosper. If you don't, your days may be numbered; at the very least, you will be doomed to mediocrity.

What do you think your number one aim in business should be, in order to best guarantee success?

Before we explore Dr. Deming's answer to this question, and how it can transform your business, let's consider the man. Who was W. Edwards Deming? Why should we value what he has to say about succeeding in business? For those who may never have heard of him, or who have forgotten the details, here's a quick overview.

"True" is better

By now, many have heard of "TQM" (Total Quality Management). It is important to note that TQM is one of many names often used in an attempt to describe pieces of the powerful, holistic system Deming created. For this reason, I have chosen to change the "Total" in TQM to "True" to better reflect the scope and genius of Deming's complete system.

A master statistician with a profound understanding of systems theory, Deming played a pivotal role in the U.S. victory in World War II by helping create the quality standards crucial to the precision manufacture of America's war equipment. However, when WWII ended, America was the only major industrial power left standing, with enormous worldwide demand for everything it could produce. So, the U.S. disregarded the very quality methods that had helped it win the war, and shifted full-speed into quantity production. Deming tried in vain to interest U.S. businesses in adopting his quality methods after the war, but his efforts fell on deaf ears. The long-term impact of the decision to focus on quantity over quality would take decades to surface.

Ironically, Deming is perhaps best known as the man who introduced quality to Japan. After WWII, Japan was a ruined nation, its people literally starving in the streets. Prior to the war, Japan had one of the worst reputations in the world for quality. Today they have the best. This was not an accident, or because of anything special about the Japanese culture. According to the Japanese themselves, Deming is the reason. In 1950, General Douglas MacArthur suggested to his friend Dr. Deming that he teach the Japanese his quality methods, to help them rebuild their war-shattered economy. Deming began lecturing to the heads of Japanese businesses in 1950, and made his now-famous prediction: If the Japanese learned and adopted his quality system, they would become an exporting nation within five years, and be well on the way to producing the world's highest-quality and most in-demand products. The rest, as they say, is history.

The original, comprehensive quality system he taught the Japanese directly resulted in their becoming a world-class business and economic power. In fact, the highest business award in Japan since 1951, equivalent to an annual business quality Nobel Prize, is named after an American: The Deming Prize. *(See "Deming Prize qualifications" at the end of this chapter.)* Emperor Hirohito would also award Dr. Deming Japan's highest civilian honor, the Second Order of the Sacred Treasure.

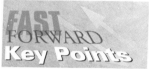

True Quality is simply the creation of systems and processes that are designed to eliminate defects and inconsistencies before they occur.

It wasn't until the early '80s, when Deming-inspired higher quality Japanese exports began to capture and dominate U.S. markets, that America woke up and rediscovered Deming, then in his eighties. The primary catalyst was a 1980 NBC News special entitled, "If Japan Can, Why Can't We?" which featured a brief section on Deming's work.

Soon, many leading American and international businesses, including Ford Motor Co., Xerox, and Proctor & Gamble, adopted the Deming approach. In fact, the leaders of Ford and Xerox directly credited Dr. Deming with saving their companies from certain extinction. For example: In 1980 Ford was losing $1.5 billion per year and had the worst reputation for quality and reliability of any American car company. Today, Ford is both the highest quality American car maker and the most profitable. Ford is in fact poised to overtake GM as the largest American auto maker for the first time in almost seventy years.

This is no accident. Deming is the reason. A U.S. News & World Report cover story named Deming's contribution to the world one of only nine "Hidden Turning Points in World History," along with events like Columbus' discovery of America, and Napoleon's conquest of Europe.

Contrary to what we've been hearing about Japan's recent economic woes, the well-known Japanese industries that adopted the Deming Method and stuck with it continue to enjoy great success. These are primarily exporting companies involved in electronics, automobile manufacturing and steel production: TOYOTA, MATSUSHITA/PANASONIC, RICOH, etc. These companies are world-renowned for healthy profits, international market dominance and quality leadership. Unfortunately, Japan's financial industry and government never adopted Deming's methods.

So, what does all this have to do with your business, you ask?

Deming's quality methods are both timeless and immediately applicable to all organizations, of every size and type. They work, like a virtual "secret weapon," to assure lasting success. The reason Deming is still so unknown to many is simple. Despite decades of stellar results around the world in every kind of business, Deming's methods challenge the dated yet heavily entrenched Western management status quo. His brilliant systems and boldly humanistic approach to enlightened management fly in the face of conventional Western management wisdom, which manages people in a top-down, fear-based manner. The Deming way manages through an integrated systems approach, the aim of which is to optimize the entire system — and everyone within it. The principle idea is to delight customers and keep them coming back again and again. This is a dramatic shift from the conventional short-term "sell, sell, sell" approach; yet every business that has adopted the Deming Method and stuck with it invariably enjoys great success — on all levels.

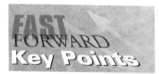

FAST FORWARD Key Points

The Deming way manages through an integrated systems approach, the aim of which is to optimize the entire system — and everyone within it.

Deming called it "profound knowledge"

The essence of the Deming Quality System is surprisingly simple. Indeed, much of it is powerful common sense. Yet like any great truth, it requires time, patience and commitment to realize its full impact. Let's start with an overview of what Deming called "profound knowledge." This consists of four interrelated and inseparable parts that act as a foundation for implementing True Quality Management. They are:

1. APPRECIATION FOR A SYSTEM. Every business consists of multiple processes that must be viewed as a whole system. A system is simply a series of interrelated processes and people whose aim is to work together to accomplish the goal of the system. The context is a place where cooperation and collaboration replace harmful competition so that everyone wins. By focusing on the whole rather than the isolated parts, organizations can actually outperform their individual assets and optimize their resources and opportunities.

2. KNOWLEDGE OF VARIATION. Variation is the voice of the system. Managers must understand how to listen to this voice and then make appropriate, continuous improvements. Too much variation in product or service is the villain of quality and success. At the same time, it is a clear indicator of where to focus attention to grow and transform a business. The regular collection and correct interpretation of relevant data (the key business "vital signs" and process results) plays a major role here.

3. THEORY OF KNOWLEDGE. There is a crucial difference between information and knowledge. Information, no matter how complete and speedy, is not knowledge. Most businesses are swimming in ever-deeper oceans of information. What is required is what Deming called *profound knowledge* — the kind of knowledge that provides highly reliable predictive power. We must learn to strategically see the whole picture, not just pieces of it. This requires a basic understanding of the importance of theory, for without theory we cannot intelligently guide and grow a business.

4. PSYCHOLOGY OF CHANGE. This helps us to understand and optimize all interactions within an organization. People are born with inner motivation, the desire for healthy relationships, a natural

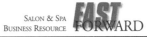

inclination for learning, a strong need for love and esteem, and a right to joy and dignity in their work. Good management must honor and support these innate factors within people, and optimize the whole business system. Internal competition between departments and people is especially destructive to optimal performance. The introduction of constructive change must include and involve all members within the system for best results. Simply put, profound knowledge provides the lens through which businesses can optimize all efforts and achieve greatest success.

Fourteen points for the transformation

Deming created his famous "Fourteen Points for the Transformation of Business & Management" to offer further guidance. These are fourteen basic ground rules that support optimum quality, which must be applied together for maximum impact. As you will see, some of these points challenge modern management beliefs and practices. This was part of Deming's genius: He was more concerned with true effectiveness than tired, misguided traditions that simply don't work well. The Fourteen Points are:

1. CREATE CONSTANCY OF PURPOSE. Create a strong "constancy of purpose" — a clear aim or vision — toward improvement of product and service, with the aim to become competitive, to stay in business and to provide jobs.
2. ADOPT A NEW PHILOSOPHY. We are in a new economic age. Management must awaken to this challenge, learn their responsibilities and take on proactive leadership for change.
3. CEASE MASS INSPECTION. Cease reliance on mass inspection to achieve quality. (Some processes where the probability and cost of error is great may be exceptions — e.g., bank proofing operations.) Eliminate the need for inspection on a mass basis by building quality into the product/service at the beginning of the process, rather than trying to "inspect quality in" at the end.
4. MINIMIZE TOTAL COST…GO FOR SINGLE SUPPLIERS. End the practice of awarding business on the basis of price alone. Instead, minimize total cost. Move toward a single supplier for any one item on a long-term relationship of increasing loyalty and trust.

5. CONSTANTLY IMPROVE SYSTEMS. Improve constantly and forever the system of production and service to improve quality and productivity, and thus constantly decrease costs. KEY: Higher Quality = Lower Costs.

6. INSTITUTE TRAINING ON THE JOB. Constantly offer continuing educational and training opportunities for all team members, both to sharpen and broaden job-related skills and to support each employee's greater potential.

7. INSTITUTE LEADERSHIP. The true aim of leadership (supervision) should be to help and support people and machines to do a better job. Supervision of management is in need of overhaul, as well as supervision of production and service workers.

8. DRIVE OUT FEAR. Drive out fear, so that everyone may work effectively for the company. Fear (of speaking one's mind, losing one's job, being disrespected, etc.) destroys innovation, trust and loyalty — essential elements in any successful enterprise. Fear also fosters destructive attitudes and adversarial fragmentation within the organization.

9. BREAK DOWN DEPARTMENT BARRIERS. Break down barriers between departments. All people in your system — people in research, design, sales, production and customer relations — must work as a team to foresee and resolve problems of production and customer use that may be encountered with your product or service.

10. ELIMINATE SLOGANS, ETC. Eliminate slogans, exhortations and targets for your work force asking for things like zero defects and new levels of productivity. Such exhortations only create adversarial relationships, since the bulk of the causes of low quality and low productivity belong to your overall *system...* and thus lie beyond the power of the work force. *(See #5)*

11. ELIMINATE MANAGEMENT BY NUMBERS. Eliminate work standards (quotas), management by objectives, management by numbers, and numerical goals for both management and workers. Setting goals without a clear method and plan to achieve them is actually counterproductive. Substitute leadership and participative management.

12. REMOVE BARRIERS THAT ROB PRIDE. Remove barriers that rob people of their right to pride of workmanship. Supervisors should be responsible for *quality,* not numbers. Eliminate annual reviews and merit ratings. (Again, as hard as it may be to believe, most of the causes of individual performance — positive or negative — are due to the overall system people work within. Also, no one person can ever accurately or fairly rank or review another. Better to move toward a more democratic 360-degree or similar feedback system, with the aim to foster greater understanding for all…never to penalize, rank or instill fear.)

13. INSTITUTE EDUCATION. Institute a vigorous program of education and self-improvement for all employees, including non-job-related areas of personal interest to them. Support the enrichment of your people at all levels, as your team is your most valuable asset.

14. INVOLVE EVERYBODY. Put everybody in the company to work to accomplish the transformation. The transformation is everybody's job…and a neverending process.

The system of PROFOUND KNOWLEDGE and the FOURTEEN POINTS provides a broad overview of the Deming Method. They are meant to inspire ideas and challenge us to ask questions, as a starting point for positive transformation. Deeper study reveals increasing opportunities for greater integration and advancement.

That one "primary aim"

So, what is that one primary aim all businesses must focus on if they hope to grow and profit? *The creation and growth of loyal customers.* All of the world's leading businesses have this one pivotal area in common: They continually focus on providing the highest quality and value of product and services that delight their customers. This increases customer loyalty — and virtually guarantees success in the process. In essence, the lower the "defection rate" of your customers, employees, and investors, the higher levels of success you will achieve. It's that simple. KEY: *Loyal* customers are the aim — not simply "satisfied." Studies have actually shown that four of five "satisfied" customers will defect, given a good enough reason. Merely "satisfying" customers is no longer enough to achieve lasting success.

It may come as a surprise, but loyal customers (and loyal employees and investors) are also your most important business asset. Loyal customers keep coming back, refer their friends and measurably grow in value over time. Consider this: A 5% increase in customer retention (loyalty) directly translates into a 50% increase in sales, on average. It costs next to nothing to keep a customer; yet it proportionally costs a fortune to attract new ones. A key outcome of the Deming Method is ever-increasing customer delight and loyalty.

Not quality in an instant

Bear in mind, the Deming Method is not an instantaneous cookie-cutter approach. It takes time, commitment, focus and work. Yet the results are huge, and multiply over time. Having a good coach can definitely accelerate the process, as it is nearly impossible to work effectively *on* any system while working *in* the system. This is especially true in the beginning stages. Regardless of which path you choose, be prepared for one of the most challenging yet rewarding experiences in business. The Deming Quality Method provides a proven, holistic formula for maximum success. It will transform the quality of your business, your life and your results. What else could you ask for in your company?

Matthew Cross is president of LEADERSHIP ALLIANCE, *an innovative consulting organization dedicated to personal and professional transformation. An acclaimed Deming scholar, his training leads companies and individuals of all types to reach and exceed their highest potentials.*

*For more information…*MCross@LeadershipAlliance.com, *or call: 203.322.1456.*

You can also visit www.LeadershipAlliance.com *for more information on the Deming Quality Method and its application to your business.*

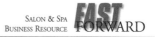
Malcolm Baldridge National Quality Award

In 1987, Congress established the Malcolm Baldrige National Quality Award (MBNQA) to recognize U.S. companies with successful quality management systems. Award criteria focus on daily business operations (e.g., process management, customer focus, leadership), and improvements in processes, structure, services and products, and the role of leadership. A successful business makes a healthy profit, has happy employees, delivers high-quality services and products, and has delighted customers.

In striving for the MBNQA, a company may systematically focus every aspect of its operations on quality and, therefore, place itself on the path to True Quality. Living by the Baldrige criteria implies running a world-class operation. Applying them to your salon will substantially improve your business (and profits), even if you choose not to compete for the award.

Baldrige scoring guidelines

The MBNQA criteria for the year 2000 address seven categories and nineteen items. *(See chart, pages 214–215)*. The scoring of responses to criteria items is based on three evaluation dimensions:

■ APPROACH (i.e., the method(s) used to address the criteria). Evaluation factors include:
1. appropriateness of the methods to the requirements.
2. effectiveness of use of methods, and the degree to which the approach:
   — is repeatable, integrated and consistently applied.
   — embodies evaluation, improvement and learning cycles.
   — is based on reliable information and data.
3. alignment with your organizational needs.
4. evidence of innovation.

■ DEPLOYMENT (i.e., the extent to which your approach is applied to all requirements of the criteria). Evaluation factors include:
1. use of the approach in addressing the criteria relevant to your organization.

2. use of the approach by all appropriate work units.

■ RESULTS (i.e., outcomes in achieving the purposes of the criteria). Evaluation factors include:

1. your current performance.
2. performance relative to appropriate comparisons and/or benchmarks.
3. rate, breadth and importance of performance improvements.
4. linkage of your results measures to key customer, market, process and action-plan performance requirements identified in your business overview.

A salon's performance system should target results according to the interests of all stakeholders: customers, staff, owners, distributors and the community. Attaining high performance levels means continuous improvement, both evolutionary and "breakthrough." Opportunities for improvement should derive from staff ideas, client surveys and other feedback; from your own research into better processes, services and products; and from benchmarking other salons or the processes of other industries.

The time investment

The decision to apply for the MBNQA in the future should be made today. Meeting the leadership criteria, developing the systems needed to implement TQM throughout your salon, and achieving and measuring results all take time. Realistically, if you commit to the MBNQA approach today, you will require a minimum of three years to apply.

Make sure you are adopting the program for the right reasons. Companies which claim 90% of their reason in applying for the MBNQA is to improve the focus on customer satisfaction, quality processes and measurable results — devoting only 10% of the effort to actually winning the award — have a healthy outlook. Remember, the journey alone is worth the effort.

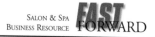
Malcolm Baldrige National Quality Award
Year 2000 Criteria Items

The following criteria for the MBNQA are a wonderful guide to enlighten salon and spa owners about the many facets of a TQM transformation.

<u>CATEGORY</u> <u>POINT VALUES</u>

Leadership..125
Organizational leadership — 85
Public responsibility — 40

Strategic Planning 85
Strategy development — 40
Strategy deployment — 45

Customer and Market Focus...............................85
Customer and market knowledge — 40
Customer satisfaction — 45

Information and Analysis 85
Measurement of organizational performance — 40
Analysis of organizational performance — 45

Human Resource Focus...................................85
Work systems — 35
Employee education, training and development — 25
Employee well-being and satisfaction — 25

Process Management......................................85
Product and service processes — 55
Support processes — 15
Supplier and partnering processes — 15

Business Results 450
Customer-focused results — 115

Financial and market results	115
Human resource results	80
Supplier and partner results	25
Organizational effectiveness results	115

TOTAL POINTS. 1000

www.baldridge.org *or* www.quality.nist.gov
E-mail: nqp@nist.gov

Baldrige National Quality Program
National Institute of Standards and Technology (NIST)
Administration Building, Room A635
100 Bureau Drive, Stop 1020
Gaithersburg, MD 20899-1020

Phone: 301.975.2036
Fax: 301.948.3716

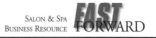
Beginning your TRUE QUALITY voyage

There is only one opinion that counts when determining the level of quality your salon provides: *the client's.* If the client isn't pleased, retention drops, attrition increases…and the salon fades away.

As more salons and spas begin the TQM process, owners are discovering that their idea of a quality salon experience doesn't always match the client's. They are quickly learning that it's time to rethink their service strategies and quality standards.

How do you define quality? A great haircut? Superb color? A happy client? If you're a *True Quality salon,* none of these traditional measurements will apply. To practice True Quality, there is only one goal: servicing customers beyond their expectations.

Expectations are important in any business transaction. Clients have expectations of the outcome of a salon visit. The True Quality salon strives to exceed them. But just as car buyers know that a Chevrolet is not a Rolls Royce, salon clients' expectations are realistic: Price does not define the level of satisfaction for the client. The Chevrolet buyer can be as delighted at the performance of the automobile as the Rolls Royce buyer.

Looking beyond technical skill

The True Quality salon experience must be designed and executed to discover and surpass client expectations. Many believe the only true way to ensure salon growth is to practice True Quality management. (Although it is part of the quality equation, superior technical skill isn't necessarily at the top of the list.)

The salon industry's True Quality performance ratio is *new client retention.* Salons average only about 30% new client retention per year — a dismal indication of the ability to meet customer expectations. On average, only three of every ten new clients think enough of their salon experience to try that salon again.

What do your clients, especially those all-important first-time clients, really encounter at your salon? Does the receptionist smile?

Is every staff member helpful? Has every stylist mastered the salon's selling system? Is the salon clean?

To put True Quality to work, the salon must treat every client as an honored guest. The client is the boss, the ultimate employer of salon owner and stylist alike. The goal of the salon is to provide each client "boss" with a wonderful experience. Whether your salon is value-priced or upscale, clients have expectations about doing business with you. Your job as a True Quality manager is to isolate and exceed those expectations.

A new way of thinking

True Quality demands a new way of thinking for salon owners and technicians. It requires putting the client first, and targeting every aspect of the service environment for improvement. Too often, client needs take a back seat to non-priority endeavors. Many salons need to learn (or relearn) to put client satisfaction first on the priority list. Disassociation from customer need directly contradicts TQM principles.

The salon industry is particularly vulnerable because of its structure. Many service technicians regard clients as simply a source of revenue, or a "head" in their chair. To begin the True Quality transformation, the salon must develop a client-first mentality. Then, other salon procedures and practices will fall into place quickly. Any attempt to implement a True Quality program will fail if client needs are not the focal point of your efforts.

Four critical factors

1. INVOLVEMENT OF TOP MANAGEMENT: Transformation will not succeed without constant support and leadership at the highest levels. Owner, key staff and the entire management team must be involved in each step of the process.
2. A SUPPORTIVE SALON OR SPA CULTURE: Culture is elusive, but is best described as the common behaviors of the salon staff. The culture of the aspiring TQM salon must support the team concept and flourish under the True Quality experience. Often, TQM requires that behaviors be altered.

3. STAFF TRAINING: People cannot perform to True Quality standards (or any new standard of performance) without proper training. They must be shown what is expected at each step, and receive continual reinforcement.

4. CUSTOMER COMMUNICATION: Constant client feedback enables you to define and understand the quality expectations of your client base. This data tells you, from their perspective, what you are doing "right" and "wrong." It provides the foundation for meeting and exceeding their expectations.

Focus groups

Direct communication is one of the best ways to determine customer expectations. Surveys can be helpful in learning what customers require and expect from your salon. HINT: Conduct a "question of the month" survey to continually monitor client perceptions. Also consider personal interviews, rating cards, external surveys and telemarketing. *(See the research guide on page 221.)*

Focus groups are an excellent forum for discovering client expectations of a typical salon visit. Vital information can be obtained by inviting a small group of clients (perhaps 10–15) to a frank discussion about the salon and its service quality.

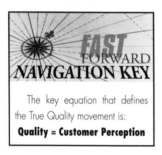

FAST FORWARD NAVIGATION KEY

The key equation that defines the True Quality movement is:

Quality = Customer Perception

True Quality begins with management's commitment to be the best. Only then can it become an integral part of the salon's vision.

TQM: How to build and sustain salon support

I f TQM is to work well, it must become an integral part of everyday business. Yet TQM literature is sprinkled with stories of failed implementation attempts. Primary reasons include:

- Lack of continued management commitment and support.
- Failure to understand that TQM is not a program or event, or something you buy from a consultant and "install" by mandate.
- Belief that long-standing problems inherent in the way business is conducted will magically disappear once TQM is announced.
- Lack of commitment to acquire the knowledge and skills needed to make TQM a viable way to manage the business.
- Inability to accept that 85%–90% of the problems in business today can be traced to poor management practices.

The support system

What can you do to successfully launch and maintain your TQM initiative? First, you will need a strong *support system.* A support system is the total environment of a person or group, an enduring pattern of continuing and inter-mittent ties. It provides emotional support, task-oriented direction, opportunities for feedback on per-formance, and validation of the staff's expectations of themselves and others.

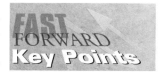

No lightning strike will cause TQM to happen, or sustain it over time.

Weaving TQM into the fabric of your salon's culture takes knowledge, time, perseverance and nurturing... a lot of nurturing.

Inadequate feedback is more likely when staff are unfamiliar with the organization's expecta-tions, and conditions are disorgan-ized. This can occur when an organization undertakes a major change in its way of doing business, such as instituting a new asso-ciate training program, or employee involvement and empower-ment practices.

A support system is not intended to prop up someone about to fall, but to build strengths and facilitate mastery of a new or changed environment. A successful support system provides a "cocoon" in which staff may try new behaviors, and receive support and encouragement in their efforts.

But there's more to a support system than feedback. Owners and managers must be personally and *visibly* involved in promoting TQM. Actions must support words. While allowing for the occasional slip-up, salon owners and managers must continually support the TQM message.

Open communication

There must be many methods of communication within a salon or spa. In addition to frequent performance feedback, staff must be "caught" doing things right, and given immediate positive reinforcement. Significant improvements must be publicized, both within the salon and outside (e.g., to clients and the media). Celebrate achievements frequently. All meetings between staff and management should include a segment on quality objectives and improvements. Use charts and graphs to show progress. Pictures, scrapbooks,

NAVIGATION KEY

TQM CHECKLIST

■ Do you provide career development planning and coaching for staff?

■ Does your compensation system promote your TQM effort?

■ Do salon operating practices support TQM's focus on clients?

■ Is the salon's organizational culture getting in the way?

■ Could your personal management style be more supportive?

■ How do you correct errors, and prevent recurrences?

■ Do you truly empower staff?

■ Do you ask employee opinions, and respond to them?

■ Are your practices for recognizing and reinforcing associates working?

■ Are personnel policies and procedures supportive?

■ Do you provide supportive developmental coaching?

■ Do you conduct internal process assessments to trigger improvement?

■ Do the salon's job descriptions support TQM?

■ Do you build effective teams, or just gather a group together?

■ Have you a well-planned, effective training and development system?

■ Do you create supplier partnerships?

■ Does your financial management of the salon sustain TQM?

video tapes and other forms of communication may also be helpful. In addition, your internal administrative policies, procedures and practices must support the TQM effort.

True Quality management is a "people process"

TQM must be carefully conceived, launched and maintained. It is not a magic wand; it is an operational philosophy. For most salons and day spas, it represents a paradigm shift — a major change in culture. The salon owner or manager leading the TQM effort must have courage and stamina. To succeed where others have failed, you must know and understand what is required to shift into fast forward.

RESEARCH GUIDE: Client data you need and how to get it	
Data you need	*How to get it*
Which salon service and product characteristics are most important to your clients?	Focus groups, direct client contact and other methods of asking "open" questions
How important is each service and product characteristic to salon clients?	Client surveys, direct client contact, etc.
What performance levels do clients expect for each characteristic?	Client surveys, direct client contact, etc.
How well are you actually providing each service and product characteristic?	Client surveys, "mystery shoppers"
Are your performance procedures under control and producing the results most important to clients...and are they constantly improving?	Internal performance measurements, salon and individual client retention rates, defect and redo rates, complaints, client feedback and other performance measurement methods

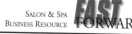
TQM: Information and analysis

The Malcolm Baldrige National Quality Award information and analysis section *(page 214)* focuses on information and data management; and company data analysis and use. It addresses a major shortcoming of many small businesses — the lack of collected and effectively used data. Considering the current affordable price-points of computers and software, every salon business can now use them to make informed decisions. Deciding *what* to track and *how* to successfully use that information is one of the most important business decisions you will make.

The MBNQA's information and analysis section evaluates the way a business uses information derived from data collection and analysis. This includes financial and operational data, and data about the marketplace and the business' clients. *How do you measure up? Try the self-assessment on the following page.*

Getting the balance right

Balance (too much versus too little) is needed when gathering and analyzing data for your business. Data becomes useful only after you have analyzed and made sense of it. For example: Sales entries only provide information for decision making when sales dollars are totaled by type of service, or when computed for a staff member and/or time of day. Comparative information can aid process improvement within your business, especially if you employ multiple technicians and offer several services.

Strategic planning

Strategic planning concerns the company's overall business plan. It guides organizations as they develop new strategies to strengthen their customer-related, operational, performance and competitive positions. For example: How does your salon perceive client needs and expectations; the competitive environment; risk factors (e.g., financial, market, technological, societal); distributor and/or supplier capabilities, and its own capabilities? How do plans translate

Self-Assessment — Information and Analysis
Rating Scale:

1 = Yes, completely   4 = Somewhat
7 = Mostly   10 = Not at all

1. _____ Your organization collects data on a few key systems and has a balanced approach to measurement, with two to three measures in each of the following data categories: customer satisfaction; employee satisfaction; product and service quality; manufacturer and distributor performance; and operational performance.

2. _____ You have designed data collection, analysis and reporting systems to support the needs of management and staff who must utilize the information to plan, make and implement their decisions.

3. _____ You have evaluated and made major improvements in your measures, data collection systems, analysis methods and effective reporting over the last few years.

4. _____ You presently collect and effectively employ competitive and benchmark data on service and product quality, customer satisfaction, distributor/supplier performance and key processes and functions. (And the data has proven reliable.)

5. _____ Your organization systematically evaluates and improves the scope, sources and uses of its competitive and benchmark data.

6. _____ Data from all areas of business performance are summarized, and results are analyzed to identify trends and opportunities for improvement.

7. _____ You can show evidence that all key business decisions and plans are based upon analysis of your performance data.

8. _____ All staff members understand the correlation between different types of measures (e.g., relationship between customer satisfaction and quality) and financial performance.

A perfect score is eight. How did you score?

Self-Assessment — Strategic Planning
Rating Scale:

1 = Yes, completely   4 = Somewhat
7 = Mostly   10 = Not at all

1. _____ Your salon conducts a thorough analysis of customer needs, competition and potential risks, and uses this information to develop short- and long-range strategic plans.

2. _____ Your salon's planning process is efficient, and plans are well-communicated to the staff members.

3. _____ You have carefully evaluated and improved the salon's planning processes several times in the last few years.

4. _____ Your salon has developed long- and short-term objectives and strategies for each major performance measure. Those objectives are linked to key salon result areas.

5. _____ You have developed specific projections illustrating how performance will compare to key competitors and other organizations. Performance is projected to be superior.

A perfect score is five. How did you score?

into action? How are planning processes evaluated and improved?

Strategic planning efforts concern key business drivers, or *key salon result areas.* These may include…

■ CLIENT SERVICE: appointment availability, waiting time, retention rates, consultations, product recommendations, salon cleanliness, salon image, checkout procedures, etc.

■ TECHNICAL SERVICE: number of redo's, their causes and prevention of recurrence.

■ STAFF TRAINING AND DEVELOPMENT: behavior, client relations, skill level, etc.

■ PROFITABILITY.

■ GROWTH.

Attempt a two- to five-year planning projection, benchmarking improvements in service quality and operational performance against key competitors. How do your strategic planning processes measure up?

Benchmarking: Reaching for "best in class"

Benchmarking is a continuous, organized process of comparing your business practices and services to salon industry and/or non-industry organizations in order to identify methods of improvement. The goal: to meet or exceed industry "best" practices.

Salons and spas with effective quality systems in place are often among the highest profit producers for their size, and will probably benefit *most* from benchmarking. Mid-level profit producers can gain valuable insights, but may get a better return on their investment by first getting themselves in better order. Lower-level profit producers, those with few or no quality systems in place, will only become frustrated with the gap between their practices and a "best in class" producer.

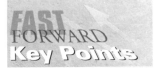

Consider benchmarking when your TQM efforts have significantly improved your business practices and services, and you want to move up to "best in class" in the industry...and, ultimately, to "world class."

What can you benchmark?

BUSINESS PRACTICES...

- Accounting system
- Staff compensation system
- Purchasing practices; supplier selection
- Client database design
- Cost ratios, direct and indirect
- Capital investments/improvements
- Tools and techniques
- Size, layout, decor
- Staffing approach: size, training, empowerment, recognition
- Advertising and promotional practices
- Use of computers and other electronics
- Rent, lease, buying practices

SERVICE PRACTICES...
- Services and products offered
- Client acquisition and retention practices
- Service quality, client satisfaction
- Salon image
- Client appointment system
- Amenities provided to client

Embrace it — Don't fear it

Some owners fear to ask others about their businesses, and to share information about their own. When benchmarking, you *do* share information with other salon owners…but only what is necessary or desired. It does involve a level of trust and confidentiality.

For example: You're in New York, and pinpoint a Seattle salon chain noted for its research and success in choosing locations for new salons. You contact them; they agree to share the key criteria they use in their site selection process. As a reciprocal gesture, you agree to relay your experience when the results are available.

Benchmarking is not "competitor analysis" or "industrial spying." It is an open agreement between two or more organizations to exchange information about their processes. Ethical and legal issues are carefully weighed, and trust is developed.

Three kinds of benchmarking

1. INTERNAL BENCHMARKING…compares one function to another within your salon (e.g., the way stylists versus manicurists attend to client needs), or in each of your multiple salons. Data is easy to collect, but the focus is limited and internal bias is possible. This approach could also cause staff issues if the data is improperly handled.

2. COMPETITIVE BENCHMARKING…compares your salon to others, either locally, nationally or worldwide. With competitive benchmarking, data is highly relevant to building your business, but also more difficult to collect. HINT: Salons outside the local market may not be true competitors, and therefore more willing to share information.

3. GENERIC BENCHMARKING...looks outside the salon industry for organizations that boast "best in class" processes and approaches which may be utilized to improve your salon. For example: You may be surprised at the number and types of businesses that benchmark with L.L. Bean, a recognized leader in customer service. When you "think outside your box," there is higher potential for discovering innovative practices. (And there is usually minimum resistance to partnering with a non-competitor.) However, translating non-industry work practices to your environment can be costly and problematic.

The steps of benchmarking

1. REVIEW, DEFINE AND REFINE EXISTING PROCESSES.

2. DETERMINE WHAT TO BENCHMARK.
   - Where do you have a critical *need?*
   - Which quality *objectives* will be aided by the data you seek?
   - What specific *data* do you want to receive?
   - *When* do you need the data?
   - *Who* will use the data?
   - What are your *expectations?*
   - What is the current *baseline* for processes to be benchmarked?

3. FORM A BENCHMARKING TEAM.
   - *Who* are the best people for the team?
   - *What* are their roles and responsibilities?
   - What *training* will team members need, and how will it be accomplished?
   - What *support* and *resources* are needed?
   - *Who* is responsible for the team's work?
   - How much *time* will be spent on benchmarking projects?

4. IDENTIFY BENCHMARK PARTNERS.
   - *Target* direct competitors, or non-competitors with similar processes.

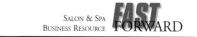
- *Target* "best practices," "best in class" or "world class."
- *Join* an existing network, or start your own.
- *Sources:* announcements of awards, media attention, professional/trade associations.

5. COLLECT AND ANALYZE GATHERED INFORMATION.
   - How will you *gather* data: direct contact with a targeted benchmark partner; in-person meetings and/or site visits; by phone; questionnaires and surveys; interviews with customers, suppliers, employees; professional and industry inquiries; publications and other media?
   - How will you *organize* and *analyze* the data? Any misinformation? Any omissions or data that just doesn't fit? What patterns emerge? What does the data tell you?

6. EVALUATE YOUR PERFORMANCE VERSUS BENCHMARKS.
   - Does the benchmark company exceed your needs and/or quality objectives?
   - Should your performance target meet or exceed your strongest competitor?
   - Is there a potential payoff for meeting and/or exceeding benchmarks? Consider the costs to achieve "best in class."

7. DETERMINE HOW UPGRADING YOUR PRACTICES WILL IMPACT YOUR:
   - *Vision,* mission and policy.
   - *Quality plans* (objectives) and critical success factors.
   - *Client focus.*
   - *Staff.*
   - *Suppliers.*
   - *Profit.*

8. ESTABLISH NEW QUALITY TARGETS.

9. DESIGN AND IMPLEMENT IMPROVEMENTS, AND A SYSTEM TO MONITOR PROGRESS.
   - What tracking, measuring and reporting systems are needed?

■ How will you review and improve the benchmarking process?

10. Do it again, and again and again.

Change is constant in business. Old methods seldom achieve new breakthroughs. To survive, you must venture into unexplored territory. Seek creative insight and new ideas by examining "best" practices, both inside and outside your industry.

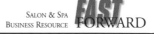
Beyond benchmarking:
From imitation to innovation

By Matthew Cross, President
LEADERSHIP ALLIANCE

You know there are things in your business you can improve. You also know that you must continuously improve in order to stay competitive and grow if, for no other reason, than to stay ahead in your market. And you know that many others have been where you are, and have found better ways to handle many of the same challenges you face. What to do? How can you gain and/or maintain the lead in offering high quality services and products that delight your customers and grow your bottom line?

One approach that has gained much popularity is benchmarking: the process of finding others in your field (allies or competitors) who are doing it better — from a specific process or service to the whole business. You then adapt their solutions to your business. *Essentially, benchmarking is copying what another business has discovered works for them, and then importing it into your business.* For instance: You identify the top five critical processes in your business and then "benchmark" them — compare your current performance levels in those same areas against another business' more ideal levels of performance — and then strive to meet or beat that level. The practice is quite popular with many businesses looking for a "quick fix" to the most pressing issues regarding the quality of the products and/or services they offer.

On the surface, this often sounds like a great idea. Why reinvent the wheel, right? Why not profit from another organization's trial and error, and take the easy road to improvement? Indeed, benchmarking has proven to be a valuable catalyst for improvement in many organizations, and can often be a stepping stone to better operations. Yet imitation is not the optimal way to build your bottom line or assure future growth.

Benchmarking copies —
Innovation creates growth energy

There is a better way to greater success, beyond benchmarking: *innovation.* Innovation requires coming up with customized answers to specific challenges. It means tapping into your staff's innate wisdom and coming up with uniquely powerful solutions that custom-fit your business. Innovation has several powerful advantages over benchmarking. These include:

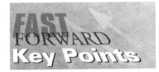

1. Innovation fosters break-through, "out of the box" solutions. Benchmarking, when uninspired, fosters imitation.

Tap into your own people's innate wisdom and come up with uniquely powerful solutions that custom-fit your business.

2. Innovation focuses on creating improvements customized for your business. Benchmarking imports solutions customized for someone else's business.

3. Innovation requires that you understand the *whole* system that leads to best long-term improvements. Benchmarking primarily focuses on getting "quick fix" results, which often compromise long-term performance.

4. Innovation focuses on going as far as you can go, and beyond. Benchmarking focuses on going as far as someone else has gone.

A good place to start any innovation process is to make a list of the most critical processes and customer interaction points in your business. Describe briefly the current less-than-optimal situations, and then ask for each one: WHAT WOULD PERFECT LOOK LIKE? Write out a short-but-detailed description of what perfect would be. Depending on the size of your business, you might simply start by addressing the following issues and brainstorming your answers on paper. Then invite other key players on your team to contribute ideas. This greatly increases your "data pool," and also strengthens your team when it is done in an atmosphere free of fear and internal competition.

Innovative beginnings

Since every journey begins with the first steps, here are some key points for getting started on your own innovation process:

- **DEFINE YOUR TARGETS:** Clarify the best innovation targets as they would apply to you and your business — not whatever level your competition has reached, or what is deemed successful in your industry. The key is to start small. Single out the top three areas in your business that are obviously ripe for improvement, and begin.

- **REMEMBER WHY YOU'RE IN BUSINESS:** Why *are* you in business? What is your aim? According to quality legend Dr. W. Edwards Deming, all businesses are really only in one business (if they want to grow and prosper): *Creating loyal customers.* Merely satisfying customers is no longer enough. Four out of five "satisfied" customers will defect, if offered the right opportunity. Building customer, employee and investor loyalty is the best investment strategy any business can make to assure its future. Do you have a clear strategy in place to create and keep loyal customers?

- **COMMITMENT:** You must commit to continuous innovation in your business. This is a vital ingredient in any effort to grow and improve.

- **SELF-EDUCATION:** Learn as much as you can about the power of True Quality management, systems improvement and strategic innovation. These critical optimization methods are powerful allies, even when applied in small steps. Perhaps best of all, they have a synergistic, cumulative effect on the whole business. This directly impacts your bottom line and future success.

- **CRITICALLY ASSESS YOUR WHOLE BUSINESS SYSTEM:** This requires both courage and honesty, and should ideally involve everyone in your business. Where do you drop the ball? Where do you experience the greatest frustrations and waste? Where do your customers experience the most problems doing business with you? While sometimes painful, the answers to questions like these often reveal the biggest opportunities for innovation and improvement.

- CONSIDER AN INNOVATION COACH: A qualified, objective coach can offer valuable insight and guidance on your innovation journey. It is usually difficult to work on improving your business systems when you are working in them. A good coach can greatly increase the velocity and value of innovation efforts.
- FOCUS ON THE SYSTEM — SALES WILL FOLLOW: Your business system, not an obsessive focus on sales targets, is the key to your success. As Dr. Deming said, "Navigating your business by past financial performance is like driving a car by looking in the rearview mirror." The key is to continuously focus on improving your critical systems, especially the *"First 15%."* According to Deming, 85% of the results you will get lie in the first 15% of any process. This means that the seeds for success are in the front end, not the back end. Sales are results, not drivers. When we identify and take care of the first 15%, growth and higher sales are the natural result.

Improve theories, systems, processes — Desired results will follow

Regarding any innovation efforts, the key is not to focus exclusively on the desired goal or results. Focus instead on discovering and applying the best improvement theories and methods, and the desired results will follow. Having an ideal target is important but, alone, is not enough to assure success. A continuously improving system combined with a clear aim is the key to hitting and exceeding any of your desired targets.

Strategic innovation is a proven "power tool" for success. For optimal results, it works best as part of an integrated approach aimed at bringing out the best in your people, processes and performance.

Summary

Benchmarking is the process of scanning your industry to find "best practices" that you can then import into your business. Essentially, it is imitating or copying another's solutions. While it can be a valuable process, there is a far better way — innovation.

Innovation is the process of discovering the best solutions for your own unique business and customers, implementing those solutions, and then tracking and continuously improving them through internal (your team's) and external (your customers' and vendors') feedback. Innovation very often leads to strategic breakthroughs in business. It also invariably leads to a greater understanding of your customer and, ultimately, to greater success.

Matthew Cross is president of LEADERSHIP ALLIANCE, *an innovative consulting organization dedicated to personal and professional transformation. An acclaimed Deming scholar, his training leads companies and individuals of all types to reach and exceed their highest potentials.*

For more information...MCross@LeadershipAlliance.com, or call: 203.322.1456.

You can also visit www.LeadershipAlliance.com *for more information on the Deming Quality Method and its application to your business.*

The Deming Prize

The Deming Prize was established in 1951 by JUSE (The Union of Japanese Scientists & Engineers), to commemorate the late Dr. W. Edwards Deming, a leading proponent of quality control in America and major contributor to quality control in Japan. This prestigious prize is awarded annually to manufacturers and individuals, in recognition of remarkable achievements in the field of quality control and improvement. It is the highest business award in Japan, akin to a "Nobel Prize for quality." Past winners have included MATSUSHITA (PANASONIC), FUJI FILM, TOYOTA, NISSAN, RICHO COPIERS, PENTEL, and FUJI XEROX. FLORIDA LIGHT & POWER CO. was the first American company to win the Deming Prize, in 1989.

NOTE: Unlike America's Baldridge Award, The Deming Prize directly reflects Dr. Deming's philosophy. It is essentially *non-competitive* (awarded to as many companies as meet its qualifications).

The following information is excerpted from "The 1996 Deming Prize Guide for Overseas Companies":

The Deming Prize application checklist

- POLICIES (HOSHIN)
  1. Quality and quality-control (QC) policies, and their place in overall business management
  2. Clarity of policies (targets and priority measures)
  3. Methods and processes for establishing policies
  4. Relationship of policies to long- and short-term plans
  5. Communication (deployment) of policies; management of policy achievement
  6. Executives' and managers' leadership

- ORGANIZATION
  1. Appropriateness of the organizational structure for quality control; status of employee involvement

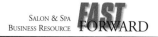
2. Clarity of authority and responsibility
3. Status of interdepartmental coordination
4. Status of committee and team project activities
5. Status of staff activities
6. Relationships with associated companies such as vendors, contractors and sales companies

■ INFORMATION
1. Appropriateness in collecting and communicating external information
2. Appropriateness in collecting and communicating internal information
3. Status of applying statistical techniques to data analysis
4. Appropriateness of information retention
5. Utilization of information
6. Utilization of computers for data processing

■ STANDARDIZATION
1. Appropriateness of the system of standards
2. Procedures for establishing, revising and abolishing standards
3. Actual performance in establishing, revising and abolishing standards
4. Content of standards
5. Utilization and adherence to standards
6. Status of systematically developing, accumulating, handing down and utilizing technologies

■ HUMAN RESOURCES
1. Education and training plans; development and utilization of results
2. Status of quality consciousness, managing jobs, and understanding of quality control
3. Status of supporting and motivating self-development and self-realization
4. Understanding, utilization of statistical concepts and methods
5. Status of QC circle development and improvement suggestions

6. Status of supporting the development of human resources in associated companies

■ QUALITY ASSURANCE
1. Management of the quality assurance activities system
2. Status of quality control diagnosis
3. Status of new product and technology development (including quality analysis and deployment, and design review activities)
4. Status of process control
5. Status of process analysis and improvement (including capability studies)
6. Status of inspection, quality evaluation and quality audit
7. Status of managing production equipment, measuring instruments, and vendors
8. Packaging, storage, transportation, sales and service activities
9. Grasping and responding to product usage, disposal, recovery and recycling
10. Status of quality assurance
11. Grasping the status of customer satisfaction
12. Status of assuring reliability, safety, product liability and environmental protection

■ MAINTENANCE
1. Rotation of management cycle control activities
2. Methods for determining control items and their levels
3. Utilization of control charts and other tools
4. Status of taking temporary and permanent measures
5. Status of operating management systems for cost, quantity, delivery, etc.
6. Relationship of quality assurance system to other operating management systems

■ IMPROVEMENT
1. Methods of selecting "themes" (e.g., important activities, problems, priority issues)
2. Linkage of analytical methods and intrinsic technology

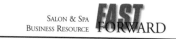
3. Utilization of statistical methods for analysis
4. Utilization of analysis results
5. Status of confirming improvement results and transferring them to maintenance/control activities
6. Contribution of QC circle activities

■ EFFECTS
1. Tangible effects: delivery, cost, profit, safety, environment, etc.
2. Intangible effects
3. Methods of measuring and grasping effects
4. Customer and employee satisfaction
5. Influence on associated companies
6. Influence on local and international communities

■ FUTURE PLANS
1. Grasp of current situations
2. Future plans for improving problems
3. Projection of changes in social environment; customer requirements and future plans based on these projected changes
4. Relationships among management philosophy, vision and long-term plans
5. Continuity of quality control activities
6. Concreteness of future plans

The Deming Prize application checklist for senior executives

■ UNDERSTANDING
1. Is the introduction and promotion of quality control objectives clearly defined and well-understood?
2. How well do they understand quality control, quality assurance, reliability, product liability, etc.?
3. How well do they understand the importance of statistical thinking, and the application of quality control techniques?
4. How well do they understand QC circle activities?
5. How well do they understand the relationship of quality control to the concepts and methods of other activities?

6. How enthusiastic are they in promoting quality control? How well are they exercising leadership?

7. How well do they understand the status and characteristics of their company's quality, and quality control?

■ Policies

1. How are quality and quality-control policies established? Where and how do they stand in relation to overall business management?

2. How are these policies related to short- and long-term plans?

3. How are they deployed for achievement throughout the company?

4. Do senior executives grasp the status of policy achievement? Do they take appropriate corrective actions when needed?

5. How do they grasp priority quality issues (priority business issues)? Do they make effective use of diagnostic methods such as top management diagnosis?

6. How well are targets and priority measures aligned with policy?

7. What kind of policies do they employ for establishing cooperative relationships with associated companies?

■ Organization

1. Is the company organized and managed in order to effectively and efficiently practice quality control?

2. How is organizational authority and responsibility established?

3. Is the allocation of human resources suitable?

4. How do executives strive to satisfy employees?

5. How well do they grasp and evaluate employees' capability and motivation levels?

6. Do they strive for interdepartmental cooperation? How do they utilize committees and project teams?

7. How do they relate to associated companies?

■ Human resources

1. How clear is the philosophy for hiring, developing and utilizing human resources?

2. How appropriate are employee education and training plans? Are the necessary dollars and time allocated?
3. How do senior executives communicate policies for quality control, education and training? Do they grasp the status of policy achievement?
4. How do they provide education and training specific to the company's business needs?
5. How well do they understand the importance of employee self- and mutual development? How do they support this effort?
6. Do they strive to develop QC circle activities?
7. How interested are they in developing human resources in associated companies?

■ IMPLEMENTATION
1. What measures are in place to ensure effective and efficient implementation and evaluation of quality control?
2. How well are quality control and other management systems coordinated?
3. Do executives grasp the status of improvements in business processes, and the individual steps of these processes, so as to provide products and services that satisfy customer needs? Are they taking necessary corrective actions?
4. How well are systems for developing new products, services, technologies and markets established and managed?
5. How are resources for establishing and operating management and information systems secured and allocated?
6. How do they grasp the contributions of quality control to the improvement of business performance?
7. How do they evaluate employees' efforts?

■ CORPORATE SOCIAL
1. Does the company structure ensure appropriate profits for a long time?
2. How do senior executives regard employer well-being (wages, hours, etc.)?
3. How do they regard employee self-realization?

4. Do they strive for co-existence and co-prosperity with associated companies?
5. How does the company contribute to the local community?
6. Does the company exert efforts to protect the environment?
7. How does the company positively impact the international community?

■ FUTURE VISIONS

1. How do executives ensure the continuity and future of quality control?
2. How do they anticipate and cope with changes in the surrounding business environment, and progresses in science and technology?
3. How well do they grasp and cope with changes in customer requirements?
4. How do they consider their employees, and help them achieve happiness and satisfaction?
5. How do they consider and manage relationships with associated companies?
6. How do they plan for the future to cope with the items above?
7. How do they utilize quality control to achieve future plans?

SOURCE: *All inquiries about this information should be directed to the publisher and Secretariat of the Deming Prize Committee.*

Union of Japanese Scientists and Engineers (JUSE)
5–10–11 Sendagaya, Shibuya-ku, Tokyo 151 Japan
Phone: +81–3–5379–1227
Facsimile: +81–3–3225–1813
E-mail: HHF03411@niftyserve.or.jp

Further suggested reading

Clare Crawford-Mason and Lloyd Dobbins, *Quality or Else: The Revolution in World Business* (HOUGHTON MIFFLIN COMPANY, 1992)

Kenneth Delavigne and J. Daniel Robertson, *Deming's Profound Changes: When Will the Sleeping Giant Awaken?* (PRENTICE HALL, 1994)

Dr. W. Edwards Deming, *The New Economics for Industry, Government and Education* (Massachusetts Institute of Technology, Center for Advanced Engineering Study, 1993)

Alfie Kohn, *Punished By Rewards: The Trouble with Gold Stars, Incentive Plans, A's, Praise and Other Bribes* (HOUGHTON MIFFLIN COMPANY, 1999)

Mary Walton, *The Deming Management Method* (BERKLEY PUBLISHING GROUP, 1986)

Things to do:

- Review Deming's "14 Points for the Transformation of Business and Management" on pages 208–210. Apply each point to your business. State in writing how you will do this.

- Consider applying the Baldrige criteria to your salon to substantially improve your business through customer focus and True Quality.

- Develop focus groups and monthly surveys to learn what your customers really want and expect from your salon.

- Develop a strong True Quality support system — a person or group of people committed to being the best.

- Attempt a two- to five-year planning projection, benchmarking improvements in service quality and operational performance against key competitors.

- Consider benchmarking when your TQM efforts have significantly improved your business practices and services, and you want to move up to "best in class" in the industry...and ultimately, to "world class."

- Be innovative: Think "out of the box," and focus on creating improvements customized for your business.

CLIENT RETENTION
Your salon's key growth indicator

The percentage of salon owners who know their business' new-client retention rate is startlingly low, perhaps even less than 10%. Many confuse retention rates with request rate, though they are *not* the same. And many have no way to track retention. Even those with point-of-sale computer systems often realize their software either tracks retention improperly, or not at all.

You cannot argue with numbers. From a technical standpoint, the

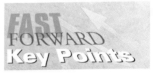

RETENTION DEFINITION

How many first-time clients return to the salon for a second visit? To whom the client returns to is not the issue...The objective is to measure how efficiently the salon is growing its customer base.

salon industry offers the consuming public extraordinarily high levels of skill and expertise. Yet, from a customer service and True Quality standpoint, salons score poorly. Industry-wide statistics show that salons *are not* retaining seven of ten first-time clients. Interestingly, poor retention remains consistent from value-priced

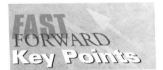

salons right up to upscale, service-intensive day spas.

RETENTION IS YOUR TRUE QUALITY SCORE. The overriding objective of every business is to attract and retain customers. First-time client retention rates are directly proportional to a business' ability to offer customer satisfaction and consistent True Quality experiences. Of course you want to satisfy clients on *every* visit, but true client retention tracking begins with the *first*. If the salon fails to meet client expectations on the first visit, there usually is no second chance. And if the salon has a 30% first-time client retention rate, don't even think about using "True Quality" to describe your business. (The only way to know if the salon is moving closer to True Quality is to track overall client retention. Once you know where you are, realistic retention objectives can be established.)

RETENTION IS YOUR SALON'S FUTURE. The rules of the salon business game have changed: Winning requires a base of retained customers who are loyal to the business rather than individual technicians working within the business. This client base is by far the salon's most important asset, as there is little resale value for used salon furniture and fixtures.

A committed retention effort will produce tremendous growth in the client list. And this growth will prove even more lucrative than an increase in average ticket and frequency of visit.

Track what's important

The traditional process of staff development focuses on hiring a stylist, providing training, and then putting him behind a chair to assist all the new clients that the veteran, request-saturated stylists cannot accommodate. He is encouraged to build a "request rate" and a loyal personal following. According to the old rules, when the stylist is booked solid with requests — he has won the game.

MENTAL TICKLE: *"Request"* tells you who is building a following and who isn't. It is your WALK-OUT FACTOR.

Request tracking has been handed down from generation to generation in the salon industry. In the old mode of salon thinking, it made sense to know how many clients were requesting each staff member. The game was to "build your clientele," and request tracking was the best measurement tool.

The problem with request tracking today is two-fold:

■ By design, it encourages staff members to divert client loyalty from the team to themselves, and is therefore counterproductive to today's teamwork thinking. IT'S OLD TECHNOLOGY...so old, in fact, that *retention* tracking completely eliminates the need to track request rates. Moreover, request tracking encourages the very followings that owners fear and guard against.

■ Request tracking fails to accurately render the salon's ability to retain clients, no matter how sophisticated your tracking procedures. New requests, repeat requests and other tracking codes fail to answer the fundamental retention question: "How many new clients came in, and how many came back?" The only measurement request tracking provides is the number of clients who ask for a specific individual. It doesn't give the *retention rate* for all those new requests (i.e., how many actually came back).

How long does it take to build request rates? How many first-time clients are lost in the process? How much salon growth potential is lost? Without tracking client *retention*, you'll never know.

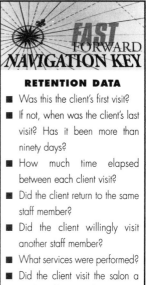

FAST FORWARD NAVIGATION KEY

RETENTION DATA

■ Was this the client's first visit?

■ If not, when was the client's last visit? Has it been more than ninety days?

■ How much time elapsed between each client visit?

■ Did the client return to the same staff member?

■ Did the client willingly visit another staff member?

■ What services were performed?

■ Did the client visit the salon a number of times before ceasing to visit the salon?

Retention builds client loyalty to the salon, and provides a highly accurate True Quality score. It's a rallying point for all salon processes — technical and interpersonal — including customer service. *No other score takes precedence.*

Why does retention matter?

Most salon owners acknowledge that client retention information is vital to growth. But when asked why, few have an immediate response. What is its practical application? How should one react to low retention — or a high 65% retention level?

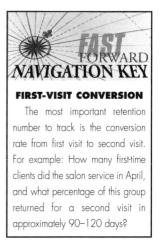

FIRST-VISIT CONVERSION

The most important retention number to track is the conversion rate from first visit to second visit. For example: How many first-time clients did the salon service in April, and what percentage of this group returned for a second visit in approximately 90–120 days?

Retention can rally staff around the "team concept," strengthen individual and team performance, help determine when to award raises, identify weak skills and services, and pinpoint other areas for improvement. "Performance" is a blanket term when applied to salon operations. We're going to look at some specific issues with Spokane, WA, salon owner Rick Phillips, and zero in on how to use retention figures to evaluate nearly every system you have in place.

How can a salon owner move retention into the spotlight where it belongs, making it the "salon battle cry"?

Most importantly, everyone has to understand what retention is. You want to develop a client base not just for today, but for the future. Once you know where you are and have made the commitment with the staff to pursue higher retention goals, you can forecast what your salon is capable of by extrapolating your current numbers.

If you know the salon's average ticket, you can project the revenue gained from an increase in the client base. You can check retail sales to see how close you are to goal. Retention numbers can even tell you where the bottom line has to be. In fact, every system in your salon revolves around retention — especially if you offer salary-based compensation. Without retention, you can't forecast the number of new clients you can see every month or calculate team bonus — you can't even tell where you want your business to go because you have no idea where it is.

Let's elaborate on the link between retention and productivity. What does retention tell you about the individual efforts of staff members?

To assess productivity, you must have a time standard. In other words, determine how long particular services should take, and hold everyone in the salon to that standard.

If you have a staff member who habitually takes twenty minutes longer to complete services than everyone else, there could be any number of repercussions for the salon. When clients get accustomed to a stylist running behind schedule, they have a tendency to tie up the phone lines at the desk by calling in to find out if, by chance, the technician is running on time. There is no way to calculate the lost dollars from appointments that don't get made because clients can't get through. Other team members may also fall behind because they are trying to help out.

But on the opposite end of the spectrum is the stylist who is very proficient and always runs ahead of schedule. Let's say this person can perform a fifteen-minute color application in seven minutes. This stylist can almost double her schedule *and* will retain more clients. She will have more time open on the book — reducing gridlock, keeping clients happy through prompt and efficient service…and those clients who call back for additional appointments get in more easily. Another important benefit of this particular situation is increased cooperation between technical and desk staff because of the easier flow of clients.

Pay evaluations are always a touchy subject. How do performance numbers tell a salon owner when it's time to reward a team member?

There is a tremendous difference between performance evaluations and pay reviews. Performance evaluations are one-on-one meetings with team members for the purpose of discussing performance only. KEY POINT: Pay is not discussed during performance evaluations.

A pay review is only scheduled after one or more performance evaluations indicate that a pay raise has been earned. (This is where cash-flow projections are essential. You cannot grant a raise before plugging the increase into your monthly payroll expenses and projecting its impact on overall cash flow.)

Key criteria used in performance evaluations are first-time and existing client retention, productivity rate and average ticket.

When a stylist's performance is consistently at or above performance goals in all categories, it's clear that he or she is contributing to overall salon growth and should be rewarded in some fashion. This could mean a raise, a bonus, time off, free education or special privileges. Of course, a technician can only operate to a certain productivity level before having to pass sales to other people, but that is the whole point of the team system — growing the salon by growing the individuals.

When you have retention and productivity numbers right under your nose, you will discover patterns of activity. Stylist strengths and weaknesses become clear within a few months.

Is there such a thing as too many clients or too-high productivity in a salon?

It's not wise to ask staff to operate at higher than 80% productivity. This will cause burn-out — stylists will get tired, and their quality of workmanship will go down. There are all kinds of ratios you can look at, but there are simply different breeds of people who work at different paces. If you put an "artist" up against someone who is perhaps equally artistic but also wants to earn money, the revenue differences can reach into the tens of thousands of dollars. Technically, their productivity levels may be the same because they have the same number of hours sold, but the stylist who works shorter appointments and can see more clients will generate a lot more money.

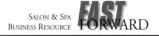

How effective is it to zero in on specific services? For example: If you call yourself "the color specialist," you don't want a 35% retention rate for color clients.

If there is a team member in your salon who focuses exclusively on haircuts and does only about 3% color, she will never reach the dollar amounts she is capable of hitting. Another stylist who does color may see fewer clients (due to longer appointments) but will bring in much more revenue. Most salons generate 80% of their business from only 20% of their clientele — these are obviously the most valuable.

There are only four areas you can concentrate on in a salon: retail, haircuts, perms and color. Day spas are a different story. But you still have to get back to your goals: How much money do you want to make? If you want your salon to operate at peak performance, you have to pinpoint exactly what each team member needs to do. You have to give them a means to the end: an accurate assessment of their retention numbers within a very narrow focus, by service and time of day if possible.

Where do you focus your marketing efforts? Is it more productive to look at clients by service or time lapsed since last appointment?

The most important thing to do when developing a marketing plan is to identify the most popular hours on the book. These don't need to be marketed because they sell themselves. Find the hours that are *not* booked and decide how to sell them. Ask yourself what you have that the clients want. What can you sell? Can you afford to run a discount on the hours you need to fill? You can always put ads in the local newspaper or in the salon to attract attention, but I don't differentiate between internal and external marketing. It's all one — your goal is to sell the hours on the book.

The first marketing front is the telephone. When a client calls, inform her of your current specials and encourage her to tell her friends. People want great quality and good value and, if you deliver these to your clients, they will stay with your salon and send new clients your way by word of mouth. Your retained base is your most important asset.

Why is it important to discuss and post retention numbers? What impact does it have on productivity and client service?

If you post retention reports and conduct monthly evaluations, you can focus on individual stylists' strong and weak points. You can track retention by service and time of day to discover why clients did or did not return. You can discuss the demographics of clientele. For example: There may have been a large number of walk-ins that need to be compensated for when calculating current retention.

The most important thing in staff discussions is follow-through. There will always be good things going on with each team member as well as things that need to be worked on. Be sure to keep thorough, accurate records so you can specify these items.

COMMUNICATION: *How should salon owners speak to staff, encouraging them to reach higher?*

This is where you really have to get back to basics. Who is the salon caretaker and team leader? Who looks out for finances? It is very important to be sure you have a base to stand on before going to the staff with anything. That is, don't try to broach issues that aren't your area of expertise. Usually, the owner will have to do the talking — reprimands, especially, have to come down the chain of command. Though issues may derive from someone else, "the boss" has to lay down the law.

Everyone wants to know if the salon is doing well, and have his or her individual contributions acknowledged. But it must also be made clear that mediocrity will not and cannot be rewarded — and that everyone is accountable as a team for the salon's overall growth.

You cannot address client retention without a detailed reporting system

The following client retention reports show all the key data that should be contained in your own reports, whether prepared by computer or by hand. Reports should be prepared for the salon *(page 255)* and for each service provider *(page 256)*.

Accurate retention calculations require that a certain window of time — usually ninety days — elapses from the conclusion of the period being measured to the present. (Three months is generally adequate to allow even chemical-service clients to return.) The basic retention formula is simply (A) the total of all first-time clients for a given period divided into (B) the number who returned within ninety days.

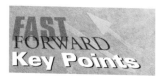

THERE IS NO DEBATE
Client retention must be tracked, tabulated, analyzed and put to work to improve salon performance.

FOR EXAMPLE: If 100 new clients visit a salon in December, and thirty return by April 1, the salon has a 30% first-time retention rate for the month of December. Client retention tracking *must* begin at the transition from first to second visit. This is where the damage is often most acute, but the greatest opportunity for growth resides.

Caution for computer users

A number of software programs use *retention* and *request* interchangeably. In these cases, the program simply yields a stylist request rate report, and offers no client retention data. Other programs offer client retention reports, but in a jumble of data that even the developers cannot decipher.

If your present software tracks client retention, ask the developers to explain *exactly* how the reports are tabulated. If the formula doesn't focus on how many first-time clients visited the salon and how many returned within a given window of time, you're not get-

Overall Salon Retention Report

Time Period Analyzed
Beginning and end dates. Monthly time periods are recommended for analysis

First-Time Client Names

Client's First Visit Date
Date of first visit when name is entered into salon database

Second Visit Date
Date client returns to salon

Salon New Retention Rate
Overall retention rate for first-time clients

First Visit Lost Customers

Multiple Visit Lost Customers

Existing Customer Data
Total Existing Customers
Existing Retained by Number
Existing by Percentage

Date Report is Generated
How many first-time clients in the time period analyzed returned for a second visit by this date — usually 90 days after the end date

Client is Lost
Indicator that client has not returned to salon and may be lost

Client Returned to Salon
Indicator that client is actively utilizing the skills of more than one staff member

Returned to Original Stylist
Client either bonded with employee or conditions exist that discourage using skills of other employees

Salon Totals by Category
How many first-time clients, who did they return to and how many were lost

Totals by Percentage

Total Clients Lost by Number

Existing Customers Lost
By Number
By Percentage

```
                        Overall Salon Retention                 Page 2
            New Clients from 12-01-1995 to 12-31-1995          04/02/96
                                                                  431P

Client Name        First Visit  Last Visit   To Stylist  To Salon  Lost
-----------        -----------  ----------   ----------  --------  ----
ORR,LINDA          12-09-1995                                        *
PAHUD,EVE          12-01-1995                                        *
PARKER,DEBORA      12-26-1995                                        *
PEETS,BOB          12-27-1995   03-07-1996                   *
PREIBISCH,MATT     12-16-1995                                        *
RICH,RYNE          12-14-1995   03-13-1996                   *
RITTLE,JONIE       12-12-1995                                        *
ROJANO,ISABEL      12-15-1995   03-19-1996       *
ROWLAND,ROXANE     12-13-1995                                        *
SCENEKL,TRISH      12-30-1995                                        *
SCHAEFFER,DORIS    12-27-1995                                        *
SCHAEFFER,MISSY    12-26-1995   12-30-1995                   *
SEAR,CODY          12-14-1995                                        *
SHULTZ,TAMMY       12-23-1995                                        *
SKAGGS,HOLLY       12-16-1995   03-16-1996                   *
SPITLER,ANYA       12-20-1995                                        *
SPITLER,RACHEL     12-20-1995                                        *
STROZZO,KAREN      12-21-1995                                        *
SWORD,DONNA        12-13-1995                                        *
THOMPSON,PAILA     12-30-1995                                        *
TORO,CHARLENA      12-16-1995                                        *
WALKER,CHERIE      12-05-1995                                        *
WEBB,PHIL          12-22-1995                                        *
WRIGHT,MORRIS      12-15-1995                                        *
XU,SHIXIANG        12-16-1995   02-27-1996                   *
-----------------------------------------------------------------------
Totals             75 New                          19         6      51
Percentages                                     25.33      8.00    66.6

First Visit Retention            33.33
First Visit Lost Customer's      66.67
Multiple Visit Lost Customer's    1.33     Total Lost %            68.00
***********************************************************************
Existing Customer Evaluation

Existing Total                  1381
Customer's Retained             1091     Customer's Lost            290
Existing % Retained            79.00     Customer's % Lost        21.00
```

Individual Technician Retention Report

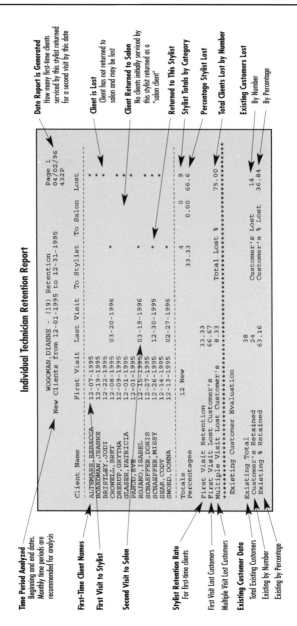

Time Period Analyzed
Beginning and end dates.
Monthly time periods are recommended for analysis

First-Time Client Names

First Visit to Stylist

Second Visit to Salon

Stylist Retention Rate
For first-time clients

First Visit Lost Customers

Multiple Visit Lost Customers

Existing Customer Data
Total Existing Customers
Existing by Number
Existing by Percentage

Date Report is Generated
How many first-time clients serviced by this stylist returned for a second visit by this date

Client is Lost
Client has not returned to salon and may be lost

Client Returned to Salon
No clients initially serviced by this stylist returned as a "salon client"

Returned to This Stylist

Stylist Totals by Category

Percentage Stylist Lost

Total Clients Lost by Number

Existing Customers Lost
By Number
By Percentage

```
                        WOGOMAN,DIANNE - (19) Retention          Page 1
                    New Clients from 12-01-1995 to 12-31-1995   04/02/96
                                                                 432P

Client Name      First Visit  Last Visit  To Stylist  To Salon  Lost
--------------------------------------------------------------------------
ALTEMARE,REBECCA  12-07-1995                                      *
BOARDMAN,JEANNE   12-19-1995                                      *
BRISTLEY,JODI     12-22-1995
CROWELL,BRET      12-08-1995  03-20-1996
DRERUP,GRYTHA     12-09-1995
GLASER,PATRICIA   12-01-1995                           *          *
PAHUD,EVE         12-01-1995
ROJANO,ISABEL     12-11-1995  03-19-1996               *          *
SCHAEFFER,DORIS   12-27-1995
SCHAEFFER,MISSY   12-26-1995  12-30-1995               *          *
SEAR,CODY         12-14-1995
SWORD,DONNA       12-13-1995  02-27-1996               *          *
--------------------------------------------------------------------------
Totals           12 New                      4          0          9
Percentages                   33.33         33.33      0.00      66.6

First Visit Retention           33.33
First Visit Lost Customer's     66.67     Total Lost %       75.00
Multiple Visit Lost Customer's   8.33
***********************************************************************
Existing Customer Evaluation

Existing Total                  38
Customer's Retained             24       Customer's Lost        14
Existing % Retained          63.16       Customer's % Lost    36.84
```

ting the retention data you need. (Use the information presented here to help your software developer understand the retention data you are looking for.)

Putting retention report data to work

The first report owners and managers should examine is the overall salon retention report *(page 255)*. This report can be as detailed as you like, but must at least contain all first-time client names, first visit dates and returned-by dates. NOTE: To analyze client retention data for December 1 through December 31, an accurate report cannot be generated until April 1.

Of the seventy-five new clients that visited the salon in December, only twenty-four returned. Fifty-one were lost. (One client made multiple visits to the salon in December but did not return. *See multiple-visit–lost-customer data.*) This salon report shows an overall first-time client retention rate of 32% for the month of December.

The report data also states that of the twenty-four retained clients, nineteen (25.33%) returned to the original stylist and only six (8%) returned to others in the salon. Owners and managers must monitor this data carefully. The True Quality objective is to increase the percentage of clients who utilize the skills of the *entire* staff. If your salon's teamwork concept is in gear, the percentage of clients returning to others in the salon should be equal to or higher than those returning to the original stylist.

An individual stylist report provides the same data as an overall salon report, but targets the retention numbers of a single employee. It therefore allows owners and managers to pinpoint retention problems with a high degree of accuracy. For example: It will be evident if the retention performance of one or two stylists is pulling down the salon's overall score. (Assigning new clients to stylists with low retention rates will lower the salon's revenue potential.) It will also be evident which stylists encourage clients to utilize the skills of the entire staff, and which are more concerned with building a personal following.

Since individual reports also list clients retained and *not* retained by the stylist, possible technical and/or customer service deficiencies can be identified. For example: Why might a stylist lose nine of twelve new clients? Examine each client's record for common patterns such as client age or gender, or particular services which may be weak.

Individual retention reports must also become a major performance factor in determining raises and possibilities of advancement. If team members don't retain clients in the salon, it is financially impossible to increase their compensation.

IMPROVING RETENTION IS A SALON MISSION. Keep retention numbers posted in the dispensary. Distribute reports and discuss performance at meetings. Maintain the urgency.

Accurately measuring client retention allows the salon to invest in its future by finding its weakest retention areas — leading to greater sales in the short-term and unparalleled long-term growth.

Make client retention the mandate at your salon

Waging the client retention battle will be a significant challenge for your salon. Will you stay out of the revolution, or raise your sword and charge into battle? Gone are the days when a steady stream of one-time clients was enough to feed a salon. Today, retained clients are the most valuable.

Your client retention weapons arsenal includes the team and their training; well-executed marketing programs; challenging yet achievable pre-determined goals of which everyone is aware; an effective way to traffic clients into the salon *and* the right chairs; an open-book policy which shows everyone the retention numbers; and a computerized system to track these new, dynamic numbers.

Make it work for the client

Bring the salon team together to focus on the most critical aspect of running a salon…the satisfied, retained client. Through this person, the salon will grow and prosper. Your salon will weather many storms if it maintains a growing client base. Mediocrity can be found anywhere, but a "take no prisoners" retention program will help your salon rise above it. Give clients exceptional customer service that they cannot find elsewhere. Eliminate reasons why they may wander away. It's time to keep them *with* you.

Today's technology will shift your campaign into overdrive. Computers can almost instantaneously process the vast amounts of information which can help grow your salon. It has never been easier to leap into the computer age. Business technology is here to stay. Stop working in the dark.

Where to start your retention program

FIND YOUR CURRENT RETENTION RATE.

- What is the salon's *existing client base* (total retained clients)?
- What is the *new client retention rate* (first-timers who return within ninety days)?
- How many *new clients* visit the salon *per month* (on average)?

■ What is the *client attrition rate* (the number of clients who "fade
   away" from the retained base due to relocation, etc.)?

   All of these figures can be generated by your computer's reporting program. Without them, you are waging a campaign with only
a fraction of the information you need.

DIRECT THE TEAM'S ATTENTION TO WEAK AREAS.

   Are only a few stylists driving clients away, or does the entire
salon need a skill and/or customer-service boost? Once you know
the problems, get to work. Focus the staff's attention on client
retention by compensating them for their ability to retain clients
(not for a misleading request rate, which will only throw you off
track.) *Put quality above quantity.*

   A client retention program can rejuvenate your salon and bring
virtually unlimited success. Retention is your True Quality score.
Turn things around. *Keep* seven out of ten new clients.

Things to do:

- If you are not tracking client retention —
   START TRACKING IT!

- Understand your software's retention reports, and the way the program calculates retention. If you don't understand the reports, call your software company's support line. If your software program doesn't track client retention:
   REQUEST THAT THE COMPANY DEVELOP A RETENTION REPORT.

- Educate your staff on the importance of client retention, and what it means to the salon's future.

- Develop a program to increase client retention. It can rejuvenate your salon and bring virtually unlimited success.
   WHAT MUST THE SALON DO TO MAKE CLIENTS WANT TO COME BACK?

- Set client retention goals and tie them into bonuses, rewards or pay raises.
   TRACK, POST AND COMMUNICATE THE RESULTS WITH YOUR STAFF.

SERVICE MARKETING & SALES

Sales are the heart of a service business

A s resistant as most salon and spa professionals are to the notion of selling, the fact is the entire industry revolves around sales. The most important items salons and spas offer their customers are *TIME* and *EXPERTISE*. Consequently, overall profitability depends on how stringently each is monitored.

Yet…many salons take few or no active steps to promote services. Potential clients are left to guess what is available, or to call and ask to hear an abbreviated version of the service menu. In some cases, salon owners and employees claim they "can't afford" publicity. Even if there is a marketing budget, it is small and easily depleted — and there's no room in the salon for any more clients, anyway. Other salons have what some would consider exorbitant marketing budgets, spending thousands of dollars per month on full-color mailers, posters and displays, and external marketing and public relations firms.

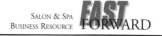
Your salon's best strategy depends primarily on the market you are trying to reach. There are a myriad of options for even the smallest of salons. In the view of many, the decision of whether to market internally or externally has been traditionally founded on the size of the salon or day spa, but this opinion is rapidly becoming obsolete. There are always potential new clients to be found in the marketplace. One's success at finding them largely depends on how well one understands the market.

Happy clients are nothing short of walking billboards for your salon or day spa business. They are wonderfully willing public relations activists. Remember, advertising costs money, so agendas must be set with care. Public relations, however, is free — it is a measure of how well clients are treated at your business and their response to that treatment. Every service session is a test.

The nature of sales and marketing

Most marketing strategies for major corporations revolve around well-researched, highly clinical and well-funded studies of market demographics, "test runs" of new services and a lot of tabulated consumer feedback. And while it would be nice for small businesses to have these luxuries, the process is often cumbersome and occasionally highly inaccurate. Small business owners often do well to emulate the practices of larger companies, but they must never lose touch with their intuition — the force which first compelled them to become entrepreneurs.

The primary goal of market research is to predict human behavior (i.e., what the consumer will respond to). The best way to predict consumer response to new services is through one-on-one interaction. When employees at all levels of the business have direct contact with clients and are able to observe reactions to services, they can more accurately predict responses to *new* services.

The goal of any business owner or employee in a service industry is to build a relationship of trust and respect with clients. This is especially so in salons and spas, where personal, often intimate, contact routinely occurs between employees and clients. In order to gain trust, service providers must approach the relationship with deference. Adversarial attitudes among the staff do little to promote sales, and can undermine public relations plans.

THERE ARE FOUR MAJOR MARKETING AREAS/DECISIONS:

- PRODUCT: The quality must be beyond reproach.

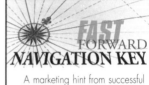

NAVIGATION KEY

A marketing hint from successful Japanese companies:

In the Western sales process, buyer and seller are often considered equals, so when one "wins" the sales game, the other loses.

The Japanese sales mentality revolves around the notion of seller as servant. Though the seller is always ready to sell, the buyer is not always ready to buy.

- PRICE: A reasonable price is part of a value package.
- PROMOTION: There are two primary options — head-to-head competition, or brand name and image development through soft campaigns.
- PLACE: The company must be "close to" customers. It is important to the ultimate value of the service. Most salon clients live within a four- or five-mile radius of the business. (Spas attract clients from further away, as they are often viewed as "destinations.") But the business must also be emotionally accessible to clients seeking an "escape."

Lessons to market by

- BUILD AND NURTURE RELATIONSHIPS WITH CLIENTS. The more you know about the market, the more likely it is your marketing campaigns will succeed. Don't let your intuition be blind.
- BALANCE MARKET RESEARCH AND INTUITION. Both are important to a successful campaign. Fact and feeling work hand-in-hand.
- MAKE BABY STEPS. If the market is unpredictable (e.g., no one in your area has offered seaweed wraps before), introduce services slowly and incrementally. There's no rush. Discovering a niche can do wonders for your business, but over-extending your resources with no guaranteed return on investment can be financially devastating.
- QUALITY IS A GOOD PLACE TO START. Image and customer service support are also crucial.
- DON'T TRY TO "OWN" THE MARKET. Imitation is easy. It won't take long for competitors to catch on to your successful ventures and sway consumer preferences.

How badly do you need it?

Learning to market and sell services effectively and profitably requires a close examination of several key salon status indicators. Before investing your salon or day spa's valuable resources (i.e., time and money) in an advertising or public relations campaign, closely examine the business' operating numbers. They will indicate whether internal or external marketing is the way to go, how many clients you want to attract and the fiscal impact on the business. Some of these numbers may in fact surprise you. They may dissuade you from setting goals which could turn out to be either less-than-challenging or too lofty to reach.

A good software program will produce all necessary reports. If the business is not automated, these figures can be calculated by hand, though it will be time-consuming.

Can any performance numbers be improved? What would you realistically like to achieve?

Understanding revenue-producing hours

The first thing to clarify in the quest for "higher numbers" is exactly what the salon can offer. How many revenue-producing hours are available for client consumption? Contrary to popular belief, revenue-producing hours do not include every hour the salon is open. A *revenue-producing hour* is a billable unit of time, during which the salon or day spa may service clients and earn money for services rendered. Lunch hours, break times and hours outside the business' normal operations are not revenue-producing hours, and should not be included in productivity calculations. All others are fair game.

HINT: Time is the most important thing a service business sells. For every hour that isn't booked,

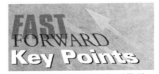

A revenue-producing hour is a billable unit of time, during which the salon or day spa may service clients and earn money for services rendered.

the salon makes no money. If revenue-producing hours were defined, and booked with existing clients currently on waiting lists, there would perhaps be less perceived need for a marketing agenda. There are a few ground rules for filling revenue-producing hours:

- WORK THE HOURS SCHEDULED. One never knows when a client may walk in. Staff who are on the schedule should be on the premises. (No more calling early in the morning to confirm the time of the day's first appointment or leaving early if there is nothing on the book.)

- ELIMINATE "SAFE" BOOKINGS. What exactly do technicians do during those extra fifteen minutes that are routinely added to their standard service times? These small breaks can easily add up to one or two *billable* hours which may be sold to clients.

- ESTABLISH TIME STANDARDS. How long should a haircut, manicure, color or pedicure take to complete? How much prep time is needed for a sports massage or vichy shower? If each technician on staff requires different lengths of time, then the business' time for sale is not being optimized. *But…*do faster technicians necessarily perform to higher standards? Continuing education and establishing skill sets can ensure all team members work at the same level of expertise and within the same time parameters, so that clients receive the best care possible.

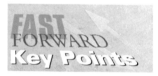

FAST FORWARD Key Points

Productivity is the ratio of hours sold versus hours for sale. The first rule of productivity management is optimization.

Optimizing salon and day spa productivity

Productivity is the ratio of hours sold versus hours for sale. Many salon and day spa owners feel that when it comes to productivity, higher numbers are better. But this is not always so. The first rule of productivity management is *optimization.*

Optimizing productivity means filling the business' revenue-producing hours — but in such a way that service technicians aren't sent hurtling toward burnout. Optimum productivity is around 80%–85%. If it runs higher, staff quickly feel the aches and pains of their demanding, unyielding schedules — and there is no room in the schedule to accommodate the new clients the salon is courting via its marketing campaigns. The key to unlocking greater productivity without greater stress is *efficiency*.

DON'T ASSUME 100% PRODUCTIVITY IS THE GOAL OF AN EMPLOYEE OR THE BUSINESS. Remember this example: A hairstylist who requires sixty minutes for a cut can claim 100% productivity if she sees eight clients per day. However, by reducing production time to forty-five minutes, she can see *nine* clients per day *and* schedule a one-hour break — all in the same number of hours. Through increased scheduling efficiency, revenues increase and stress levels decrease. Making this happen requires across-the-board skill sets *(see chapter 3)* to ensure that all technicians operate at peak levels.

The power of average ticket

Increased sales numbers are the tangible result of streamlining revenue-producing hours and crunching productivity figures. Simply defined, a salon or day spa's average ticket is the total sales revenue generated over a specified period of time, divided by the number of client tickets issued during that time. This easily attained figure is crucial to business growth. It is a specific and measurable indicator of service and retail sales and, therefore, of staff performance.

When all elements are taken together, the average ticket offers a reliable benchmark for the value of a client visit. Broken down into its constituent parts, it can yield the business' retail-to-service and service-to-service percentages, and individual performance statistics for each technician. There is no better indicator of where to focus your marketing efforts.

But, increasing the average ticket for a salon is not as simple as selling more products to clients. With the standard 100% mark-up on retail product, salon profits *will* rise, but so will costs. For each increase in retail sales, the *cost of goods sold* increases.

On the other side of the equation is services. In salons and spas that pay a commission on service tickets, the cost of producing services is tied directly to the number of services rendered. No mat-

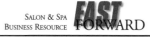
ter how many haircuts a stylist performs or facials an esthetician gives, a fixed percentage of revenues is automatically allocated into the business' *cost of sales.*

When a salon is on salary, payroll costs are somewhat fixed, in that they do not fluctuate with the level of sales. Employees' production time is already paid for. This is where a salon business can really profit through a sustained increase in average ticket — and disburse bonuses at the owner's discretion to deserving technicians. *(An in-depth comparison of compensation strategies can be found in chapter 13.)* Cross-marketing services throughout the salon or day spa and promoting ancillary services such as conditioning treatments, chair massages and mini-facials can produce a marked increase in the overall average ticket.

However, before flooding technicians' schedules with appointments they may not really have time for, one must consider the feasibility of the business' current pricing structure.

Pricing services: A fool-proof formula for profit

The pricing structure in many salons and day spas, much like other operating procedures, is based purely on guesswork and "what the other guy is doing." But more and more owners are discovering that this is not the most profitable method of pricing services. After all, you're not running the other guy's business. It's critical to keep an eye on the competition, but if you don't know *your* salon or spa's cost per hour to produce services, how do you know you're making money? YOU DON'T.

When setting service prices, consider:

- WHAT IS BEST FOR THE CUSTOMER? Do clients offer feedback on whether prices seem too high or too low? Is multi-level pricing confusing? Do clients receive value for the services they purchase? Do they prefer *a la carte* or packaged services? Service businesses must make the customer purchase process easy.

- WHAT ARE THE BUSINESS' OPERATING COSTS? If you are a business owner, you know how to read a profit and loss statement (P&L). The P&L outlines all salon expenditures necessary to provide services to consumers. The TOTAL *cost of sales* includes *cost of sales* (service payroll, payroll taxes, cost of goods sold, professional use products) and *general and administrative, or G&A, expenses* (administrative payroll and taxes, benefits, advertising, bank fees, rent, utilities, etc.). Because they are relatively fixed over a significant period of time, G&A expenses tend to drop as a percentage of sales when productivity rises. If service providers are paid salary, this percentage will also diminish; if they are paid commission, payroll can erode the sales margin.

- WHAT IS THE PRODUCTIVITY RATE? Generally, higher productivity results in a lower cost per hour to generate sales. Get clients off waiting lists and into the salon if there are technicians with available time. Post productivity rates weekly.

- WHAT WILL THE MARKET SUPPORT? This is where one must look

Continued on page 274

What does it cost to produce a service?

	EXAMPLE	**YOUR FIGURES**
1. REVENUE-PRODUCING HOURS AVAILABLE for sale (A)	860	

The total number of hours each production employee has available for sale for an average week. (Only saleable hours...exclude lunch and other down time.) Multiply by 4.3 weeks to find total monthly revenue-producing hours.

REVENUE-PRODUCING HOURS SOLD (B)	559	

All hours actually sold in a week. Multiply by 4.3 weeks.

2. SALON PRODUCTIVITY RATE (B ÷ A)   65%

> _____ **Key figure NUMBER 1**

The salon's "efficiency score." How well is the salon utilizing its people and payroll resources?

3. COST OF SALES (C) $10,000.00

Production payroll, payroll taxes and professional use products and materials.

Less COST OF GOODS SOLD...RETAIL (D)	− $1,500.00	− _____
COST OF SERVICE SALES (C − D = E)	$8,500.00	

4. COST OF SALES for ONE hr. of Service (E ÷ B = G) $15.21

> _____ **Key figure NUMBER 2**

5. GENERAL & ADMINISTRATIVE Expenses (F) $7,000.00

Include all non-production payroll (management, front desk coordinator, receptionist), payroll taxes, and all other overhead expenses that must be factored into selling price.

6. GENERAL & ADMINISTRATIVE COST for ONE hour of service (F ÷ B = H) $12.52

> _____ **Key figure NUMBER 3**

7. TOTAL COST OF SALES and G&A for ONE SERVICE HOUR SOLD (G + H = I) $27.73

> _____ **Key figure NUMBER 4**

$27.73 is the hourly amount the salon must produce in sales to cover all costs. This hourly cost should be viewed much the same way as you view the product cost for a bottle of shampoo. This hourly cost is the number you will mark up to reach your service price.

WHERE DOES THE PRODUCTIVITY RATE FIT IN? The higher the productivity rate, and the more efficiently the salon uses its resources, the lower its cost percentages. The above example uses a 65% productivity rate. Optimum productivity is approximately 80%. Beyond that, client retention begins to decline as the salon nears capacity.

Calculating your profit margin

PROFIT MARGIN is the difference between selling price and cost. If you want a profit margin of 15%, *divide* your *cost* by 85%. (Why 85? Because 100 – 15 = 85.) Don't make the common mistake of simply adding 15% to cost to determine your selling price. You will not achieve the full 15% profit margin that way.

SERVICE TO MARK UP . . . . *Half-hour* haircut and style

COST *(1 hour, letter I on previous page)* . . . . $27.73 x .5 (1/2 hr.) = $13.87

PROFIT MARGIN *(desired profit)* 15%

SELLING PRICE *(minimum to ensure profit)* . . . . $13.87 ÷ 85% = $16.32

SERVICE TO MARK UP . . . . *One-hour* perm

COST *(1 hour, letter I on previous page)* $27.73

PROFIT MARGIN *(desired profit)* 15%

SELLING PRICE *(minimum to ensure profit)* . . . . $27.73 ÷ 85% = $32.62

SERVICE TO MARK UP . . . . *One and a half-hour* foil color

COST *(1 hour, letter I on previous page)* . . . . $27.73 x 1.5 = $41.60

PROFIT MARGIN *(desired profit)* 15%

SELLING PRICE *(minimum to ensure profit)* . . . . $41.60 ÷ 85% = $48.94

out for the other guy. It's alright to charge a little more or less than other salons in the area, as long as clients don't perceive it as a gimmick. Don't price yourself out of your market.

SET PRICES AND STICK TO THEM. There are a limited number of circumstances under which a salon or spa should lower prices. Occasional specials can boost business, and offering price reductions for packages and series purchases only makes sense, but bartering prices under most other circumstances simply says to the consumer that your services were not worth the initial cost. This can undermine the talent of the staff and the reputation of the salon. Don't do it.

Due to increased operating costs, however, prices will occasionally have to be raised. Be direct, forthright and *gentle* with clients. They certainly understand cost-of-living and operating expense increases. Be objective in presenting the new pricing structure.

"Dos and don'ts" of price changes

✓ **Do** deal with the increase openly and comfortably.
✓ **Do** practice responses to clients' questions with staff.
✓ **Do** tell clients about changes before their next appointment.
✓ **Do** continually ask clients how much they value services.
✓ **Do** fix anything that devalues services before raising prices.
✓ **Do** ask clients regularly for feedback on the new prices.

✗ **Don't** avoid talking about an upcoming price increase.
✗ **Don't** get defensive with clients that balk at the adjustment.
✗ **Don't** rely on a front desk sign to advise clients of changes.

Budgeting your advertising dollars

As with any new project or agenda, the first and most important step in developing a marketing campaign is to run it through the cash flow. Advertising is the most common method of paid media marketing. A common salon budget is 3%–5%; 5%–10% is not unusual in more aggressive ones.

To ensure effectiveness, plan for a 5%–8% budget, allocating approximately 70% of these funds to paid advertising. The balance can be used for special events (e.g., price promotions, photo shoots and community or charity events) which will generate good public relations.

Internal versus external marketing

So the money is set aside for a marketing agenda. You are determined to attract more new clients over the next year than the salon has ever drawn before. But should the money be spent internally or externally? Analyze the marketplace and your business' needs. Focus on two primary issues:

■ Are your current clients "ideal"? Do they fit the image you want to project in the community?

■ Is the client base strong and stable? Or do most customers visit only occasionally — maybe even only once?

Internal perspective: A stable customer base provides an automatic advantage. It is a firm foundation to build upon. Chances are, your salon or day spa has a core group of raving fans who never stray. Doing more business with this group is profitable in two ways. You can certainly gain a greater share of their personal disposable income. And consider this: Up to two-thirds or more of new clients can be, and often are, generated through referrals. If your current clients are "ideal" and you want more just like them, concentrate on internal efforts.

External perspective: Marketing externally in a focused, deliberate manner will better attract the type of client the salon wants to add to its base. These clients must fit the business' image and mar-

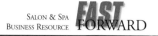

ket niche. Employing a thorough but targeted external marketing agenda can reposition the salon or spa in the community. It's an opportunity to transform the image of the business into one that will draw a different caliber of client. CAUTION: Do not alienate the current retained base. They are your greatest source of stability, even in the slowest of times.

Client retention must be priority number one

Each time a new customer visits the salon or spa, the business has a chance to add to the retained base and increase its corresponding revenue potential. Attracting the consumer and selling your services is not a one-shot deal. *Customers must come back.*

What are the business' growth goals? If the salon or spa's retention rate is low, will it be worthwhile to invest in a marketing agenda? If new clients are attracted but then lost, your business will grow no more quickly than the competitor's that may attract fewer clients but retain more. Under these circumstances, it may be more sensible and cost-effective to concentrate on improving retention levels than to invest heavily in advertising. Ad dollars can be channeled into promotional campaigns designed to increase retention, such as client feedback forms and telephone calls, care packages and special offers.

Attracting new clients – Strategies that work

There are several strategies for developing an effective and profitable marketing campaign for salon and day spa services. *(See chapter 10 for in-depth public relations strategies.)* Targeted marketing is one of the best methods of bringing in new clients. In order to target a market, however, one must first understand it. There are two crucial areas to explore: demographics and psychographics. *Demographics* concerns the absolutes of the marketplace: age, sex, education, income, occupation, race, marital status, geographic location, home ownership, credit card usage. *Psychographics* concerns softer statistics: interests, hobbies, favorite recreational activities. A targeted marketing campaign will focus on several different methods of contact.

- DIRECT MAIL: With proper research, it's possible to develop mailing lists for almost any market segment desired. For information, visit the local library and/or contact your chamber of commerce. There are also organizations from which the information may be purchased. For example: DIGITAL ASSET MANAGEMENT, INC. of Stamford, CT, (look for DAMI at www.thinkdirectmarketing.com) allows subscribers to search a massive database of business and consumer listings — including addresses and telephone numbers — from their desktops. DAMI's data is provided by ACXIOM CORPORATION (look for www.acxiom.com). The lists are continuously updated. Subscribers pay $50 to $200 per year for access to DAMI's database. There are also a number of less-thorough free searches available.

- E-MAIL LISTS: Internet access is booming in businesses and households. Standard operating procedure for greeting clients should include gathering their e-mail addresses, as well as addresses of friends they feel would be interested in the salon or spa's services.

- GIFT CERTIFICATE MARKETING: The quintessential gift for the person who is at a loss for birthdays, anniversaries or holidays is

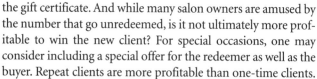

the gift certificate. And while many salon owners are amused by the number that go unredeemed, is it not ultimately more profitable to win the new client? For special occasions, one may consider including a special offer for the redeemer as well as the buyer. Repeat clients are more profitable than one-time clients.

- CONVERTING RETAIL SHOPPERS: Salons and spas with large retail areas and a lot of walk-by traffic can potentially do very well with retail, but their service sales can also be exemplary. If product draws potential new clients into the business, post information on the displays about the services during which each of the products is used. If you employ a retail specialist, educate him or her on every service, so that information can be communicated to shoppers.

- NEWSLETTERS: Keep current clients abreast of goings-on in the business, introduce them to service promotions and invite them to "bring a friend" through a regularly distributed newsletter. It can be mailed to selected clients, distributed through e-mail or made available at the salon front desk.

- NEWS RELEASES: Carefully worded releases promoting salon services can reach large segments of your targeted market if they are conscientiously placed. Which local periodicals do current clients read? To which television and radio consumer programs are they loyal? If you want to gain a greater share of the demographics represented by your current base, use their preferences as a starting point for reaching the rest.

- DONATE SERVICES: Raffles, charity auctions and community events are all wonderful forums for showcasing salon talent. They are also great for public relations. Consider sponsoring a salon event such as a cut-a-thon to attract new clients.

- BUSINESS PARTNERSHIPS: Impress potential new clients by distributing business cards and offering special promotions on services in other businesses. For example: Winners of trivia or other contests in local establishments will be excited about a complimentary shampoo and cut or half-hour massage. It's a *treat* — and they will return to the salon or spa if their anticipated customer service standards are met or exceeded.

Increasing referrals is the most effective marketing method for small businesses. Clients already familiar with spa services are their best promoters. They can speak one-on-one with others about the overall salon experience and feelings evoked during services. They will only do this if they perceive that their friends will receive value for their investment. *However:*

Price is rarely the most important factor in a consumer's decision to buy. People will pay more — generally 10%–15% — if they feel the price is supported by the level of quality received. In reality, 65% or more of customers who are "satisfied" or even "very satisfied" with services, including the price, may choose not to return to your salon. Satisfaction simply isn't enough. Salon and spa owners must become aware of how clients *feel* and what they expect from their visit — and then build those experiences into their long-term salon business goals.

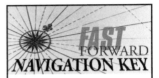

Increasing referrals is the most effective marketing method for small businesses. Clients already familiar with spa services are their best promoters. They can speak one-on-one with others about the overall salon experience and feelings evoked during services. But they will only do this if they perceive that their friends will receive value for their investment.

Building value into services is a tremendous marketing tool. It encourages referrals and solidifies existing relationships. And it is not complicated. Profit should be the *goal,* but not the *focus.*

- CUSTOMER FIRST. Concentrate on the consumer's needs, not your own. Salon and spa service providers are, after all, *service providers.* Living up to your title is a huge first step.
- BUILD LONG-TERM RELATIONSHIPS. Clients who know the business well are likely to experiment with new services and feel more free to recommend them to others.
- BUILD BUSINESS CHARACTER. Does the salon or day spa have a position in the community? A reputation? An image? Take every opportunity to make the business into what you want clients to perceive it to be.

- **THINK HARD.** Pour thought, not dollars, into the business. Throwing money at problems doesn't make them go away; in fact, it often worsens them. Take time to take care of clients and offer unparalleled service.

- **PERFECTION?** Don't drive yourself or the staff insane with notions of the "perfect" client experience. Perfection is an eternal goal — one that can never be reached. Encourage the team to be the best they can, but don't set expectations too high.

- **SHARE IDEAS.** To really stay on top of trends, converse with other small business owners in the area. There's no need to trade master strategies, but great service ideas *can* come from others.

SEASONAL OPPORTUNITIES are also critical for sustained growth. Taking advantage of Valentine's Day, Mother's Day, Secretaries' Day and Christmas as gift certificate and general marketing opportunities will draw a lot of first-time business into the salon and prompt veteran customers to try new services.

- **SPECIALIZE STAFF AND SPACE.** If the salon is going to attempt a serious sales push for the holidays, devote a styling, manicure or temporary station to a display. Make it colorful and position it so that it immediately grabs the attention of anyone entering the salon. Ask a receptionist or other desk staff member to work exclusively at the display, answering client questions and taking orders. **HINT:** The display should be set up away from the desk, to prevent traffic problems.

- **MARKET CORPORATELY.** Offer discounts on bulk gift certificate purchases for local businesses, or offer a complimentary certificate or service for the purchaser. Promote Secretaries' Day through a mailer. Explain that such gifts are well-received by employees, and can even increase work productivity.

- **CREATE A THEME.** Decorate, play seasonal music, use banners, wear the colors of the season…anything to display the salon's spirit and get clients excited about being there.

Selling one-on-one

Before they can generate *client* excitement about new services, the staff must become excited — and communicate the feeling to every customer who telephones or walks through the door. The problem is, the stigma of sales in the salon and day spa industry has psychologically tied the hands of many service providers and front desk personnel.

Leaving reactive...becoming proactive

The person who answers the phone in a salon or day spa is equivalent to a customer service representative (CSR) in a larger corporation. Some salon owners already refer to front desk positions as *customer satisfaction* positions. First contact is critical. Employees need certain tools to help them get past their repulsion to sales. As front-line communicators with clients, receptionists, bookers and coordinators should have several objectives to guide their interaction with consumers.

- ASK QUESTIONS. What better way to uncover opportunities? Current and potential clients only call salons when they have a need. Don't let them hang up without discovering what it is.

- BE A GREAT LISTENER. Learn to accurately interpret client responses. Sometimes "I'm not sure" means "I just need a nudge." Sometimes it doesn't. Ask questions to find out.

- BE ORGANIZED. The front desk can be devoid of the smallest speck of dust, but if it's covered with notes scrawled on slivers of paper, and no one can find a client's service records, the impression made is not favorable. To ensure service consistency, formulate scripted responses to situations that have proven troublesome in the past.

- FIELD (AND OVERCOME) CLIENT OBJECTIONS. Softly and gently: "I realize you usually see Stylist A, but he is unavailable at the time you requested. You can feel comfortable seeing Stylist B because..." When clients know the reasons behind changes, they are more receptive and understanding.

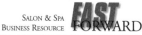
It is not enough to outline interaction and sales goals for staff, however. Whether they work the desk or the service floor, they require coaching to help change their attitudes about sales. To many, an attempt to upsell a service is an intrusion into the customer's time, or even a betrayal of trust. This attitude derives from the fact that people don't like to *be sold* — but they do love to *buy.*

- CHANGING ATTITUDES. The most important idea to communicate to staff in sales-oriented positions is that selling is helping. It's not about being pushy or arrogant. It's about offering solutions to clients' stated needs. The right sales skills will often enhance employee/consumer relationships because they allow salon staff to offer more assistance to clients than before. There is no betrayal of client trust.

- NECESSARY TOOLS. Is the salon's desk and reception area organized efficiently so that staff has the time and space needed to converse with clients? Are traffic jams a frequent problem? BLINKING RED LIGHTS: If customer access through the phones is an issue, the prospect of selling services is unpredictable at best. Are there enough people on staff to handle call and traffic volume? *(If you are considering a booking room, see chapter 5.)*

- ACCESS TO INFORMATION. You can't sell it if you don't know it. Everyone with access to the phones or in a marketing position should experience every service the spa has to offer. Who says homework is no fun?

Determine the client's level of interest…Make the sale

According to Charles D. Brennan, Jr., author of *Proactive Customer Service,* customers progress through three stages in their decision to buy. The goal of a business' marketing effort is to get as many consumers as possible to stage three.

- OPPORTUNITY: Clients recognize an unsatisfactory situation (e.g., my roots are starting to show). They realize that it *can* be changed, but have not yet made contact with the salon.

- NEED: They recognize the situation *should* be changed, usually for a specific reason (e.g., this color just isn't me, my spouse doesn't like it). There is still no commitment to action.

- CHANGE: They become proactive because they perceive that the situation cannot be allowed to continue (e.g., okay, I can't look in the mirror any longer).

There are five steps salon employees can take to move clients to the *change stage*. Because they are all service-oriented, they are low-impact sales methods. They are all conversational items, targeted at making clients feel comfortable.

- MAKE THEM TALK. Do this by asking probing questions, to which they must respond with more than "yes" or "no." Many clients listen to their salon or spa technicians more avidly than to their therapists.
- ADDRESS SPECIFIC PHRASING. Don't be afraid to ask, "Does *considering* mean you've decided?" Learn where the client stands.
- CONSIDER CLIENT HISTORY. Which services does this customer usually purchase? Has she expressed interest in others?
- EXPAND THAT LIST. "You usually get a pedicure and massage when you visit. What else interests you?"
- "DO YOU WANT TO TAKE ACTION?" It's not only a service provider's prerogative to ask this question, but it's expected by clients. If the question is not asked, hopes for future sales could be lost. They want to hear your concern and your solutions. Just don't start offering solutions until you have a commitment of action from the client.

PRESENTING THE SOLUTION: *The customer is interested in what a product or service can do, not in what it is.* There are three actions necessary to confirming a client's interest in your salon's services.

- ASSURE. Be confident in telling customers that you know how to solve their problems. Explain the process which will resolve their stated needs.
- EXPLAIN. How do a service's benefits address the specific needs voiced by a client? Don't be generic. (The benefit is what the client is really purchasing. A feature is an element of the service which enables it to deliver the benefit.)
- REVIEW AND CONFIRM. Wrap it up with enthusiasm.

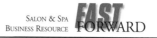
Internal marketing – Strategies that work

The key to successful internal marketing is efficiency. The sales process must be streamlined so that clients have every opportunity to learn about and experience services. It starts at the front desk and, at various stages, involves every person in the salon.

THE ABILITY TO IDENTIFY POTENTIAL CLIENTS is the first step in an efficient sales process. Whether they are new clients attracted to the salon by one or more external marketing resources, or they have been clients for years, every person who arrives for services is a "potential" client. They are the primary market of in-salon sales efforts.

THE CONSULTATION is the second step. Consider it a fact-finding mission in which one gathers information by asking questions. For example: What do you want the results of this service to be? Are there other services you are interested in? Have you ever tried a regimen of home maintenance? Why did you choose this spa for your facial treatments and massages? Have you tried other spas in the area?

SHARING KNOWLEDGE is the third step. Tell clients how to achieve the results they have stated they want. For example: I can personally do this for you…My co-worker can do this…These are the products you need…This is why these services and products will work for you. Be sure to state *what, when, why* and *how much.*

ASKING FOR THE SALE is the final step of efficient selling. There is no other way to achieve the desired result. At this point, it isn't as much about sales as about resolving a client need.

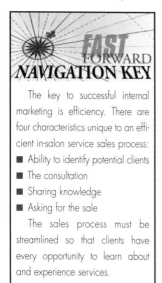

NAVIGATION KEY

The key to successful internal marketing is efficiency. There are four characteristics unique to an efficient in-salon service sales process:

- Ability to identify potential clients
- The consultation
- Sharing knowledge
- Asking for the sale

The sales process must be streamlined so that clients have every opportunity to learn about and experience services.

Your sales attitude

- WHO NEEDS CONFORMITY? Do it your own way. It's important to have a number of points to cover with each client — *it's called a consultation* — but be unique in your individual presentation.

- ARE YOU COMMITTED? Commitment requires the ability to see a purpose in one's actions. That purpose should be two-fold: *growth* of the salon or spa's bottom line through client *service.*

- TAKE THE INITIATIVE. Feel free to introduce new services to clients. Don't ever assume they don't want to change.

- KEEP YOUR PERSPECTIVE. There are always clients who will "browse" salons for the best services and prices. You want to turn these browsers into long-term customers. Many of them will be receptive to long-term relationships. Learn to recognize them. Selling is an interaction between individuals; it's critical to maintain a professional relationship, but one must also get to know clients.

- YOU'RE GETTING FUZZY. Learn to keep your focus. If the goal is to solve customer problems, you have to be 100% tuned in.

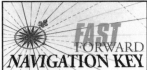

NAVIGATION KEY

Establish a routine: At a particular point during *every* service performed in the salon, begin the customer inquiry:

- Get their attention.

- Describe the benefits of the services being performed and recommended.

- Suggest a purchase of a package or an ancillary service.

- Cite examples of satisfied clients (perhaps the very one who referred them to you).

Maintain a professional appearance and demeanor — and, no matter what, BE CONFIDENT.

- THINK POSITIVE. Everyone has emotions. To market and sell efficiently, one must learn to not get caught up in them. Negative emotions markedly reduce one's ability to communicate.

- BE ENTHUSIASTIC. Genuine belief in the ability of a service to improve a client's quality of life shows in one's eyes and voice. There is no better way to gain trust than through sincerity.

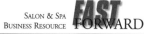
Interest questions and ending questions

Experienced salespeople identify three main types of questions they ask clients — all geared toward gaining insight into what makes them tick. Because once you know what makes them tick, you know how to relate and sell to them. Inexperienced salespeople use the same methods, although they may not have the verbiage or lingo to describe them.

- GENERAL QUESTIONS: These are broad and far-reaching. The goal is to get a glimpse of clients' philosophy or beliefs.
- SPECIFIC QUESTIONS: These are more targeted, aimed at learning particular facts. As such, they may be misconstrued as challenging. Use caution.
- FRAMED QUESTIONS: Constructed by incorporating an idea one knows to be inaccurate in order to elicit new information.

DEALING WITH OBJECTIONS AND QUESTIONS becomes simple when they are treated as requests for more information. Maintain composure. *Identify* the client's concern, *validate* it rather than avoiding it and *resolve* it through a patient, thorough explanation of why your suggestion will work.

END WITH A QUESTION. Don't get over-anxious about developing the ideal closing technique. Offer suggestions that make sense to clients. Ask when they would like to schedule an appointment. Set a date. Asking clients "What do you think?" demands a response and puts the ball squarely in their court.

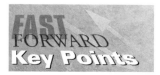

If you find yourself listening to your own voice during much of the client's visit, shut up. Ask questions. Empathize with client responses, offer personal examples, but remember — it's all about the client.

The client database: Mining for gold

Salon and day spa owners are often quite proud of the number of names stored in their business' databases. But how many of those names belong to *active* clients? And how many belong to clients who are actively visiting *other* salons or spas? Why, if the information is literally at your fingertips, does the business not mount continual campaigns to regain their loyalty?

Every client who walks through the door must be queried for name, mailing address, phone number, e-mail address, birthday — any important marketing information they are willing to provide. Most salons ask these questions via "new client forms" which also inquire about medical conditions, prescriptions, pregnancy or other factors that must be considered during services. The information can then be entered into the database during down time.

EVERY CLIENT WHO HAS VISITED THE SALON OR SPA IN THE PAST DID SO FOR ONE OF TWO REASONS: She made a conscious, considered decision to do so because something about it appealed to her, *or* she was influenced to come by someone to whom it had previously appealed. Either way, you have "appeal" working for you. *Use it.*

When asked, clients will offer any number of reasons why they have not returned. Most can easily be corrected or counteracted. But there's no way to know what to fix until someone asks. Contacting dormant clients is a relatively inexpensive way to stir up the client base. It is an effective marketing method because everyone contacted has prior knowledge of the salon.

Many customers can be regained through simple postcard mailers or e-mail messages. Let them know they are not forgotten. Offer special one-time discounts on services if they return within a specified time or spend a certain amount on their next visit. The few dollars sacrificed on the recovery service will be made up many times over when the customer's loyalty is regained.

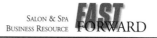

Team selling: It's not a one-person effort

O ne reason sales is often so emotionally draining is that it is viewed as a solitary process. In salons and day spas, technicians are accustomed to being responsible for their own numbers; anything else is not in the job description. Many owners recognize the merits of teamwork and believe that they encourage it in their businesses; nevertheless, they still see the individualistic, build-my-own-book mentality dominate their salons. Why? Technicians are *taught,* in school and "the real world," to look out for number one. In order to implement a true teamwork imperative, one must first unteach these ideas. There are numerous ways to introduce the teamwork concept to staff; regular *team* meetings and a shift in terminology are two of the most effective.

- MEETINGS ARE NOT COMPLAINT SESSIONS. They are state-of-the-business expositions. The most effective method of underscoring the benefits of teamwork and trust is to *take the first step.* An owner must trust employees before the sentiment can be reciprocated. Show you trust the staff by explaining, with numbers and examples, *why* cross-promoting services will benefit them and the salon. Share information openly, as a group, so that no one feels alienated.

- START SAYING "WE." Most salon and day spa owners are accustomed to being the center of their own worlds. The business is theirs, clients think there's no one better and employees are construction projects, requiring time to build and mold. Though the business may consume an extraordinary amount of time and effort, many owners are not really in touch with the goings-on in the break room. Rather than attempting to do everything yourself, get the staff involved. They *will* respond.

- THE TECHNICIAN BESIDE YOU IS NOT YOUR COMPETITION. If salon sales goals are to be met, the resources of the entire team must be utilized. If you are not completely comfortable applying multi-dimensional highlights, advise the client that she will be "thrilled" with the results Stylist B achieves with the process. It's not about what one "can't" do; it's about achieving the best results for the client. HINT: Lack of skill should never be used as an excuse to send a client to another technician — but the client's satisfaction, if necessary, should.

■ NO ONE CAN BE EVERYTHING TO EVERYONE. Salon and day spa technicians often feel they should be able to fulfill clients' every wish — and if they can't, they are somehow failing to meet expectations. Ironically, clients usually don't see it this way. They would much rather be referred to another technician with the time and skill available than to put additional stress on you.

Until steps are taken to make staff aware of the benefits of team service and cross-promotion, the idea will never take root. Solve the *what's-in-it-for-me* dilemma by discussing the points listed above.

Everyone plays a part

Not only must technicians develop the self-assurance to feel confident in referring clients to other technicians, but the front desk and/or booking room staff must be aware of the competencies of every team member. Clients must be matched to the service providers most technically and psychologically equipped to productively interact with them. A good environment in which to learn about each other is the team's regular meetings.

Every sales strategy outlined in this chapter will work for every position in the salon or day spa, including the reception area. In fact, the front desk is especially crucial because clients' initial impressions of the business must be positive. A pleasant phone manner, knowledge of the business' systems and procedures, experience with services and product, and the ability to converse with clients in order to ascertain and meet their needs are all necessary skills. The desk, like the salon as a whole, is a sales center.

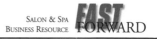
Ten action strategies

1. Classify your current customers into three segments:
   TRANSACTIONAL
   CONSULTATIVE
   PARTNERING
   Decide how you want to treat each group.

2. Develop a systematic referral program.

3. Pick a "guerrilla" marketing activity.

4. Develop a "capabilities statement."

5. Consider the benefits of a regular salon newsletter.

6. Make your business card a powerful "billboard" to promote your business.

7. Develop a program to increase your client retention rate. A 5% increase in retention can mean up to a 90% increase in profits.

8. Develop a program reminding customers to visit the salon more often.

9. Get your staff involved in marketing.

10. Analyze the "moments of truth" in your business when customers form their impressions.

SERVICE MARKETING AND SALES

Things to do:

- Know your productivity rate. Where are you now?

  HOURS SOLD ÷ HOURS AVAILABLE

- Develop a program to increase productivity through optimizing the salon or spa's revenue-producing hours:

  WORK THE HOURS SCHEDULED

  ELIMINATE "SAFE" BOOKINGS

  ESTABLISH TIME STANDARDS

- Implement a system to increase average ticket. Find out where you are now, and set goals for:

  UP-SELLING

  RETAIL SALES

  ADDING ON SERVICES

- Figure your cost per hour for each service. Use the formula on page 272.

- Calculate your desired profit margin. Use the formula on page 273.

- Develop an advertising budget and stick to it. *It must fit into the cash flow.* Determine where your advertising dollars will be spent.

- Implement a referral program. It's the most effective marketing method for small businesses.

- Build a one-on-one selling system. Internal marketing strategies start at the front desk and, throughout the client's visit, involve everyone in the salon.

RETAILING LIKE
THE PROS

*Shifting your retail business
into fast forward*

T hirty years ago, salon retailing was in its infancy. The haircutting boom was just working up a head of steam and
REDKEN was virtually the only professional product company with a selection of products packaged for retail. As baby
boomers flocked to salons for their precision cuts and blow-dries,
shags, angle cuts and bobs, client visit frequency shifted from
weekly to every four to six weeks. The "natural look" took off like a
runaway train; the wash and set fell into a coma. And professional
salon retailing was born.

As more and more salons jumped on the haircutting bandwagon, manufacturers and distributors responded with illumi-
nated signs and decals for salon windows, a larger product and size
selection, and better point-of-purchase materials. Some manufacturers began offering their own retail displays.

Salon clients liked professional products. Owners liked the extra income from their new profit centers. Distributors loved the added sales volume and the potential of salon retailing. Stylists loved the products, but most turned to "artistic" mush when it came to prescribing, recommending and selling — and most still do.

Today, there are powerful forces at work in the salon industry that, for better and worse, are shaping the very nature of professional salon retailing. Intense competition has brought a new level of sophistication to professional product manufacturers' marketing, merchandising, advertising and packaging strategies. The acquisition of professional manufacturers such as REDKEN, SEBASTIAN and AVEDA by major corporations is altering the playing field and raising the stakes at the highest levels of the product pipeline.

Prime-time television and print advertising campaigns have catapulted a handful of major professional product brands into the consumer consciousness. Professional products are now a part of mainstream consumerism. Without challenge, consumers believe that professional products are of higher quality and outperform their over-the-counter (OTC) counterparts. In fact, consumer passion for professional products is so strong that it fuels the dark side of salon retailing — product diversion. Some unscrupulous souls even go so far as to manufacture counterfeit professional products.

So where are the professional recommendations?

Through it all, the true potential of salon retailing still lies in the professional recommendation — yet this is one area where the industry barely gets a passing grade. The dilemma is interesting: Diverters and counterfeiters will risk costly fines and legal battles, even jail, to satisfy the consumer appetite for salon products… while salon professionals cling to "I'm an artist, not a salesperson" thinking. Some even use diversion as an excuse not to recommend products for home use.

HERE'S THE REALITY: Salon professionals' failure to recommend products to clients while they are in the salon or day spa drives clients to make retail purchases — including diverted and counterfeit professional products — through traditional OTC outlets.

Rejecting the personal and financial rewards of retailing is surrendering a key revenue-producing segment of the professional salon and day spa business to the OTC and mass-merchandising market. This is a shortsighted and costly mode of uninformed thinking.

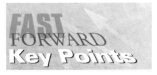

Fast Forward Key Points

Rejecting the personal and financial rewards of retailing is surrendering a key revenue-producing segment of the professional salon and day spa business to the OTC and mass merchandising market…a shortsighted and costly mode of uninformed thinking.

Nope…you're not there yet

The product side of our industry and the ability to move significant amounts of merchandise through salons, with profit margins that far exceed those of consumer products, has elevated professional salon retailing to the ranks of "big business." But just because salons have attractive retail areas and displays doesn't mean they're in the business of retailing. Today, it's hard to find a salon that doesn't have a significant investment in retail floor space, displays and inventory. Yet, many of these salons struggle to see their retail sales represent more than 10%–15% of total revenues.

Why is retail sales performance so lackluster? In a nutshell, it is due to the lack of a systematized approach to retailing. Salons are notoriously *inconsistent* in their customer service delivery. The professional product recommendation is an inseparable part of that experience. Failure to recommend professional products for home maintenance is nothing short of a breach in the customer/salon professional relationship.

The difference between a salon which generates 10% of gross revenues from retail and one which boasts 28%–30% is system design. As before: You manage systems, not people. Design your retailing system to achieve the results you're looking for, and continuously perfect the system — and retail performance will improve dramatically.

If your salon culture is one in which employees are free to decide whether retailing fits their "artistic" demeanor, sales will suffer.

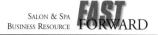
Without a system to guide the process, the fear of rejection so often associated with retail selling is difficult for most individuals to overcome. The consistency of the system and the results it produces quickly help employees jettison their retailing fears and mental roadblocks.

If you want to "retail like the pros," your salon's selling system must be tested, practiced and perfected until the desired results are achieved. Compromises within the system, such as stylists offering professional recommendations to only two of ten clients, will have a negative ripple effect throughout the salon if left unchecked. In this case, managing the system calls for coaching and training.

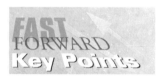

Key Points

The difference between a salon which generates 10% of gross revenues from retail and one which generates 28%–30% is system design.

"Percent of sales" or "percent of service"?

To avoid confusion, it is important to establish a common frame of reference for discussing the financial aspects of retail sales in the salon/day spa environment. Over the years, manufacturers, distributors and salons have intermixed formulas and terminology to the point of confusion for owners, staff, accountants, bookkeepers and consultants.

Some factions in the industry have created a standard based on retail sales as a percentage of service revenue. This is an interesting calculation that, on the surface, appears to offer a clear picture of where retail sales fit in the salon's overall revenue picture. Some owners and managers use this calculation as a performance goal for individual staff members. For example: "Your retail sales must represent 15% of your service sales in order to qualify for a retail sales commission."

WHAT DOES THIS CALCULATION REALLY TELL YOU? Unfortunately, not much. In fact, it yields a distorted and incomplete picture of retail sales in relation to overall performance. Since the formula only shows the ratio of retail to service sales, it naturally shows a *higher percentage* than when retail is calculated as a percentage of total sales. In the example below, retail is 24% of service sales ($4,453 ÷ $18,578 = 24%).

RETAIL AS A PERCENT OF <u>SERVICE</u>

Service Sales	$18,578	
Retail Sales	<u>4,453</u>	<u>24%</u>
TOTAL SALES	**$23,031**	

There is an inherent downside to this calculation. First, it is a ratio of only two revenue categories. It overlooks any relationship to other revenue categories, such gift certificate sales. Second, and most importantly, the ratio has no connection to the total combined sales of the salon — the most important ratio to know.

It is much more beneficial to know, in dollars and percentages,

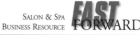
the contribution of every revenue leg to total sales. The ratio between two revenue legs (e.g., retail to service) is immaterial. The ratio of retail sales to *total* sales is important. In the example below, we calculate service sales as a percentage of total sales ($18,578 ÷ $23,031 = 80.7%). Next, we calculate retail as a percentage of total sales ($4,453 ÷ $23,031 = 19.3%).

RETAIL AS A PERCENT OF TOTAL SALES

Service Sales	$18,578	80.7%
Retail Sales	4,453	19.3%
TOTAL SALES	$23,031	100%

In this calculation, retail sales account for only 19.3% of total sales. This is the actual, no smoke-and-mirrors contribution of retail to total sales. *It is almost 5% less than the ratio of retail to service sales.* It may be impressive to use the 24% of service figure, but it can be misleading and inaccurate.

Always a percentage of total sales

What percentage of total sales does payroll represent? What about rent, spa services, gift certificates and retail? Whether you are examining expense or revenue categories, the percentage they represent of *total sales* is the one you want to know — and diligently track.

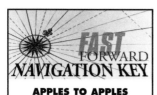

NAVIGATION KEY

APPLES TO APPLES

When discussing retail sales percentages with others, clarify that you calculate retail sales as a percentage of total sales. Ask how they calculate their retail sales percentage.

Remember, if they use a ratio of retail to service sales, that percentage will always be higher and misleading. More importantly, it fails to show retail's true contribution to total salon sales.

Determining your retail potential

Although retail has become a significant sales contributor at many salons and day spas, the sophistication of retail merchandising industry-wide is still at grade school levels. True, salon retailing has come a long way since it was brought to life in the early '70s. Today, consumer advertisements featuring professional salon products are commonplace. Packaging is better than ever, and many retail display and merchandising tools are as attractive as those found in the finest specialty stores.

So why is salon retailing still in elementary school? Because retailing is a process involving an array of management decisions: space allocation, financial investment, product movement analysis, creative display planogramming and design, promotions and — lest we forget — recommending and selling. Salons have a lot of catching up to do to realize their full retail potential.

Imagine for a moment that you own a 5,000 square foot specialty merchandise store. Think about all those aisles, shelves and displays — all those thousands of products. Think of the planning, product selection, inventory control and presentation decisions that have to be made in order to fill your store in the most efficient and appealing manner possible. Everything is on the line. If you make poor purchasing decisions, overstock slow movers or fail to buy enough of the hot new products — you'll "feel the pain" of lost sales and discounted inventory that will bring little or no profit. The everyday world of the retail merchandiser is very different, and infinitely more aggressive, than the service environment at salons and day spas.

Salon retail merchandising is greatly influenced by the high-speed pace of change in the consumer market. Professional manufacturers and distributors are driven by stiff competition. They are learning fast, and teaching their new merchandising techniques to salon owners. For them, the unanswered question is how quickly salons and day spas can master the retail merchandising process.

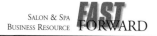
Retail potential remains a moving target

The emergence of retailing salons with names like ULTA[3], TRADE SECRETS, BEAUTYFIRST and others, proves that professional product retailing is a business unto itself. When approached with a retail merchandising and selling mentality, the results are truly impressive in comparison to most independent salons, where service expertise reigns supreme.

It's not unusual for retailing salons to generate 40%–60% of total revenues from retail. This success, coupled with cries of "foul" from the independent salon ranks, has led manufacturers of professional brands to establish purchasing and selling guidelines for retailing salons. Most have imposed a 50% service-to-retail ratio. If retail sales account for more than half of total revenues, the line will be pulled. Pressure to meet the 50% service-to-retail ratio was cited as one of the factors that prompted BEAUTY WAREHOUSE — now operating under the name BEAUTYFIRST — to revamp and reconfigure their stores with a new emphasis on service.

The success of AVEDA's Lifestyle Stores is another fine example of *focused* professional product retailing. Outstanding high-profile locations and a high-end approach to display and merchandising is reaping big rewards for these specialty stores. And AVEDA's Concept Salons are built around an exclusive single-line relationship between salon and manufacturer. The clear objective is to build a strong brand identity through an exclusive network of salons. And the concept of single-line, exclusive salon relationship seems to be paying off. Many AVEDA Concept Salons boast retail sales performance that ranges from a low of 18% to a high of 38% of total revenues. That's well above the national average of 10%–12%.

SEBASTIAN's Grand Salon program is yet another example of a focused, tactical approach to professional product retailing. Through the program, SEBASTIAN shares equipment and merchandising display costs…in exchange for contracted retail space, annual purchase quotas and exclusivity. They will even pay up to $10,000 in product credits to offset the salary of a full-time retail specialist.

Retail potential is a function of focus

But a salon needn't become a retail store, SEBASTIAN Grand or AVEDA Concept Salon in order to achieve impressive retail performance. The key is the ability to focus on the process of selling professional products in the salon environment. Many salons try to be all things to all people by imitating retail stores and stocking their display shelves with multiple brands. The common justification is, "We must have the products clients ask for." But applying broad-based retailing principles to the service-driven salon environment can be costly. Salon technicians' consultations and product recommendations can sharpen a salon's retail focus and significantly narrow its inventory. This focus will improve sales, efficiency and profits. It is a cornerstone of True Quality thinking. You can't progress without focus.

A high-traffic salon in a busy mall or strip center has the critical mass to support a retail store concept and offer a broad selection of product brands and sundry items. Their focus can be wide; their volume of business may support one or more retail specialists. But this approach can backfire in a lower traffic service-driven salon, where the focus should be narrow to avoid overstock, and the complexity of trying to support too many brands.

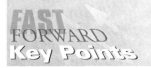

Many salons try to be all things to all people by imitating retail stores and stocking their shelves with multiple brands. The common justification is, "We must have the products clients ask for." The new thinking says, "If we consult with and recommend product solutions to clients, we can significantly narrow our inventory."

So, what's your retail potential?

Frankly, the sky's the limit — as long as you don't exceed that 50% service-to-retail ratio set by most major manufacturers. Salon retailing is still evolving and manufacturers are inventing ever-more focused, sophisticated and exciting retail programs for salons. It's a safe bet that you'll see more exclusive brand-based efforts like SEBASTIAN'S Grand program and AVEDA'S Concept Salons. Unfortunately, so much effort is going into merchandising and marketing that little is left for developing the consultative selling skills of technical staff. *That's where the real potential is.*

Imagine the salon's retail sales if every service customer — not *one* of ten, but *ten* of ten — arrived at the check-out desk with a recommendation for two or three products. It must become a customer service mandate. Until product recommendations and retail selling become part of the customer service process, technical staff will continue to view retail as a non-essential option. *Retailing is a process — not an option.*

Key ratios to measure retail performance

As with any other performance data, the power of the following ratios will not be realized if not clearly communicated to staff. Retail professionals feed performance objectives and data to staff. They play the retailing game *every day* to win — and to win, the team must know the score. In this regard, monthly meetings and quarterly reviews just aren't enough.

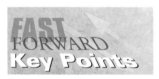

FAST FORWARD Key Points

Retail professionals feed performance objectives and data to staff. They play the retailing game every day to win — and to win, the team must know the score.

Use the following key ratio calculations to set retail goals and monitor performance for individuals and for the salon or day spa:

Retail as a percent of total revenues
FORMULA: Retail sales ÷ total revenues
Average retail ticket
FORMULA: Total retail sales ÷ number of retail tickets
Retail tickets as a percent of total tickets
FORMULA: Retail tickets ÷ total tickets
Retail customers as a percent of total customers
FORMULA: Retail customers ÷ total customers

Know your retail inventory turns

I nventory turns, or stock turnover, is a fundamental principle of retailing success. It measures the number of times during a given period — usually a year — that the average amount of retail stock on hand is sold. Though usually computed on a yearly basis, it may be calculated for any period desired.

When it comes to managing inventory costs, salons and day spas have a long way to go. Runaway retail inventory costs are commonplace because there is often no association between the cost of inventory and how much is sold. Make monitoring inventory stockturn a must. *Turn your inventory four or more times per year. Watch your retail profits grow.*

The rate of stockturn is most commonly determined by dividing the average inventory purchase cost into the cost of the merchandise sold. Quite frequently, however, it is computed by dividing the average inventory at retail price into the net sales figure.

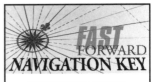

INVENTORY TURNS

To succeed in retail sales, inventory costs and inventory turns must be monitored and managed. If inventory costs are allowed to "free-float" as the result of uncontrolled retail buying practices, inventory will become bloated and the number of turns will decrease.

Additions to retail inventory must be carefully planned and budgeted. Stick to your budgets to avoid overstocking. Discontinue or keep minimal stock on any slow-moving items. *Control your costs.*

When computing inventory turns, observe two cautions:

1. Sales and average stock figures must be *comparable* (i.e., both should cover the same operating period, and be stated either in terms of cost or retail prices).
2. The average stock must be *representative* (i.e., it should accurately reflect the average size of the inventory for the period it covers).

The following three methods of calculating the rate of stockturn assume certain figures: A salon begins the year with **100** bottles of shampoo costing **$5** each, and retailing for **$10** each. During the year, more bottles of shampoo are purchased; at year's end **60** bottles remain in stock. During the year, **600** bottles of shampoo were sold for net sales of **$6,000** and a cost of **$3,000**. The annual rate of stockturn may now be calculated as follows:

THREE FORMULAS TO CALCULATE INVENTORY TURNS

1. Opening inventory at COST (100 x $5)...$500
   Closing inventory at COST (60 x $5).......................................<u>300</u>
   800
   Average inventory at cost (800 ÷ 2) 400
   Cost of goods sold (600 x $5) $3,000
   STOCKTURN RATE ....$3,000 ÷ $400 = 7.5

2. Opening inventory at RETAIL PRICE (100 x $10) $1,000
   Closing inventory at RETAIL (60 x $10) ....<u>600</u>
   1,600
   Average inventory at RETAIL (1,600 ÷ 2)..............................800
   Net sales $6,000
   STOCKTURN RATE ....$6,000 ÷ $800 = 7.5

3. Opening inventory in UNITS...100
   Closing inventory in UNITS...<u>60</u>
   160
   Average inventory in UNITS..80
   STOCKTURN RATE.............................600 ÷ 80 = 7.5

Advantages of rapid stockturns

The advantages of a rapid rate of stockturn are obvious. By limiting the investment in inventory, expenses such as interest, taxes, insurance on merchandise, and display and storage space are all reduced. Return on inventory investment improves exponentially.

CAUTION: Many believe there is a direct relationship between stock turnover and profit, and that a retailer can boost profit by increasing the turnover rate. But... *Whether profits increase with stock turnover depends entirely upon the methods used.* For example: A salon may increase stock turnover by reducing inventory while maintaining the same sales volume. This may be achieved by eliminating slow-moving items or by dropping entire product lines. And increased profits are not sure to result from reducing stock, even if sales volume holds steady. Purchasing in small quantities may result in increased handling and shipping costs and eliminate opportunities for quantity discounts. And if slow-moving lines are sold at a discounted price, the profit margin is eroded.

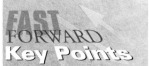

Satisfactory inventory turnover is the result of good merchandising and, therefore, a measure of the alertness and ability of management.

An increase in stock turnover is not always the best strategy to increase profits. Profits are the end result of a collection of sound retailing practices. Concentrate on careful buying, judicious pricing, a well-balanced stock, effective sales promotion and properly trained personnel. Higher inventory turns — and profits — will follow. Satisfactory inventory turnover is the result of good merchandising and, therefore, a measure of the alertness and ability of the management.

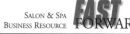
Fear of selling is universal: Beating the demons

A ll the product knowledge and "pep talks" in the world will not overcome the deep-seated distaste, even fear, that many people harbor about sales. To overcome such seemingly insurmountable obstacles requires the expertise of a professional salesman and educator who can offer a unique perspective to salon employees. The fact is, sales happen every day, in any number of circumstances. You just have to learn to recognize that you have the ability to become a salesperson.

According to Art Savage, president of BUSINESS COMMUNICATIONS GROUP in Annapolis, MD, the problem is multi-faceted. The list of barriers to successfully building personal selling skills among professional service providers is filled with feelings of inadequacy, poor self-image and downright fear of failing.

FAST FORWARD Key Points

What's been forgotten is that people buy products and services from other people.

What if I just don't like it?

People who are unaccustomed to personal selling can usually feel more comfortable and proficient at it once they recognize what is holding them back. Selling skills can be acquired and fine-tuned when individuals realize they are not alone, when they understand the following facts of selling:

- Turndowns are inevitable, but they make people stronger.
- Canceled appointments aren't always disasters.
- Stalls and objections can be overcome with creative selling.

In the recent past, many service marketing consultants advised clients to devote energies and budgets to mass-marketing tools such as advertising and public relations. *What's been forgotten, though, is that people buy products and services from other people.* Says Art, "The most important knowledge is of human behavior, being able to uncover customers' needs — and relate your services to them."

It's critically important to get your clients to talk, rather than talking endlessly yourself. Art explains, "Learn how to stop talking, to hear what people are saying. Customers will tell you a lot about themselves, and this helps you sell. Sometimes training fills you full of product knowledge — and the customer doesn't always want to hear that. Look for problems. Identify the problem and then offer the solution." He concludes, "Once a client says, 'Can you help me?' you've got him." The diagnosis and recommendation are up to you as a professional salon service provider.

Breaking the success barrier

According to Art, there is no such thing as *status quo*. There are only two options when it comes to your "success barrier" — that invisible barrier which holds every person, not just salon employees, back: You either tear down your wall of limitations or throw up more barriers to stand in your way. Each time you decline to offer your expertise to clients, you build your wall.

To tear down the wall, salon employees must set future goals — tangible, monetary goals as well as psychological goals based on their levels of self-esteem and assertiveness. Says Art, "A goal is nothing more than a jackhammer. Each time you set a goal and act upon it, you are chipping away at your success barrier. As each brick is removed the barrier wall becomes weaker. That is why success breeds success. The toughest part of tearing down your wall is removing the first brick."

Understand your clients

No salon owner needs to be told that today's clients are more savvy than ever before, and know what they want before they set foot in the salon. Says Art, "Today's buyers buy for their own reasons…not the seller's. They are sophisticated decision makers." However, they still

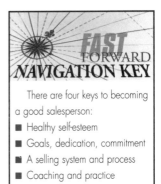

FAST FORWARD NAVIGATION KEY

There are four keys to becoming a good salesperson:

- Healthy self-esteem
- Goals, dedication, commitment
- A selling system and process
- Coaching and practice

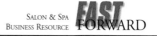
need and desire your professional advice and assistance.

One strategy for communicating with clients: "Stop selling features and benefits and start providing ways for customers to avoid or overcome their 'pain.' Talk about investment instead of cost," Art suggests. But salon employees must also be careful to avoid a particularly self-defeating situation: talking too much. Says Art, "If you hear your voice 70% of the time in a selling situation, just shut up. Get the clients talking and they will tell you how to sell to them."

Sales Sensitivity Index

How effective are you at:

- Being willing to solicit "add-on" business from current clients
- Trying to sell ideas to peers
- Believing selling is an honorable activity
- Making decisions
- Selling oneself as assertive
- Handling rejection
- Getting others to make a commitment
- Organizing one's time
- Presenting ideas to a group
- Being a good listener
- Having a healthy self-concept
- Handling defeat

Are your employees servicing customer needs, or just working the appointment book?

As with any other profession, there is an inherent danger of boredom in the salon industry, of falling into *static* mode. This is especially true of stylists and technicians who have either too little or too much to do.

Those who wait all day for a walk-in may not be at the top of their game when a client finally appears. Conversely, those whose schedules are always packed with the same clients may have great client retention skills, but also face a certain risk: There comes a time when you know the schedule by heart. In both scenarios, there is a need for variation, for something new and exciting.

No salon can operate long or profitably once the team falls into "stand-and-cut" mode. Salon staff's personalities are as unique and varied as the services they offer. They need a forum in which these personalities can be seen and responded to by clients.

THE ANSWER: *The client consultation, which promotes interaction between staff member and client, and culminates in the professional product recommendation.*

Salon management must institute an effective client consultation procedure. Don't trust that clients will remember every question they thought of in the car. Staff must have a standard list of questions to get the ball rolling. The content of those questions will depend on the services and products your salon offers.

Introducing a consultation procedure to staff not only ensures client needs are met, but also lays an operational groundwork. The team must understand there is more to a salon career than standing behind the chair. They must take responsibility for meeting client expectations and stop the "free-falling" so common in the workplace. The consultation and recommendation are great starting places for salon owners to incorporate accountability into their team's job descriptions. Eventually, the salon should run smoothly without the presence and supervision of the owner.

Create a new attitude about selling...
create a "selling system"

Everyone knows how to sell. It's part of life. Some people just do it better than others. Some people love the challenge of the "sales game." They love discovering people's needs and satisfying them with the services and products they have to sell. They understand that everybody wants something, that everybody has needs and that everybody buys sooner or later. They take rejection in stride and consider it part of the selling process — they expect to hear *no* before they hear *yes.*

But many others find sales difficult. For them, approaching others and initiating a sale is uncomfortable and unsettling. They do try, but the first "no" they get sends their airborne sales efforts crashing to the ground. The rejection is simply too much to overcome. Owners can set sales quotas, bonuses and rewards, but stylists who fear selling will never sell. *The winners will always be those who love getting to "yes."*

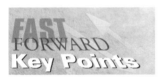

FAST FORWARD Key Points

Amateurs sell — professionals provide solutions. Salons sell services and products if the staff prescribes them.

The missing link

Why do certain stylists get so busy while others watch in awe? Why do the same stylists always win the sales contests? They win because they have unconsciously developed a selling system of their own over time. Good, bad or indifferent... *it works.*

Every successful business will quickly credit its success to a "selling system." Companies invest millions of dollars every year to develop and refine training programs and weekly sales meetings to keep salespeople focused. The salon owner's mission is to develop a selling system the entire team can use, which guides the efforts of the staff to a common goal.

By now you may be thinking, "But I sell haircare services and products — not copiers and fax machines." There is no difference. You and your team must utilize your professional training and expertise to discover customer needs and recommend the necessary course of action to satisfy those needs. A copier salesperson does the same thing. So does your doctor, dentist, lawyer, plumber, electrician, car mechanic and computer technician. Everyone in business is charged with the task of determining and satisfying needs. Salons are no exception.

Repositioning selling

To develop a selling system, selling must be repositioned within the salon environment to remove its negative associations. Not so long ago, professional product distributors were referred to as *beauty supply houses.* Their salespeople were called *dealers.* About thirty years ago, an effort began to reposition them in the marketplace and upgrade their image. Today, beauty supply houses are most often referred to as distributorships where salons receive not only products, but education, and technical and business support. Their salespeople became distributor sales consultants who offer not only products, but inventory control, retail merchandising and other essential skills. It's still selling. It's just a more modern and professional approach to the process.

Assume you told your staff they no longer have to sell. (Listen to the collective sigh of relief.) Suppose you explained to them that the salon will assume all sales responsibilities for services and products through marketing, advertising, in-salon promotions and other means of exposure. Staff responsibility will focus on determining each client's needs, and prescribing the appropriate services and products to satisfy those needs. To achieve this, the salon will provide the staff with a "system": tools to efficiently probe for client needs, and prescribe services and products.

IT'S A MATTER OF SEMANTICS. Whether you call it "selling" or "prescribing," the objective is the same — to create a sale. Stylists react more positively to prescribing than to selling. If that's what works, use it.

Changing attitudes

Staff react negatively to selling only because they are uncomfortable with the process. It's a new behavior that requires a certain level of proficiency. It also requires a certain level of self-esteem and self-confidence. It is fallacious to assume that some individuals are natural salespeople. They just have a higher tolerance for the failures and rejections they encounter as they learn to sell. And the faster they learn, the more they sell and the sooner they achieve their financial and career goals.

Once employees understand the selling process, they can reap the personal, professional and financial rewards it can deliver. It begins with the reinforcement that selling *can* be rewarding.

SELLING, PRESCRIBING, CONSULTING — IT'S ALL THE SAME. There isn't a salon client who wouldn't appreciate the extra guidance and recommendations a stylist can provide to enhance his or her personal appearance. The client may respond with "I don't think so," or "I'll think about it for next time." Maybe the client will say, "Sounds great…let's do it." The point is that your salon's service technician did his or her job as a professional, helping a client improve his or her appearance.

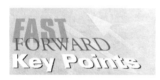

Selling can and will be fun for salon and day spa staff when management replaces sales negatives with sales positives.

Selling can and will be fun for salon and day spa staff when management replaces sales negatives with sales positives. Changing stylists' attitudes about sales is the first step in developing your salon selling system.

The team approach

The foundation of a true selling system is the collective effort of the salon team. There is no place for the back-room manager in a sales-driven salon. A single negative influence can upset the salon's forward sales momentum. Keep naysayers under control.

The salon environment is perfect for team-based sales efforts. Once the staff is trained and proficient in their portion of the selling system, you'll quickly discover the revenue-generating capability at your command. Remember, sales motivation and management is an ongoing process. Your team will need an extra boost of encouragement from time to time…and so will you.

Plant the selling seeds

Begin working with your staff to reposition their views and attitudes about selling. Your mission is to redirect their perception of selling by presenting and discussing the process and the rewards it can offer. Remember, the word *sales* never has to enter the picture. The caliber and sophistication of your staff will dictate a course of action. Points to discuss can include:

- How selling is the key to achieving professional and financial success.
- How selling can be fun and rewarding. There is no greater feeling in sales than getting a "yes."
- How clients appreciate a stylist's guidance and recommendations even if they don't buy today, or in the future.
- How developing selling skills can do wonders for developing one's self-esteem and self-confidence.

There is no mystery to selling. It's simply a process of defining and filling needs.

Probing questions that lead to "yes"

robing is nothing more than asking questions and involving a client in a conversation that will allow you to determine his or her needs. Knowing which questions to ask and when to ask them leads to the ultimate "yes." Following are some probing guidelines. Ask questions…

- that allow you to maintain control of the conversation.
- on a broad range of possible client problems which you can help solve. Narrow the focus until you discover specific needs.

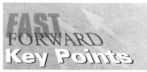

- that continue to produce *yes* answers, until reaching the final *yes* for the services or products you believe they need.

There is a big difference between telling staff to sell more and giving them a "selling system" with procedures designed to achieve retail sales results.

- that arouse positive emotions and move the client toward the purchase. EXAMPLE: "Wouldn't you like to have hair that feels thicker and has more body?"
- to isolate client objections, and prevent unimportant objections from getting out of control.
- in direct response to objections. "Is there a reason you hesitate with color?" You're not trying to trick a client into buying — you're trying to help the client make an educated decision on a service you believe will benefit him or her.
- to determine the benefits the client will realize with the service or product.
- to acknowledge a fact about the benefits of the service or product. When clients state facts, they sell themselves.
- to confirm whether you may proceed with the service, or if you should continue to the next step in the selling process.
- to help the client rationalize his or her decision to proceed with the service or buy the home maintenance system.

Don't get stuck on closing a sale. If you probe efficiently for needs, and offer opportunities that will help solve customers' problems, closing occurs automatically.

Fine-tuning retail merchandising

Retail has recently taken a dramatic turn. Companies which had never retailed (such as WARNER BROTHERS and COCA COLA) opened their own stores. These companies have some basic qualities in common with retailers: product selection, competitive pricing, pleasant shopping environment and a lot of shoppers. They created an atmosphere of wonderful, well-lit displays, large open areas and *themes* to support their goods for sale. Today's consumer is comfortable in this type of atmosphere. To succeed in retailing, salons must create such environments. There are a few fundamentals to follow:

Inventory control

Some salon owners believe their computer will completely manage and control inventory, but the reports produced by most salon software systems are only as good as those who interpret the information. Efficient inventory control demands precise and frequent analysis of product movement — to ensure you don't run out, that fast movers receive extra attention and that slow movers are minimized or eliminated if necessary. Bi-weekly inventory analysis is essential in formulating a plan of action for either increasing or reducing inventory.

Most salon owners know what sells, but not what doesn't. If a dozen units of product are in stock but only two have sold in the past six months, is it profitable to carry that product any longer? The sales consultant and salon retail manager must decide whether to eliminate that product altogether or lower its inventory level. It's better to sell out slow moving items through special merchandising efforts or return those products and reinvest in one that will move more quickly (and ultimately make money for the salon).

INVENTORY CONTROL IS A GAME. As in chess, inventory is constantly moved and adjusted to maximize its selling potential. For example: A specialty shampoo that deep cleans hair suffering from chlorine build-up is a natural product for summer merchandising.

If it works well, you will have a pre-tested merchandising plan ready for next summer. Your inventory control system should include this promotion and ensure that sufficient product is on the shelves during the summer months.

HINT: Too much product on salon shelves can crush the cash flow and choke profits. Find the right balance and mix…and keep products moving. Here are some suggestions to get you started:

■ STICK WITH TWO OR THREE CONSUMER-DRIVEN PROFESSIONAL PRODUCT LINES. Consumer buying patterns will tell you which products to stock. The bottom line is profits.

■ HAVE AN IN-SALON STAFF MEMBER WORK WITH SALES CONSULTANTS to monitor and control inventory movement, and the salon's merchandising efforts.

■ DON'T CARRY PRODUCT LINES because they are well-advertised. There's more to successful retail merchandising than big advertising budgets: sales training, product knowledge, in-salon promotions, signage, displays and creative merchandising materials. Remember, the professional recommendation remains a salon's most powerful merchandising tool.

■ AVOID COMPANIES THAT DO NOT TAKE BACK PRODUCTS. If it doesn't sell, nobody wins. Make sure you're not stuck with an inventory you can't turn over.

Product display tips

■ Face labels forward. Don't make customers "work" to find their favorite products.

■ Leave a one inch gap between products. It's easier for customers to identify products, and allows room to remove it from the shelf without disturbing the display.

■ Place the price on the bottom of the product, where the customer can easily find it. HINT: *No price means no sale.* In general, a customer will not ask the price — and will not buy.

■ Lighting makes a world of difference. It frames the display area, making it easier for customers to focus on items. Consider leaving the retail display case lights on at night after closing.

■ Display products by category. Place shampoos in one section, conditioners in another, etc. This makes the shopping experience much simpler for the consumer.

- Basic retail housekeeping includes dusting and neatly arranging the products every day. No one wants to buy dirty or dusty products. Move products to the front of the shelf every day.

- In-salon promotional displays should be consistent in message and presentation, whether in the window, retail display area, styling stations or backbar area. Tie all of them together to reinforce the promotion and the products.

- Company props such as banners, national print advertisements, monthly specials and tent cards can all add to your promotional themes and sales impact. Some companies that use television advertisements will provide supporting materials for in-salon use. This provides a strong tie-in to your salon's efforts.

Retailing and merchandising are still evolving at salons, and there is still much to master before true retail success is realized. Continuously monitor your inventory strategies — both successes *and* failures — and salon retailing will become easier to predict, track and profit from.

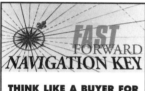

FAST FORWARD
NAVIGATION KEY

THINK LIKE A BUYER FOR A SPECIALTY STORE

When it comes to retailing, most salons and day spas are specialty stores. If the bulk of customer traffic is generated by service sales, think like a *specialty retailer*. Attempts to emulate OTC retail stores with a wide array of similar product lines will do more to drive up inventory costs than retail sales.

The emphasis should be on exclusivity, product knowledge and the professional recommendation.

Mastering the "Five P's"

Your salon's overall retail marketing strategy is composed of a target market (in most cases, the salon's client base), and a retail marketing mix (designed to satisfy that target market at a profit). *The five P's make up your retail marketing mix.*

- PRODUCT...Includes both goods and services. Broadly defined, product includes physical goods, *and* merchandise variety and selection. Your customer service system, return policy and True Quality management processes are all tied into product.

- PLACE...Includes the three primary areas of salon merchandising activity: the location, the use of space within the facility and the physical distribution system.

- PRICE...Has a direct and measurable impact on profit. Price is not simply "how much you charge." It can be controlled, and used to dramatically influence buying decisions and value perceptions. Display price openly; don't make clients ask.

- PROMOTION...Often misunderstood and poorly used, this process extends far beyond advertising. It includes contests and deals, personal selling, and public relations. All must work together to successfully communicate the value of professional product to customers.

- PEOPLE...Extends beyond personality and image. Your "people process" includes matching staff to the expectations of customers, thorough training and product knowledge, consultative selling skills and a commitment to True Quality. The professional recommendation is the most powerful people tool.

Using the *five P's* to fine-tune your salon's merchandising program will teach you to focus on the primary factors that will most directly influence your decisions and sales potential.

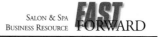
Creating strategic distributor alliances

Today's "tactical consumer" demands more than many beauty salons can provide. Intense market fragmentation, non-traditional forms of competition and vacillating buyer preferences are mandating radical and widespread change at all levels of the industry. Innovative industry leaders are responding in non-traditional ways. Manufacturers are researching consumer demographics, and psychographics and other soft data — often in place of product research and development.

Distributors, grappling with a lack of sales productivity, are questioning the most basic aspects of sales. Many distributor attempts to move from a "transactional marketing" (vendor) relationship to a "co-marketing" (partnering) relationship with salon and spa accounts are stifled by traditional (order-taker) sales consultants who cling to the adage, "There's never anything new about selling." Nevertheless, a new breed of salon consultant is bridging the distributor-to-salon gap, and replacing the order-taker.

Brand versus generic salespeople

Consider the sales consultant who parks right in front of the salon. (Order-takers usually park where the salon owner can't see them arriving.) Upon entering the salon, he recognizes a competitive product representative at the reception counter. Following protocol, he acknowledges the situation, politely excuses himself and begins to leave. "Wait!" exclaims the salon owner, "He's just taking an order. I'm ready for our strategy session. Come on back to my office." Can you imagine the look on the first sales consultant's face? *That* is the difference between a brand and generic salesperson.

Profile of the new breed of salon consultant

■ CONFIDANTE

Outstanding sales performance depends on consultants' ability to "think" (not just see) from the salon owner's point of view, and go beyond a superficial reading of immediate customer needs. They see each salon as a different market, and seek a deeper understanding of the owner's current and desired position. They are skilled at capturing information. More importantly, they know how to interpret what they hear. They understand that a mutually productive relationship goes beyond taking orders.

■ ADVISOR

The next generation salon consultant will have such command of the salon owner's business problems, concerns and goals that he or she will be empowered to act on behalf of the salon owner. This is where the salon owner draws the line between a trustworthy salesperson and a salon *consultant.* A salon consultant has achieved this status when he hears a salon owner say, "If you believe it is the right thing to do, then I want to do it!"

■ STRATEGIST

Salon consultants have the ability to look at the salon from the salon clients' point of view. They leverage all available resources to continuously build a competitive advantage for the salon. They act on behalf of the salon without undermining the owner.

■ MARKETER

Marketing "information" and marketing "expertise" are distinguished by the degree of involvement of the salesperson. Many *order-takers* (in fear of being stereotyped) are quick to pick up on timely marketing lingo to mask themselves. They present themselves and their new buzz words as an information resource. The salon *consultant* applies proven marketing principles to solve the explicit needs of the salon. Behavior defines the intentions of a salon consultant.

■ TRAINER

Today's salon consultant is skillful at training both the salon owner and staff on more than business principles which can help the salon as a whole. They "customerize" technical, personal and professional training with the understanding that, "Each salon training workshop is nothing more than an audition for the next."

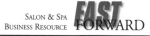
Get the most from your salon consultant

1. LEARN YOUR SALES CONSULTANT'S EXPERTISE BEFORE YOU LEAP. Spend more time with the salespeople calling on your salon; qualify their abilities. You cannot capitalize on their strengths if you don't know what they can do for you. Today's salon consultant will meet your expectations. If you want more, expect more!

2. ESTABLISH A GAME PLAN. The fundamental objective of any business-to-business relationship is to advance the partnership. As a strategist, the salon sales consultant understands the necessity of a mutually developed and agreed-upon game plan. The salon owner establishes the objective; the sales consultant conceives the plan.

3. WORK BY APPOINTMENT. Schedule regular meetings in order to advance the partnership. A salon does not evolve overnight, so don't try to reinvent your business in one meeting. Begin with a problem-solving session to identify your most pressing business needs. Follow up with strategic planning, decision making, implementation, tracking and measurement. All are good topics for business meetings. Regardless of the agenda, never forget the purpose: *Advance the situation.* Things don't remain static in today's business world — you either climb or slide.

"Next generation" salons, distributors and manufacturers are rapidly emerging — all in response to the increasing demands of the tactical consumer. Each must evolve and adapt to the forces of change. In essence, the new salon consultant is here to provide what the salon owner needs most: business expertise. The salon sales consultant is employed by the distributor, but works for the salon owner.

Profile of a successful professional retailer:

NATURAL BODY DAY SPA & SHOPPE

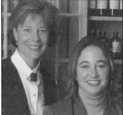

Owners: Patti Beggs and CiCi Coffee
Location: Atlanta, Georgia
Retail: 50% of total sales

PATTI BEGGS (LEFT) AND CICI COFFEE.

N ATURAL BODY DAY SPA & SHOPPE began with an inspiration. In 1989, Patti Beggs was a flight attendant. Her inspiration came from the combination spas/shops so common in Europe. It wasn't long before Patti and CiCi Coffee, the two founding principal partners of NATURAL BODY, opened their own spa and shop — a one-room affair on Highland Avenue in Atlanta, Georgia. Today, they are a rapidly growing enterprise, and NATURAL BODY is the parent company of a number of fran-

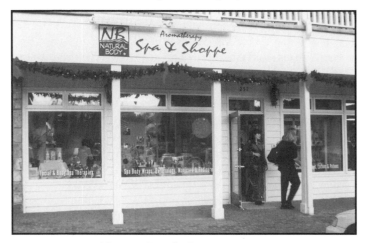

NATURAL BODY'S CHRISTMAS FACADE.

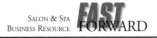
chises. They have also acquired a third partner, Arn Rubinoff, a franchise attorney.

NATURAL BODY concentrates exclusively on spa services. Hair services were once available in the Buckhead (Atlanta) franchise, but the business threatened to become more about clients' outward appearance than their inner health. Patti avows that franchising NATURAL BODY in a hair salon will be successful only if a "delicate balance" between making clients look good and feel good is maintained.

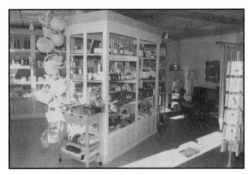

AN ELEGANT AND WELL-STOCKED RETAIL AREA.

She and CiCi were also concerned about disrupting this balance when they first decided to expand into multiple locations, but it was the only way for NATURAL BODY to reach more people. The greatest challenge throughout the company's history has not been to avoid chaos, but to turn it into a positive influence. Says Patti, "Chaos levels fluctuate and there will always be disturbances. But they can be your primary source of creativity. You have to embrace them and then grow from them."

Fiscal and emotional growth

To rally the staff through chaotic times, Patti and CiCi hold monthly meetings, during which everyone discusses the growing needs of the business. An unchanging goal at NATURAL BODY is to grow by at least 5% over the previous year's numbers.

Meetings are mandatory, often held at lunch time on slower days; they are always fun, built around learning and sharing. A frequent topic of discussion is salesmanship. According to Patti, many hand and foot technicians need help learning to share their knowledge with clients, while estheticians are generally more accustomed to selling (hence, one group can assist the other in an important area). All communication is open and honest, and the main thrust of the meetings is team building, so the staff has been supportive of programs and changes implemented at NATURAL BODY.

Management meetings are held weekly. Each location is managed independently, though under the NATURAL BODY corporate umbrella. Patti's extensive responsibilities include maintaining their private label, therapeutic and skincare lines, as well as overseeing marketing and public relations. CiCi keeps the business' financials in order and monitors retailing, while Arn acts as corporate attorney. Says Cici, "We want to start getting the owners together even more often to stimulate interaction and motivation."

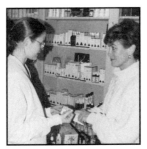

Lead therapists are also included in the management team. Lead therapists conduct initial interviews with potential new team members and lead their basic training. They work with the other managers to coordinate sessions, always maintaining a high level of hands-on training and inter-

RECOMMENDATIONS ARE A "NATURAL" PART OF THE SELLING PROCESS.

action. NATURAL BODY boasts its own training facility, but the team will travel or bring in outside assistance if necessary. Says Patti, "If we don't have expertise in something, we go out and find it."

Marketing for NATURAL BODY was almost a matter of happenstance in the beginning. Patti and CiCi relied heavily on client referrals, and got some press coverage from the Fund for Animals (because the spa sells cruelty-free products). News of the growing business also spread to magazine editors by word of mouth. Then, in 1996, a huge breakthrough occurred. NATURAL BODY was selected to provide spa services for Olympic athletes at the village in downtown Atlanta. Says Patti, "It was quite an honor. All the services were done *gratis,* but it provided great PR."

Patti and CiCi now target the spa's advertising dollars at the holidays, promoting gift basket and certificate sales. The retail space within the spa is designed for comfortable client browsing. In fact, many clients not scheduled for services make retail purchases. Says CiCi, "Service sales usually slow down in winter, but retail goes up substantially." They have also put together a catalog to showcase their line of products.

The steps to team playing

- SKILL SETS: Team members at NATURAL BODY must complete basic spa and operations training sets, which usually require between two and four weeks to complete. For example: Massage therapists begin with basic courses exploring the use of hot compresses and move through seaweed wraps right up to advanced courses on manual lymphatic drainage. Certification at each skill level is required for advancement.

- SCOREBOARDS: NATURAL BODY posts the spa's overall score on numbers such as service, retail and gift certificate sales, productivity and retention. Patti and CiCi are "easing in" to individual scoring. These numbers are shared only at one-on-one meetings which take the form of a formal or informal "quality check." (Quality checks are conducted at least once per quarter, and sometimes more frequently, depending on an employee's job description and performance.)

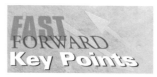

FAST FORWARD Key Points

Increasing the average ticket is very important at NATURAL BODY. Patti says, "It is all about suggestions. Therapists must tell clients about services and products."

Increasing the average ticket is very important at NATURAL BODY. Patti says, "It is all about suggestions. Therapists must tell clients about services and products."

- COMPENSATION REVIEWS ARE NOT PRE-SCHEDULED: According to Patti, timing depends on "what's going on" with a particular therapist. Evaluations consider the value therapists offer clients, which is apparent in the amount of home-care product clients purchase and how well they grasp the product's value. Therapists should be efficient and effective with client care and generate a lot of "all-around" business. (For example: If a team member has a great personality but works slowly, what's the best way to increase speed?)

The value of therapists' client care and service is also reflected in hard numbers. Number of new clients seen, retention and productivity are all easily monitored by generating a set of computer reports. Says CiCi, "Facts don't lie. I can't imagine growing the business without a good computer system."

- PERFORMANCE EVALUATIONS AND REVIEWS ARE HELD MONTHLY. At the time of the evaluation, each team member receives a worksheet showing whether a bonus has been earned and exactly what the bonus is based on. "We call it profit-sharing," says CiCi. "When pay is attached to it, the idea of meeting goals becomes more interesting. We have gotten great feedback, even a suggestion to distribute paychecks in unsealed envelopes so they can be used again."

The profit-sharing principle at NATURAL BODY is based on service sales, retail percentage of total sales, retention, spa maintenance and cleanliness, continuing education and activities outside the spa. The percent of bonus earned is calculated on a "curved" scale. CiCi explains, "The highest producer earns a 100% share of the pool. Everyone else earns a percentage of that."

The wheels of management

NATURAL BODY has little trouble finding therapists to fill technical positions. The difficulty is filling management and receptionist positions. Says Patti, "We need people who love caring for people."

The actual hiring process at NATURAL BODY is highly intuitive. Receptionists and therapists are required to interview twice; resumés must show people skills, customer service experience and initiative. However, Patti says, "You just know when you know someone is right for the spa."

As for sharing the wealth of responsibility at NATURAL BODY,

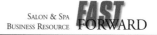

Patti says, "It's extremely difficult for a woman to delegate anything. It's not about control — it's a feeling of wanting to be sure everything is done appropriately. The ability to delegate comes with having a strong management team."

Patti believes that management is "one of the hardest jobs in any business. It takes instruction, but it is a learning process. Plus, there are no cubbyholes at Natural Body. We have chaos, but we make room for it. Every day, we work on the chaos of the business."

Retail sales management checklist

Nancy Flinn offers some specific management guidelines for building retail sales.

- Measure the current level of retail sales by month and quarter. Define them as a percentage of <u>total</u> salon sales. Records should be kept of units sold and dollars generated. Separate sales by each brand and type of brand stocked.

- Establish reasonable rates of retail sales growth by month and quarter for the next twelve months. Goals should be broken down to define the expected sales performance of each person who will sell retail products.

- The internal design of the salon must reflect your commitment to retail sales. Retail sales are stimulated by attractively displayed and merchandised selling environments. Focus on the front of the salon, styling stations and main desk.

- Select the retail brands and number of each brand's individual items which will complement your salon's image and clientele. Base the selection process on an analysis of products previously stocked. Establish a minimum sales level, and don't carry brands that perform below that level. Have your key distributors and manufacturers develop alternative plans for your consideration. Positioning of the products, their price point and your decision to carry your own private label should be considered when setting sales goals.

- The staff must be educated and motivated to sell retail. Staff should be made aware of management's retail goals and their expected role in achieving the goals.

- In-salon training programs must include client consultation and product knowledge. Product knowledge should encompass all products sold in the salon or spa, *and* by major competitors.

- The staff should participate in an incentive program to increase retail sales levels. The program should be designed

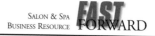

to run over a one-year period. At least quarterly — but ideally, monthly — there should be group recognition of individual and, when appropriate, team performance. Distributors and manufacturers often offer advertising and promotional programs to increase retail sales. Co-develop yearly event and/or activity grids that allow you to plan in-salon programs at least a few months ahead.

■ PROGRESS SHOULD BE ANALYZED AT LEAST EVERY THREE MONTHS. If not progressing as forecasted, make changes that will help you achieve your desired goals. Staff "behavioral" changes are generally the most important element in goal achievement. Often, a consistent management focus on increasing retail sales is more effective than increased incentives in helping staff commit to selling retail.

■ ANNUAL RECAPS AND PLANNING. At the end of the first year, there should be a formal recognition of the past year's achievement and the establishment of goals for the new year.

Things to do:

- Know your retail sales as a percent of *total sales.*

- Determine your retail potential. Where are you now — and where can you be?

- Understand and clearly communicate to staff the key ratios which measure retail performance.

- Know your retail inventory turns. Use the formula on page 304.

- Create a "selling system" by replacing sales negatives with sales positives, and providing solutions to clients' problems.

- Fine-tune your retail merchandising through efficient inventory control and proper product display.

- Master the *five P's* of retailing:
  PRODUCT
  PLACE
  PRICE
  PROMOTION
  PEOPLE

- Develop relationships with your distributors and sales consultants. Learn about your sales consultants' expertise, establish a game plan and work by appointment.

- Review the retail sales management checklist on page 329–330, and apply each item to your business.

10

PUBLIC RELATIONS

It's time to get the right word out

GUEST CHAPTER BY:
> Larry Oskin, President
> MARKETING SOLUTIONS, INC.

Quality public relations programs are not extra costs of doing business. They are designed to ensure your long-term salon success, and are therefore an investment in the future. A strategic PR program will earn tremendous rewards and client loyalty for years to come. Though you cannot expect overnight success, PR is a valuable marketing element that must be treated with professionalism, care and respect. It requires a long-term commitment. One or two press releases a year is not sufficient for success. *A quality PR program never ends.*

THE MOST IMPORTANT PR STRATEGY IS TO HAVE ONE. Salons that earn consistent exposure through creative, strategic PR objectives, calendars and action plans will reap the rewards of successful media relations. The first steps in public and media relations can

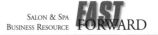

be tricky, sometimes even scary. Preparation is key, especially if you have never attempted PR before. Your leadership skills and salon vision will be put to the test in coordinating the many elements of a successful PR campaign.

Public and media relations

Public relations is…the business of inducing the local community, the nation and the industry to respect your salon, its team and the overall professional beauty business through the creation of news, promotions, community involvement and media exposure.

Today, public relations should be more broadly thought of as "media relations." It consists of much more than mailing press releases to editors in the hope a story will result. There are terrific opportunities for PR through local, regional and national magazines; radio and television shows; and the newspaper media. But you will need to create a PR plan before "pitching" the media.

Do you need PR positioning?

It is important to make headlines. Today, you need to do much more than simply open your salon for business. A strong media relations program will help your salon become known as *the* most respected beauty resource in town. Start blowing your own horn!

Public relations will become one of your most powerful and cost-effective marketing strategies if local, regional and national media are effectively used to build awareness, credibility and a professional salon reputation. Public and media relations should become the foundation of your salon's marketing plan.

Salon symptoms and challenges

Compile a list of reasons why you need public relations and media exposure before creating strategic PR objectives and searching for solutions to major business growth challenges.

- Do you have a distinctively unique and attractive salon — that no one seems to know about?
- Are total salon sales flat or sluggish compared to last year's performance?
- Will you soon introduce a new day spa or an additional location that requires and deserves media attention?

- Does your salon offer new and unique services of which clients are not aware?
- Do you want to increase new first-time client opportunities?
- Does your salon have high client turnover, and need better client retention totals?
- Do you need more salon professionals and technicians to recognize the salon as the most prestigious place in town to work, and to inquire about and apply for positions?

A critical difference

Public relations is not paid advertising! You may pay a fee to a professional public relations agency for the creation of a public relations program, but the resulting stories in newspapers and industry trade publications do not require payment for the space occupied. Therefore, there are no guarantees with PR. The final story angle and editing lies within the hands of the editors.

Likewise, a sales or promotional event is *not* public relations. Community involvement programs and charitable fundraisers can often lead to tremendous PR exposure, yet these types of marketing activities are more properly labeled as salon promotions.

THERE ARE FOUR PRIMARY PUBLIC RELATIONS CHANNELS:

- Local consumer outlets
- Regional beauty trade resources
- National and international beauty trade outlets
- National and international consumer beauty and fashion resources

Strategic PR objectives and goals

Create and prioritize a list of five to ten public relations objectives. The objectives should be synergistic with your mission statement, vision statement and your annual marketing program. Decide upon and detail the unique salon products and services you want to promote.

DEFINE ACCOUNTABILITIES. Develop action plans for each PR objective, assigning various projects to yourself and the staff. Where possible, set up specific, quantifiable and measurable goals for each PR objective. *Sample strategic PR objectives:*

- Build consistent, unique name brand awareness for your salon, utilizing the trade name and logo. The salon mission statement is your guiding force.
- Develop a professionally prepared salon PR media kit, including reprints of published articles.
- Develop a comprehensive PR calendar to maximize all haircare, nailcare, skincare, spacare, retail and gift certificate sales.
- Position yourselves through local, regional and national consumer media as the top fashion-forward, artistically talented and creative salon team in your city.
- Position your salon through the national and international beauty trade media as one of the top fashion-forward, artistically talented and creative salon teams in your country.
- Generate a steady stream of high-quality new clients and referrals through media exposure.
- Position total image makeovers and beautycare spa packages as two of your top PR position statements.
- Partner with the community at large, targeting at least one local and national charitable cause each quarter of the salon marketing calendar.
- Enhance professional salon staff recruitment and retention.
- Promote the entire team, and each of their unique specialties.
- Research, hire and facilitate the work of an external marketing and PR agency to professionally represent you and your team.

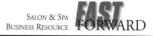
Develop a unique salon marketing niche

Establishing a targeted salon business niche will make publicity easier to attain. Stay on the cutting edge by developing a list of unique salon service advantages and promoting them in your new public relations programs. You need to be distinctive, rather than simply another salon. For example: You may strive to be known as a "progressive haircolor salon," a "children's salon," or a "holistic day spa." A unique marketing niche will become your PR magnet.

PR calendar

An annual public relations calendar and accompanying action list will help you systematically manage a complete PR program. Determine specifically what you want to promote each month and season of the year, based upon the media's needs, your marketing calendar and, ultimately, the salon clients' seasonal needs.

Plan well in advance to promote seasonal beautycare trends, spa services, gifts of beauty, makeovers, innovative new services, hair fashions and total image beautycare services. Request annual editorial calendars from every publication and media company you plan to target, and always attempt to meet their calendar needs.

Local or national media exposure?

I f you are launching a campaign of your own or plan to work with a local public relations agency or publicist, plan to work first with local media. You should have two goals:

■ DEVELOP A BRAND NAME.

■ GAIN EXPERIENCE WORKING WITH THE MEDIA.

Take advantage of your local PR agency's best assets and existing contacts. The news and beauty media are always hungry for quality editorial and fashion features...but surprisingly few salons attempt well-planned, long-standing PR programs. It *will* place you apart from and ahead of the competition.

Over time, a consistent public relations program will generate a media track record which positions your salon as *the* local professional beautycare resource. You will command more respect from local editors and television producers than other nearby salon, spa and beauty store owners who claim to be newsworthy resources. Provide creative, resourceful ideas to your media contacts, so they will come back for more in the future. Local PR will bring in new clients, and make your regulars even more loyal. It will help the salon sell its services and products.

What does national exposure buy?

National consumer and beauty trade media exposure buys more local and national media exposure...and offers a unique level of prestige, position, name awareness and credibility. Local editors are besieged by everyone who wants media attention. However, salons that achieve some level of national notoriety have in effect "proven themselves," and local editors will put their ideas on the top of the pile, due to their earned credibility.

National consumer and beauty trade media exposure is extremely powerful. It will bring you fame and, more importantly, the consumer exposure will attract many new clients. National beauty trade exposure will also draw new salon professionals to your salon or day spa.

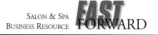
Begin your search for a publicist or public relations agency by looking for the authors of PR stories in beauty trade publications. These agencies are listed in the AMERICAN SALON GREEN BOOK and the MODERN SALON SOURCE 2000 directories. Ask respected professional beauty trade editors and publishers for recommendations.

Salon industry publicists and marketers already know many of the national beauty magazine editors. Encouraging relationships between these salon industry PR professionals and your local media contacts is important.

There is tremendous value in approaching the national beauty *trade* editors to build your salon's credibility and reputation with the media. Local and national *consumer* beauty editors have great respect for salons that gain national prominence within their own trade publications. A sound PR program starts with both the national and local beauty trade media, moving to the highly competitive consumer media once you have earned a reputation.

Hiring a professional agency

Agreements and retainers

Most local and salon industry-specific public relations agencies will work only on an annual retainer agreement, and rarely on a project-by-project basis. Retainers require a mutual long-term commitment, but usually create a more comprehensive and affordable PR program for salons that have the budget.

Annual retainer agreements are paid monthly. Base retainer fees usually start at $2,000 to $3,500 per month. Beyond that, one should expect to pay all out-of-pocket expenses such as telephone, fax, postage, delivery services, photography and printing. Before thinking you cannot afford it, consider the value of this investment in relation to your entire marketing and advertising program. Filling a full-time position with a staff marketing director would be just as costly, and the person hired probably would not have the salon industry experience or contacts of a professional agency.

WHATEVER IT TAKES: Retainers are a sensible investment for a serious long-term approach to salon marketing. Agencies on retainer will usually do "whatever it takes" to do a first class job. Whether designing graphics, writing newsletters or pitching the media, they will be your best representatives, often representing salons more professionally than the owners can do themselves.

RETAINERS VERSUS INDIVIDUAL PROJECTS: It may be more expensive in total dollars but, in the long run, an annual retainer is more cost-effective than working on a project-by-project basis. You can prioritize the PR company's work and keep everything under control. Instead of merely pitching your releases, they will utilize their media contacts to bring numerous PR opportunities your way.

There is a big difference

Most local medium-to-large city advertising and PR agencies often charge at least $5,000 to $10,000 or more on a monthly retainer. These companies may also charge 15%–20% more in

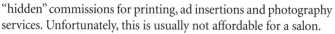
"hidden" commissions for printing, ad insertions and photography services. Unfortunately, this is usually not affordable for a salon.

■ EXTRA CHARGES: Printing and photography may be your most expensive add-on PR investments. For example: A professional photo session with a salon industry hair, makeup and spa expert may cost $1,500 to $2,500 or more per day, plus the cost of models and wardrobe. Printing costs will vary with the job; a PR media kit may cost several thousand dollars, though you may use it for several years. Reprints will be $100 to $200 per set, depending upon whether you provide camera-ready art and half-toned photographs.

Check references

Good references are much more important than a cost savings of $25 per hour or $250 per month on a retainer agreement. Review the areas of expertise, success stories, credentials and client list of *any* potential freelance writer or public relations agency.

Return on investment

Professional second- or third-party representation makes a salon appear much more credible. (CONSIDER: You don't like it when clients cut, perm or color their own hair. The same holds true here.) Put your public relations in the hands of a professional. Even if you hire someone to work part-time every week and month, it could represent a large cost-savings over working on a per-project basis.

Don't expect an overnight success story with your marketing, advertising or public relations plans. It takes time. And be careful…cheaper PR isn't always better. Like anything in business today, you will get what you pay for. Make your program an investment you will be proud to share with everyone.

■ STOP THE PRESSES: PR is not just a short-term or single-event publicity gambit. Media relations must be an ongoing, never-ending commitment to building your salon's success.

How to build name brand recognition

Energizing your salon through community awareness and public relations exposure is important for attracting both clients and staff members. You cannot afford to remain "the best kept secret" if you want to grow and succeed. With salons in virtually every major shopping center today, you must utilize a sound public relations campaign to maintain a competitive edge. You must continually create exciting *buzz* about your salon and its team.

Powerful public relations doesn't happen by chance. You must first create a sound strategy, with specific pre-determined objectives and goals. Study the opportunities and challenges of local consumer PR, as well as those of national consumer and beauty trade exposure. You must understand the limitations and guidelines of professional media relations, before becoming over-zealous in your expectations.

The media are always looking for exciting news. Create the opportunity for beautycare PR features through *calendar options:*

■ List several potential feature story ideas per month, and then decide which to pursue.

■ Plan to develop each story idea well in advance of media deadlines, but keep its news value timely.

Most PR stories need to be submitted (with photos) to the local media at least one month prior to any calendar or seasonal date. Stories such as makeovers can be promoted any time of year, but with distinct seasonal themes. Regional magazines and some television talk shows require at least two to four months of advance planning.

Public relations action plans

D etermine whether you and your staff are capable of managing a salon public relations program — or if you need to hire a freelance publicist, local PR agency or nationally respected beauty trade marketing services agency. Then, assign selected projects to staff members with public relations experience or to external PR resources, while you manage the overall program.

Use an *action list* to avoid last minute knee-jerk approaches that may offer weak results. The action list should include a preplanned time line to assist in meeting necessary deadlines. Though various projects on your PR calendar may overlap, each should have someone in charge of it, and specified mini-deadlines to ensure timely planning, implementation and facilitation.

Media releases and kits

A complete salon media kit is vital to your success with media contacts, investors, and potential staff members and clients. A media kit is a collection of materials used to convey the salon's message and tantalize the editor, writer or television producer. In the salon industry, a PR kit can promote a business, introduce team members, and highlight accomplishments or awards. (Such kits are sometimes referred to as "backgrounder kits.")

Even though it is often best to leave the creation of your public relations kits and media releases to professionals, one should learn as much as possible about preparing and formatting releases and cover letters. Media kit design should be limited only by the power of your imagination.

Key elements to consider:

■ THE SALON STORY: Include a professionally written and printed story explaining your salon's unique position, its services, products, staff, awards and achievements. This should be a one-page history of the salon, including a brief description of recent charitable work, previously published articles and photos, and your slogan.

- BIOGRAPHIES: Include single-page summaries of the accomplishments of each key member of the salon team, from owners to artistic directors. Spa directors, haircolor directors and others may also be added. Biographies should include the salon logo, address and telephone number, and each person's title and photograph. If there are more than five people, consider using half-page biographies.

- BROCHURES AND SERVICE MENUS: Include sample copies of your salon brochure, newsletter, marketing materials, fact sheet and business cards.

- PR REPRINTS: Always include copies of any previous media attention and published articles.

- PHOTOGRAPHS: Always include professional quality photographs such as exterior and interior shots of the salon; creative hair-, nail-, skin- and spacare service photos; and makeovers, when possible. Include a few extra fun photographs of the team or of special events. Often, 35MM slide transparencies are preferred.

- MEDIA KIT FOLDER: The presentation should be attractive, perhaps incorporating gold foil labels embossed with your logo that can be affixed to a colorful folder.

- COVER LETTER: A personalized cover letter ("pitch"), informing editors and producers when the story is to be released, should accompany each release — especially if you're promoting a special salon event for a specific date. This will ensure timely news value. Indicate whom editors should contact for further information. List your name, title, address, phone, fax, and e-mail and web addresses on the top of the first page.

- THE RELEASE: Start with a newsworthy or clever headline. It must be strong; the first sentence should clearly state what the story will be about. Make releases short and sweet. Try to keep each to a single page.

- SURPRISE EXTRAS: Small gifts, promotional items, logos, confetti and extras may be included. However, make certain they are related the announcement.

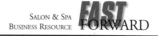
Target media lists

A *target media list* should include all local and regional newspapers, magazines and other publications. Don't be afraid to add some radio and TV talk shows, as well as broadcast news reporters who occasionally cover fashion features. Add the names of various beauty, women's, lifestyle, business and news editors. Your local library maintains annually updated directories of these contact names.

Check regularly in the local media for stories on beauty, fashion or women's businesses, written by both regular and freelance writers. These should be on your media list. Also include professional national beauty trade magazines, so you can share public relations success stories with other salon professionals. Keep your target media list fresh through continuous updates.

Exploring the costs of salon PR

Costs associated with public relations should be considered *investment spending*. Even though media exposure is free, and very different from paid advertising, PR takes a time and budget commitment to be successful.

■ INVESTMENT VERSUS COST: The costs associated with ongoing PR are not easily translatable into a specific return on investment. You don't have to engage in salon marketing, advertising or PR to attract new clients or keep the clients you already have. However, without these critical business investments, you may someday find yourself out of business.

Budget guidelines

How much money should be invested? Most salons budget at least 3%–8% or more of total sales for marketing, advertising and public relations programs. A PR budget usually falls within the marketing budget. Thus, it could represent one-third, one-half or even up to two-thirds of the total marketing budget. Though we recommend it be at least one-third, this budget guideline is a personal decision of the salon owner. The only wrong decision would be to have no budget allocations at all.

Local freelance writers and publicists

Local freelance writers and publicists usually sell their services on a project or hourly basis. Though freelance writing is different than freelance PR services, freelancers' costs will run at least $25 to $100 or more per hour, often falling between $50 to $85 per hour. Freelancers will sometimes have a minimum fee of a half day, especially with new clients.

Public relations costs in large metropolitan cities may be higher. Writers' guidelines suggest a charge of $100 to $150 per page or per hour on a press release. Writing and designing a simple media kit will probably cost at least $500, perhaps up to $2,500, depending upon the extent of the project. For example: A single grand open-

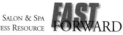
ing press release from a freelance writer may only cost $200, while facilitation of a complete grand opening media kit with mailings to key media targets and follow-up calls will cost at least $2,500.

Whether you pay postage and long distance toll charges to reach the national media yourself, or pay them as an expense to a contracted salon industry PR specialist, the costs will be the same. These charges will also be incurred with local publicists. Your cost savings will lie in the fact that local publicists are easily accessible. However, local resources may not know how to approach national consumer beauty editors, and it is unlikely they would have relationships with the national beauty trade media contacts.

Variable costs

There are numerous financial variables to consider before calculating the total cost of using a local or a salon-specific freelance person. First, will you provide the necessary information for the writer, and will you do the mailings? Will the writer need to do any research or assist you in setting up a photo session? Do you need publicists to research your target media list and facilitate mailings with personalized cover letters to each editor, or will you do that yourself? Will you conduct follow-up telephone calls on your own, or will you take advantage of their valuable network of editorial and media connections?

Public relations sources

Salon freelance writers and publicists

These talented people understand the professional salon industry niche, even if they are not conveniently located in your neighborhood. Surprisingly, their costs per hour and per project are equivalent to local freelance resources. A single press release page will still run $50 to $100, or up to $250 or more, depending on the assignment. (A charge of $50 to $100 per hour is normal.) Salon industry freelancers charge by the estimated time it takes to research and create each project, as do local resources.

THE DIFFERENCE: Industry freelancers may not have existing *local* media contacts, but they do have *national* consumer and beauty trade contacts.

Salon PR and marketing agencies

Professional public relations is an art. Those who are successful at it create images, build awareness and stimulate exposure while creating both news and feature stories. An investment in a professional external PR resource is an important consideration for your future. It is difficult to professionally represent yourself. It is even more difficult to find a publicist or marketeer that really knows the professional beauty business.

There are a number of well-respected PR and marketing services agencies in the salon industry. Public relations agencies usually handle PR only, and do it extremely well. Full-service marketing agencies will help you create PR opportunities — plus advertising, marketing, promotions, special events, graphics and newsletters. Some offer business and marketing consulting services as part of their retainer packages.

■ USE PR AFTER THE STORY PRINTS: Getting attention from the media is important, but not as important as how you use that feature story or the television talk show *after the fact*. Not everyone will see your article or watch the news. Create in-salon window or wall posters that say, *"As seen in…"*, with a colorful framed reprint of the story.

- WALL OF FAME: Remember, it is not important that everyone see your story in the news or on television the month it comes out. Frame examples of media exposure and post them on your salon's "wall of fame." This gallery will impress clients for years to come.

PR: In the know

■ Personalization of stories, cover letters and follow-up calls works in attracting PR exposure; mass-produced form letters do not work as well.

■ Be careful not to bombard editors and media contacts with useless information and trivial ideas.

■ Realize that editors think in terms of exciting news and trend statements. Don't complain if they get your story or quote wrong or if your first mentions are minuscule!

■ Never criticize an editor for a mistake. If you do, it may be your last media exposure with that publication.

■ Never burn bridges with the media.

■ Follow up successful publicity and feature stories with a personal *thank you* note.

■ Never expect to make your salon an overnight success through PR. You'll build your salon's PR reputation one story at a time, just as you build your salon clientele one success story at a time.

■ If you take the time to properly build your media reputation, the editors will soon be calling on a regular basis!

This special guest chapter was written by Larry H. Oskin, president of MARKETING SOLUTIONS, INC., *a full-service marketing, advertising, public relations and consulting services agency specializing in professional beauty, salon and day spa businesses.* MARKETING SOLUTIONS *is headquartered in Fairfax, VA. For further information, call 703.968.0400 or e-mail at* mktgsols@aol.com.

Specialized Experts Who Can Create Your PR Program

AGENCY	HEADQUARTERS	TELEPHONE
Esche & Alexander	Oceanside, CA	760.414.3370
Anne Hardy PR	New York, NY	212.496.6585
JR & A Marketing & Creative Services	Los Angeles, CA	310.286.9940
Norma A. Lee Company	New York, NY	212.750.2012
Marketing Solutions	Fairfax, VA (Washington, D.C.)	703.968.0400
Morehouse Communications. Inc	Cleveland, OH	440.846.6022
Munshower Communications	Studio City, CA	818.734.2010
Vi Nelson & Associates	Chicago, IL	312.944.1262

FREELANCE PR WRITERS	HEADQUARTERS	TELEPHONE
Bersch, Suzanne	Montclair, NJ	973.233.9449
Chiger, Sherry	Stamford, CT	203.358.4386
Hill, Suzette	Roswell, GA	770.649.7598
Jewett, Barbara	El Paso, IL	309.527.5060

Things to do:

- Compile a list of reasons your salon or spa needs public relations and media exposure.

- Create and prioritize a list of five to ten PR objectives. The objectives should be synergistic with your mission statement, vision statement and marketing program.
  Decide which products and services you want to promote, and develop an action plan for each PR objective.
  Assign various projects to yourself and staff members.

- Develop a unique salon marketing niche. What makes your business different from the competition?

- Plan an annual public relations calendar. What will you promote each month?

- Build name brand recognition through community awareness and public relations exposure in order to attract both new clients and staff members.

- Develop a public relations media kit to promote your business.

WORLD-CLASS CUSTOMER SERVICE

How good do you want your salon to be?

T o move your salon toward true customer service excellence, you'll have to dig through years of preconceived notions, poor work habits and inefficient operating systems until you reach the very core of *why* you're in the salon business.

Begin your quest for service excellence with a question: JUST HOW GOOD DO YOU WANT YOUR SALON TO BE? The way you answer will say a lot about who you are, your business philosophy, performance expectations...and the price you're willing to pay for success.

Mediocrity is easy to achieve in business, because it requires only

FAST FORWARD Key Points

Without a customer service system, a client's perception of quality can vary significantly, depending upon which staff members he or she comes in contact with.

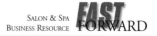
minimal attention to detail, supervision, planning and skill development. As with everything else in life, the *effort* of doing things right yields the best results. It comes down to the price you're willing to pay for discipline, standards and skill development.

This chapter touches the heart of the salon business — customer service. On the surface, one would think customer service to be rather straightforward. It's easy to say, "We're going to treat our clients like royalty." But what does this statement really mean to you, your staff members...and your customers? Do a little research. There are many opinions of what "treating clients like royalty" means. If you want to achieve customer service excellence, you must detail your service standards, and develop a system to ensure you and your staff continuously meet those standards.

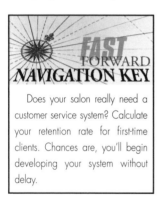

NAVIGATION KEY

Does your salon really need a customer service system? Calculate your retention rate for first-time clients. Chances are, you'll begin developing your system without delay.

Just how good you want your salon to be? Clearly, there isn't a salon or day spa owner alive who wants to deliver mediocre service. Yet, there is an abundance of salons and spas offering mediocre and inconsistent service...only because they lack a customer service system. Ask yourself another question: Does the level of service and attention the client receives vary from one staff member to the next? If your salon doesn't have a customer service system, a client's perception of service quality can vary significantly, depending upon which staff members he or she comes in contact with. Simply put, service quality is left to chance — and you're losing customers and sales because of it.

Achieving service excellence may seem like a lot of work at first, but it's probably more *fun* than the way you're doing business now. Service excellence means giving customers what they want — pleasant, satisfying and memorable salon experiences. It requires leadership, self-discipline, new communication skills and hard work, but it's fun and tremendously profitable.

Building a customer service system

A salon customer service system is a combination of plans, processes and practices designed to deliver (at a profit) the salon's services and products in ways which develop loyal clients. It is the practical extension and application of your salon vision and purpose. Because your system describes in detail the level of customer service it is committed to delivering, it will be an integral part of your mission statement. In the intense, personal nature of the salon environment, a customer service system is at least of equal importance as technical skill.

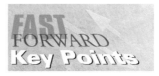

Service excellence takes research, planning and plenty of fine-tuning — and it all begins with a commitment.

Why develop a customer service system?

When customer service systems are neglected, client retention drops below acceptable levels. (MENTAL TICKLE: A salon's client retention rate is its True Quality score. So is its customer service quotient.) An industry-wide first-time client retention rate of only 30% clearly indicates that many salons operate every day with no systems to ensure service standards are met.

To get a better picture of just how important a customer service system is, compute the costs of delivering less-than-exemplary service. *Examine the chart on page 362.* How many clients of each level do you have? What does it cost to replace lost clients? What does it cost to redo services? Do these clients come back? What does it cost when competitors whittle down your share of the market? What do you lose when appointments are confused, or clients forget to show up?

IF THE SALON DOING WELL NOW, how much *higher* might profits and sales grow with an effective salon customer service system in place?

Mining your computerized database

D etailed information is a customer service necessity. Building a service system based on unsubstantiated opinions and beliefs creates more problems than it solves.

Today, more and more salons depend on computers to store and analyze client data. A good system should meet the following requirements:

■ Ability to store a wide range of data (e.g., client, staff, distributor, operations, inventory, cash management).

■ Data is easy to input, update and retrieve.

■ Expandable database to meet growing salon needs.

■ Data and database operation is understandable to staff.

■ Programs and database can be linked to other systems (e.g., point-of-sale, accounting, banking, payroll).

Advantages of computerization

1. CENTRALIZED SOURCE OF DATA...

■ for analyzing client service type, sales, frequency and trends.

■ to balance client exposure to different staff members.

■ for analyzing trends relative to types of customers serviced and client satisfaction levels.

■ to identify profit-producing services and products.

■ to identify relationship of staff skill competency to client satisfaction and profit.

■ to correlate promotional efforts to sales levels through market segmentation (e.g., geographic, income level, age, gender).

■ accessible, yet safeguarded against improper use.

■ difficult for a departing or disgruntled staff member to download information (especially client lists).

■ to help staff members better serve clients, and receive positive reinforcement for their input in the system.

2. PROVIDES CLIENT-ORIENTED INTERACTIONS SUCH AS...

■ appointment reminders and scheduling.

- anniversary and birthday promotions.
- market-segmented promotions.
- staff refreshers (consultation reminders) before client contact.

3. PROMPTS SALON DECISIONS AND ACTIONS REGARDING...

- cash management, via categorized sales and staff performance statistics.
- inventory management.
- staffing requirements and additions.
- staff training and development.

Salon customer service system benefits

- Potential competitive edge.
- Enhanced client perception of salon's attention to clients.
- Potential for increasing service and product sales.
- Enhanced staff perception of salon's effectiveness and care for its staff.
- Salon growth and prosperity.

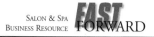
Implementing a salon customer service system

Planning: Surveying and assessing satisfaction and needs

CONSIDER THE CHART ON PAGE 362. *At what level are your clients now?* If they are mostly at level 2, your customer service system needs serious improvement. The first step is to collect the basic client data necessary to maintain contact and initiate feedback. If you are not yet computerized, now is the time.

If most clients are at level 3 or 4, and you are striving for level 5, the salon probably has a basic customer service system in place. Concentrate on obtaining more in-depth client information, fine-tuning your system to better analyze the data and using the data to more effectively manage customer service.

CLIENT PROFILE DATA SHOULD INCLUDE:

- contact information (e.g., name, address, phone, fax, e-mail).
- preferred days and times for appointments.
- type and frequency of service.
- product(s) purchased.
- client demographics (e.g., birthday, occupation, household income, children).
- client's interest level in the salon (e.g., service improvements, new services).

Define when, where, how, and by and from whom client data will be collected. Define how and by whom it will be accessed, analyzed, maintained, updated and used to contact clients.

Formal tools for collecting data include assessments and surveys, focus groups, and one-to-one structured interviews. A client satisfaction survey can yield valuable data for improving the client service and products offered. An effective survey requires:

- a pre-defined purpose.
- carefully structured questions or statements.
- a well-balanced presentation of topics and questions.
- no biased opinions from the salon.

- a plan for recording, analyzing and using the data collected.
- a commitment to use the data gathered to improve a service or product. (Clients must not perceive their efforts to be useless.)

COLLECTED DATA MUST BE USED TO IMPROVE SERVICE QUALITY. Effective use requires communicating the information to staff members for use, as well as analyzing the salon's performance and client base for specific market segments (e.g., geographic areas, client types, service clusters) to target for improvement.

Core competencies: Service skill standards

The core competencies of staff are vital to any service system. Determine the competencies (such as knowledge, skill and attitude) needed to develop level 5 clients. Hire only persons with these competencies, or those who can develop them with training.

PROVIDE TRAINING FOR ALL STAFF on the salon's values, vision, mission and objectives — and their roles in making each a reality. Provide training on client interaction, staff empowerment (to ensure client satisfaction), and specific techniques and technical skills to ensure quality service.

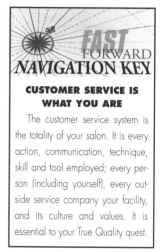

FAST FORWARD NAVIGATION KEY

CUSTOMER SERVICE IS WHAT YOU ARE

The customer service system is the totality of your salon. It is every action, communication, technique, skill and tool employed; every person (including yourself), every outside service company your facility, and its culture and values. It is essential to your True Quality quest.

Processes: Directing and controlling operations

Communication takes many forms, both *written* (e.g., promotional materials, advertisements, letters, surveys) and *oral* (e.g., requests, conversations, queries, speeches). It can also include body language, which often relays quite a different message than the accompanying verbal remark. *Listening* is vital to communication. Training staff members to become active listeners is critical in capturing "hidden" messages from clients.

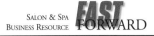
Consider a formal *complaint recording and resolution process* to capture additional information for your client profile database. This will provide two important types of information. First, you can track the resolution of a complaint, ensuring that the client is satisfied. Second, you can determine problem patterns and frequency, actions taken to resolve them, time to resolve, etc. This information should heavily influence your service system.

Another item often implied but seldom documented (or promoted) is an *unconditional guarantee.* Many business owners fear clients will take advantage of an unconditional guarantee. Yet the percentage of "cheating" clients is small. And the image of excellence perceived by a level 4 or level 5 client translates into a far greater payback than a few unjustified claims. Of course, your salon should already deliver top quality service and products before publicizing an unconditional guarantee.

WHAT IS YOUR CLIENT-LEVEL GOAL?

Five levels can be used to define your clients.

Where are your clients now? At what level do you want them to be?

IS THE CLIENT...	IF SO, THE CLIENT IS...
1. Dissatisfied?	Probably departed forever
2. Marginally satisfied?	Casual (any salon will do)
3. Basically satisfied?	Borderline, uncommitted
4. Delighted?	Retained, a return client
5. Committed...an advocate?	Loyal, loves your salon and tells others

If your goal is to have most of your clients at level 4, with many at level 5, your customer service system will play a vital role in achieving that goal.

Jill Griffin: Building salon customer loyalty

Client satisfaction is the traditional mantra of progressive companies, but a new focus has recently emerged — client *loyalty*. What's the big idea? Long-term customers generate the revenues which sustain your salon. It's time to take care of the people who take care of you.

Jill Griffin of THE MARKETING RESOURCE CENTER (and author of *Customer Loyalty: How to Get It, How to Keep It*), discusses the trend toward finding and keeping clients…and what it means to have truly loyal customers.

How can a salon turn a non-buyer into a raving fan?

Look at your customer development process stage by stage to discover how to *grow* clients. This turns the wheels, and creates sales and profits.

THE SIX CLIENT DEVELOPMENTAL STAGES ARE:
1. "Suspects" to prospects
2. Prospects to first-time customers
3. First-time customers to repeat customers
4. Repeat customers to clients
5. Clients to advocates
6. Reactivating inactive customers in the customer or client stage

These six steps recognize that people become loyal in stages, over time. Many salon owners will say, "But we call first-time customers *clients.*" You may call them clients, but they haven't yet truly earned that title, as shown by their purchase patterns. A first-time customer is still only a "tryer" to a salon and its staff.

Where do salons go wrong with prospects?

Many lack programs to turn a *first-time* customer into a *repeat* customer. Most salons merely break even, or even lose money, on first-time customers. It's crucial to move a first-time customer into higher stages of loyalty, where the real financial returns are. Many businesses, including salons, believe that if customers buy once, they will automatically buy again. Consequently, the average business spends five times more marketing to new customers than taking care of the ones it already has.

The behavioral patterns of loyal clients generate sales and profitability for the salon. A client advocate who leaves your salon is a far greater loss in terms of profitability than a first-time or repeat customer.

The average life span of a salon client is five to seven years. The lifetime value of a client is substantial; it warrants an investment. Salons that master customer loyalty skills can extend the expected lifetime of a client with relatively little effort (versus other businesses with fewer relationship-building opportunities).

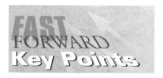

FAST FORWARD Key Points

A Harvard Business Review study states that if the average company could reduce customer defections by as little as 5%, it would boost profits by as much as 25%–85%.

SPECIFIC THINGS TO DO: Maintain an up-to-date database, including client purchase histories. Any database program will start the process. The salon industry has incredible financial potential because of clients' predictable repeat purchase cycle. They go *somewhere* every six, eight or ten weeks for salon services. Too few salons take advantage of database marketing.

Since there are so many opportunities for customer contact, are clients considered "disposable"?

Certainly that mindset is there, and I feel that everyone in the salon needs to be educated about the gains associated with a loyal clientele. A misconception I frequently encounter is that all customers are created equal. They're not. Each salon has clients who are more profitable than others. *Remember the 80/20 rule.* Eighty percent of revenues are generated from 20% of a business' clients.

Some salon teams have no clue who the most profitable clients are. Owners wonder whether to share this information in staff meetings. *Absolutely.* Let your staff know who the long-term and profitable players are in your salon.

And reward the upper echelons. If you rank the client base according to who is most profitable, chances are you will find they are the most loyal as well. We suggest special offerings for client birthdays, client purchase anniversaries or a salon birthday celebration for long-term clients.

What is the relationship between customer loyalty and customer risk?

Customers know what a bad perm or bad color is like, so when they find someone who performs a service to their satisfaction, they are reluctant to go elsewhere. But there will always be price shoppers who look for coupons in the newspaper when they need a service. Three months later, when they need another perm, where do they go? *Back to the newspaper.* Salons should proceed with caution with mass market coupon offers. By definition, you will attract price shoppers. Your ability to make them loyal customers is about one in a million. Many discount salons question their customer loyalty rate, but their marketing programs attract the very people who will not be loyal.

However, I am uncomfortable with hard-and-fast rules that say "never coupon." Even with high-end salons, savings certificates have a place when used appropriately. You need to find a niche, and be specific about whom you are targeting. THE MARKETING RESOURCE CENTER advocates *cross-promotion:* partnering with non-competitive businesses.

For example: Assume you have a client who works for an upscale firm. A cross-promotion would offer that firm's employees a special purchase privilege at the salon for a given month. It brings those people in (at a savings) for the first time. The salon must then transform first-time customers into repeat customers by building trust and broadening the services they buy. The more services customers buy, the less likely they are to leave. They can be "hooked" on loyalty-building services such as perms or color. You're less likely to get them in for these the first time.

It is in the salon's best interest to use the *hook* principle to turn these people into users of multiple services. They are a very specific market that has *already* been attracted.

Why does a customer stop buying from a business?

Most customers defect for "no special reason," which translates into benign neglect, and false belief that certain customers "belong" to the salon. Salon owners who think this way spend money on attracting new customers instead.

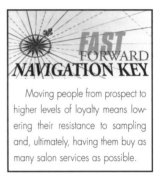

FAST FORWARD NAVIGATION KEY

Moving people from prospect to higher levels of loyalty means lowering their resistance to sampling and, ultimately, having them buy as many salon services as possible.

In my seminars, we talk about customer loyalty — beginning with attracting new customers. Inevitably, a hand will go up and a salon owner will say, "Our problem with this type of promotion is that our regular customers become angry because there's nothing for them." And they're right — you're not doing anything for them. They deserve rewards and recognition. When you graph promotional costs for these salons, virtually nothing is spent on the most valuable clients.

How can you tell when a customer is loyal?

Customer loyalty is a buying behavior. A loyal customer…
- makes regular repeat purchases.
- purchases across product and service lines.
- refers others.
- is immune to enticements from the competition.

The common denominator is that they produce dollars for a salon. *That's* why loyal clients are so valued. First-time or repeat customers do not meet these four points, but clients and advocates typically do. Clients become easier and more cost-efficient to service over time because you know what they want. Your profit margin can be much higher. At the suspect or prospect stage, the salon must do more expensive things to get them through the door.

When is a repeat customer not a loyal customer?

Business owners must secure a *share of customer,* not just a *share of market.* If a customer comes into a salon for services, but buys product from a beauty store, the salon has not won that customer's complete loyalty.

Think of customer spending habits as a pie chart. What percentage do they spend at your salon, and what do they spend elsewhere? The goal is to maximize your share of customers. Today's customers are time-deprived. They like exclusivity, where all of their services can be taken care of in one place.

What steps can be taken to build a loyalty-driven culture in a salon or spa?

We must start by raising salon and spa staff awareness about the value of loyal clients. Every staff member is a profit generator for the salon. But some people are not motivated by profit. We advocate not talking about profit at all, but about *loyalty* — because with loyalty comes profits.

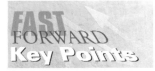

Salon and spa owners must tell the staff "what's in it for them" when the salon has loyal customers. Loyal customers ensure a continuous flow of business. They create opportunities for personal and professional growth, income stability and security for the entire team.

Many people define a loyal customer as one who buys from you again and again. I find that a loyal customer will <u>not</u> buy from your competitors.

Jill Griffin, author of Customer Loyalty: How to Earn It, How to Keep It, *conducts loyalty marketing seminars nationwide and works with a range of clients from Fortune 500 companies to law firms and small businesses. For more information regarding Ms. Griffin's consulting services, call 512.469.1757. Web site:* www.loyaltysolutions.com.

Share of customer…

New thinking: One-to-one customer service

To earn long-term customers who look to you for all their professional salon needs, you must deliver more than high-quality services and products. You must satisfy them completely, whether your salon is value-priced or a high-end day spa. If one element of the service experience fails to create value — from first contact to follow-up satisfaction calls — the salon/client relationship is compromised.

Salon culture: Team members add value or cost

VALUE-ADDED IS CULTURE-DRIVEN. It's as much a state of mind as a way of doing business. You cannot create or dictate value-added through rules or mandates at staff meetings. Creating a value-added environment requires changing your salon culture.

In his book, *Value-Added Customer Service,* Tom Reilly drives home some simple yet powerful points:

■ A value-added service culture is one in which everyone feels and acts accountable for satisfying clients. When the organization's people care about satisfying customers, they just naturally behave according to that attitude.

■ Employees either add value to what your business sells, or they add cost. Value-added begins with an attitude of service, and the behavior is "free." There is no cost to adding value-added behaviors to your business.

■ Employees' worth increases in proportion to the value they add through their service behaviors and performance. Do you encourage and reward the right behaviors?

Reilly's concept that team members either add value or cost to what you sell establishes the absolute basis for creating a value-added culture. For example: A stylist sees by her client's body language and facial expressions that she dislikes her new hair color but is reluctant to talk about it. The stylist can choose to ignore the problem and wait for the client to express her dissatisfaction, or take responsibility for satisfying the client and say, "I see you're uncomfortable with the results. Your satisfaction is most important to us. Tell me your concerns so we can address them." Too many clients don't complain — and don't come back.

In a value-added salon culture, the stylist will naturally put client satisfaction first in this value-added "moment of truth." The client sees commitment, caring and collaboration. Trust and loyalty are established. Ignoring the problem may mean losing the client forever — and thousands of dollars in revenue and referrals. *The right behavior is free. The failure to act is costly.*

New thinking: "Share of customer"

A VALUE-ADDED CULTURE EVOLVES WHEN A BUSINESS SHIFTS FROM "SHARE OF MARKET" THINKING TO "SHARE OF CUSTOMER" THINKING.

Every business, every salon, wants to attract more customers. But today's glut of mass market advertising makes it difficult and costly. Intense competition has spurred a sense of urgency in salons to discover new marketing and value-added strategies to set them apart from the crowd. For most, especially large salon day spas, a

CALCULATING A CLIENT'S LIFETIME VALUE	
Average client ticket	.$42
Visits per year	.7.5
Client life cycle	.6 years
Cost to retain client during life cycle	.$120
(based on $20 per client per year)	
Total individual lifetime value	**.$1,770**
Average new clients from referrals	.5
(family members, friends, co-workers, acquaintances)	
Total lifetime value of referrals	.$8,850
Total client lifetime value	**.$10,620**

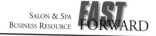
value-added culture is the most powerful and differentiating strategy they can ever hope to master.

Share of customer thinking runs contrary to traditional share of market thinking. Instead of marketing services and products to the masses, you collaborate with customers to discover and satisfy individual needs. The prime objective is to gain the maximum share of each customer's professional salon service and product business. This one-to-one approach is driven by your salon's intimate knowledge of each customer. It capitalizes on every bit of information in your records and computer database, enabling you to find your best customers and blow them away with incredible value-added service and delivery.

How much share of customer?

Do you really know how much service and product your best customers will buy from your salon? There are some very impor-

FOCUS ON NEW CLIENTS	
Bring in 50 new	$2,250
Retain 10 existing clients	$200
Total marketing cost	$2,450
Total customers	60
Annual sales projection	$8,190
(based on annual per-client sales of $315 with a 32% first-time client retention rate)	

FOCUS ON CLIENT RETENTION	
Bring in 10 new clients	$450
Retain 100 existing clients	$2,000
Total cost	$2,450
Total customers	110
Annual sales projection	$31,500
(based on annual per-client sales of $315 with a 55% first-time client retention rate)	

tant differences among your customers. Your database offers the biggest clues to answering the following four questions:

1. WHICH CUSTOMERS ARE YOUR MOST VALUABLE, AND WHY? Not all customers are valuable customers. It could be that 80% of your business comes from 20% of your best customers. Find out who they are and develop special value-added programs that cater just to them (e.g., preferred/frequent buyer cards).

2. WHICH ONES WILL GIVE YOU MORE BUSINESS BY REFERRING OTHERS TO YOU? Your clients' family members, friends, working associates and professional relationships all represent potential new business. Explore new strategies to get clients involved in growing your salon (e.g., bonuses for new business).

3. WHICH OF YOUR CURRENT CUSTOMERS ARE NOT WORTH CATERING TO AT ALL? Every salon owner knows that some customers are high maintenance and low profit. Sometimes it's in the salon's best interest to fire a customer.

4. WHICH PROSPECTS WOULD YOU LIKE TO CONVERT TO CUSTOMERS? Once you know who your best clients are, you have a profile to help you find more.

The value-added paradigm

The old mass market approach spent more time attracting new customers than servicing and growing existing ones. One-to-one marketing is the wave of the future. Value-added service will differentiate the "winners" from those who fail to recognize the need for change.

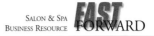
Customer service consistency
works in real life

A client's most important visit to the salon is the first. The experiences of that visit will influence the decision of whether to become a faithful customer or to go somewhere else. Consequently, it is important for salons and spas to develop procedures to assure each new client of better-than-satisfactory service. Technical and interpersonal skills must be employed in tandem. Many salons have learned how to do this. Here, salon owners detail their first-time client service procedures.

HOW MANY SALON OWNERS CAN HONESTLY SAY: "Everything we do is about retention"? Kay Hirai of STUDIO 904 in Seattle, WA, can and does. The STUDIO 904 team developed and implemented a client satisfaction policy they call LSPA. Adhering to their *Listen, Share, Permission, Action* rules has earned great retention benefits for the salon by ensuring consistency in each client treatment.

Says Kay, "One important thing we do is hold 'quality circle' meetings which begin fifteen minutes before the salon opens. Everyone is paid for the time — or counted tardy if late." At these meetings, the coordinator reviews the day's schedule (each technician is provided a printout) and new customers are discussed. "We try to give as much information as possible to the designers and technicians: by whom the new clients were referred, whether they are another client's relative. We are very aware and communicate well with each other so clients can get the attention they deserve."

John Robert DiJulius, of JOHN ROBERT'S HAIR STUDIO & SPA in Mayfield Heights, OH, concurs. "We have a total of about forty items that we go through every time a client walks through the door," he says. "We believe that the first visit starts on the phone. A client develops a first impression from the way the phone is answered. We always offer directions, ask if there is any other way we can be of assistance, and confirm appointments within twenty-four hours."

- Royal treatment: First-time clients in both STUDIO 904 and JOHN ROBERT'S wear white drapes.
- Scripted consultations: Upon entrance and exit at STUDIO 904, clients are asked questions such as *Are you happy?* Subjective questions yield more useful feedback than those that can be answered *yes* or *no*.

Another requirement at JOHN ROBERT'S is to offer clients additional appointments (e.g., a manicure in addition to haircut). The simple process of asking yields a 10% positive response rate, and introduces new clients to a spectrum of services.

Our guarantee...

A guarantee policy is a good idea for any salon. STUDIO 904 takes it a step further: *The Customer Trainer Program,* Kay explains, is designed to "keep customers in the circle." How does it work?

If a client is unhappy with a service, she may choose to become a participant in the program. She is invited to attend the team's Wednesday morning training classes and have her hair recut at no charge.

The benefit for the salon is not only in technical skill, but also in

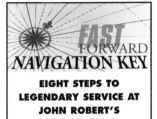

FAST FORWARD

NAVIGATION KEY

EIGHT STEPS TO LEGENDARY SERVICE AT JOHN ROBERT'S

1) FIRST PHONE IMPRESSION: Exchange information; explain staff education; make appointment; offer additional appointments; give directions.

2) FIRST VISIT: Client greeted within 8–10 seconds; new client cards; operator notified; salon tour and refreshments.

3) CONSULTATION: Use portfolio every time; conduct a needs analysis; offer service and retail recommendations.

4) SHAMPOO: 3–5 minute stress relief treatment; explanation of product used; all new clients in white cape.

5) TECHNICAL SERVICE: Properly executed; professional conversation; lesson on how to maintain and duplicate style; product recommendations.

6) EXCEEDING CLIENT EXPECTATIONS: Makeup touch-up; jewelry cleaning for manicure and spa services; complimentary bang trims; free blow-dry lesson; referral incentives.

7) END OF FIRST EXPERIENCE: Compliments all around; display recommended products; schedule next appointment; new client package (service menu, newsletter, business cards).

8) CONTINUED CUSTOMER CARE: Thank-you, birthday cards; phone follow-up; newsletter; client appreciation events; community work; constant positive PR.

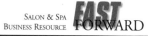
client relations: In such an intimate setting, clients "really talk," says Kay. STUDIO 904 also conducts customer callbacks. Says Kay, "It would be impossible to call all clients. We'll call every fifth one to get a random sampling for feedback." Questions cover employees' technical *and* social skills. It's just one more way a savvy salon owner can boost all-important retention numbers.

Fast-forward to team service

When it comes to teamwork, humans can learn from nature. CONSIDER: When geese fly in "V" formation, they can travel 73% farther than if each flew alone. Their honks encourage the leader to press on. When the leader can no longer maintain the pace, it drops back into formation. Another quickly moves up, and the flock continues on...*without skipping a beat.*

In the business world, no operational tenet has undergone more scrutiny and reengineering than teamwork. It's all part of the quest to be more efficient, more productive, more True Quality...and more customer-service driven. Terms such as *empowered* work groups, *quality* teams and employee *part-ners* are the order of the day. All of today's modern business practices are brought into play, including open-book management, process management, skill-based pay and team-based incentives. It doesn't matter if you're an auto parts manufacturer, a fine restaurant or a salon, staff must be involved in growing the business.

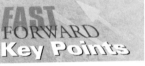

For team service to work, everyone must be responsible for every hour the salon has available for sale

The KEY POINT on this page challenges the perceptions of many salon owners: How well do their businesses really service clients as a team? There is a night-and-day difference between a salon's perception of team service, and the levels practiced in other industries that relentlessly pursue True Quality.

IF YOU'RE HAVING TROUBLE WITH THIS, ANSWER THESE QUESTIONS: Is each and every member of your staff, from coordinator to shampoo assistant, completely focused on growing the salon and pushing the numbers in the right direction...sales up and expenses down? Is there a "whatever it takes" commitment to customer satisfaction? Is everyone responsible for every hour the salon has available for sale — not just for their own chair or station?

Seven-step game plan:
Shifting from individual to team service

When you are ready to embrace team service in your salon, you will need an effective plan to make it happen. Designing your plan around these seven steps will benefit everyone (the staff, clients *and* you) through higher productivity and uncompromised customer service.

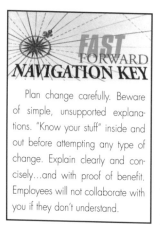

NAVIGATION KEY

Plan change carefully. Beware of simple, unsupported explanations. "Know your stuff" inside and out before attempting any type of change. Explain clearly and concisely...and with proof of benefit. Employees will not collaborate with you if they don't understand.

1. Understanding and consensus

Before team service will work in your salon, everyone must understand it. It's not simply an idea of sharing clients. There are many underlying factors that support team service: increased productivity and client retention, better service, salon growth, career growth. To move ahead, employees must agree that the salon needs team service. They must be shown how requests and stylist followings actually hinder growth. It takes more than a staff meeting, a memo or a drive-by announcement. As with any big change, educating the team must be an ongoing process.

2. Commitment to the cause

A single naysayer can destroy a team service environment. In addition to understanding, there must be commitment from *everyone* to the major objectives: client retention and productivity. These two items are the principal reasons for making the change to team service; they will grow the salon. Create a written *team service contract.* Post it in the dispensary to keep the commitment alive.

3. Redefine the customer service platform

- Make the skills of the entire staff accessible to every client.
- Educate the team: Waiting lists symbolize gridlock, inefficiency, poor service, lost sales…and, very often, lost clients.
- Accommodate customers when it's convenient for them — not when it's convenient for employees.
- Balance workloads to reduce staff burnout and boredom.
- Improve quality: Send clients only to skill-certified technicians.
- No client or service sale ever leaves the salon if hours are available for sale and the client will see another technician.

4. Create team service systems

The switch to team service must include revamping and standardizing critical salon systems. Team service can only work if these systems support the new environment. For example: Rethink the way the telephone is used to sell appointments. What does the reception team tell clients if they can't get a convenient appointment? Are they left frustrated by a lack of options, or are solutions explored?

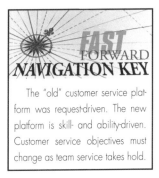

The "old" customer service platform was request-driven. The new platform is skill- and ability-driven. Customer service objectives must change as team service takes hold.

USE THE TELEPHONE TO START THE TEAM SERVICE BALL ROLLING. Make clients aware of their option to utilize all the salon's skills. Explain how your salon is different, how teamwork provides a more thorough service. Showcase your skill certification program to build their confidence.

CONSULTATION SKILLS ARE IMPORTANT. Every new client consultation must detail the team service concept. Clients need to know from the start that your salon is committed to True Quality, and will service their needs as a team.

HINT: "Double-team" consultations to give clients a broader perspective of the business' capabilities, and first-hand exposure to team service. Most clients are reluctant to see other staff only

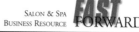
because they are unaware of their skill. Double-teaming and introductions can go a long way.

SKILL CERTIFICATION IS PART OF TEAM SERVICE. Training and team service go hand in hand; if clients are expected to try other technicians, the team must be trained and certified.

CLIENT INDOCTRINATION. If you don't already give new clients a tour of your salon…start. Familiarizing clients with the salon gives the coordinator a chance to introduce the staff. It's another great opportunity to reinforce the team service concept.

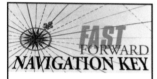

NAVIGATION KEY

The team service concept won't fully mature for several months. Throughout that period, maintain daily team reminders and updates on progress. Share all client feedback. Praise accomplishments and learn from mistakes.

5. Goal setting

What do *you* want to achieve through team service? Ask your team *their* goals. Clearly define each; then, track progress toward reaching them. Post the results on a scoreboard in the dispensary. Show the team how to compare goals to actual results. Update the scoreboard weekly, and celebrate successes frequently. The more the team is rewarded, the faster goals will be achieved.

6. Getting the word out

Create a team service column in your newsletter. Make it a focal point during consultations. Reinforce it on the telephone answering system. Advertise it. The message must be loud and clear. Clients looking for a change or for convenience will respond favorably. Team service is an effective client retention and sales tool.

7. Follow-through and maintenance

No matter what, remember one thing: *The change process is difficult.* People need encouragement and clear direction. If you encounter resistance or fail to reach team agreement: step back, clarify your approach and start again. In time, true team service will take hold and become part of your salon culture.

Team service contracts

A team service contract cements the concept of growth through teamwork, for both staff and clients. It's a written commitment for reaching defined goals.

The staff contract states exactly what the team is shooting for. Make it a team effort: Staff will adhere to a contract they help develop. When it is complete, hang it in the dispensary or staff break room. Visit it often. Maintain the drumbeat.

The client contract informs clients about the benefits of team service, and invites them to experience the options and conveniences it creates. Again, gather staff input. When the client contract is complete, make sure every client learns about it. Frame it for the front desk, include it in your service menu and print it on your business cards.

Use these templates to develop your team service contracts.

TEAM SERVICE CONTRACT FOR SALON STAFF

In its purest form, True Quality means continuous improvement and unconditional customer satisfaction. True Quality also means efficient use of resources, and teams of dedicated individuals focused on growing the business — going halfway just doesn't make the grade.

Unlike other salons, the skills of our entire staff are available to all clients. We regard waiting lists as a sign of inefficiency and lack of teamwork. Each and every team member takes responsibility for every hour on the appointment book. Our clients' schedules are more important than our own. As long as there is time on the schedule and the skill is available, we will accommodate their needs without inconvenience or delay.

We do not allow personal egos or clienteles to interfere with the service and satisfaction of our clients. We regard and service every client as a salon client. Always…without exception.

Client retention is our True Quality score. Our productivity rate is our efficiency score. Our commitment to team service is the centerpiece of our True Quality commitment.

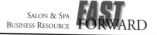
Team Service Contract For Salon Clients

Unlike other salons, we practice the highest form of team service. This means that the skills of our entire salon are available to you. We don't lock you into one stylist. We don't keep you on a waiting list. Meeting your salon service needs and busy schedule is our top priority. Not every stylist or salon technician is a master of all skills. We each have areas of expertise that, when combined under our guidance, offer you a palette of personal image-enhancement skills that are truly unrivaled.

To ensure consistent service quality and technical skill, each and every staff member must complete our in-salon skill certification program. That means you can always have confidence and peace of mind, knowing that you are in the talented hands of a skilled-certified team member. You will always have a fresh perspective, and you will always receive the utmost in True Quality salon service and attention — unconditionally guaranteed.

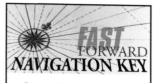

NAVIGATION KEY

Existing clients are accustomed to your <u>old</u> culture — not your <u>new</u> team service culture. They must be reindoctrinated and educated on the benefits of team service.

Failure to reindoctrinate existing clients will impede team service efforts and could cause old behaviors to resurface.

Invest the time and effort to adapt these contracts to your unique salon or spa environment. The process of creating these contracts will go a long way in defining the *governing values* of your business.

Educating clients on team service

You must have a team service *client education plan.* Unless clients know what team service is, they will not accept it. The salon or spa team must explain to clients why they should take advantage of the skills of the entire staff. If you teach clients well, the effort will be rewarded.

The scope of the salon or spa's client education program may mean the difference between True Quality customer experiences and mediocrity. Flying by the seat of your pants invites mediocrity. But if you choose to pursue teamwork and team service, you must plan thoughtfully and deliberately.

HINT: You actually need *two* plans for educating clients on team service: one for new clients, and one for existing clients.

New client curriculum

New clients need to be taught everything. All they know of the salon, they've heard from friends and co-workers, or seen in your advertising. So until they hear it directly from the team, they won't completely understand the "special" features. Create your team service education plan using the following standards:

■ The salon coordinator welcomes clients, tours the salon and introduces the entire staff; and offers a gift bag filled with samples, the salon menu and other information…including the team service contract.

■ New clients should complete a questionnaire asking their name, phone number, physical and e-mail addresses, and two questions: *"Why did you leave your last salon?"* and *"Do you know that the skills of our entire staff are available to you?"* The first question may reveal that they left because they couldn't get a convenient appointment with "their" stylist. These clients are ideal team service candidates. The second tells you if clients are inclined to try team service. If they say "no," they probably don't understand the benefits. It's time to educate. If they say "yes," education is still required, but to a lesser extent.

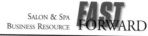
- Technicians conduct a consultation, inviting others to assist. This encourages client/team interaction.
- The technician explains the salon's service concepts. It must be detailed and effective, without sounding rehearsed: "Let me tell you a little about our salon. We are a True Quality salon, which means we are dedicated to making sure you are completely satisfied with everything we do. We also practice team service, so we can better assist you on *your* schedule. We keep detailed records so that any staff member may provide the service you desire. Plus, our in-salon training program ensures that, as a team, each member meets specific skill requirements. You may schedule appointments at any time, with any technician. Does team service interest you?" Ending with a question guarantees a response. No matter the response, explain team service benefits.
- When the service is complete, but before the client leaves the chair, team members should compliment the final results. Recommend future enhancements or services at this time.
- Remind clients that they can schedule their next appointment with any technician. Suggest one or more by name.

Existing client honor class

Existing clients should be handled differently. They are comfortable with the way the salon is. *It's why they come back.* Don't spring big, unexplained changes on them. Here's one possible plan to educate existing clients:

- Technicians should explain team service benefits (just as for new clients) during the consultation and service.
- Present it casually. Reassure clients they can see any stylist they want, so they now have even more options.
- They may need an incentive to try other stylists. Try a multistylist discount.
- After the service, encourage clients to take advantage of team service in the future.

It will take time for many clients to adopt team service because they have been taught to see only one stylist. Now you are training them to see something new and better — team service.

Things to do:

- Build your customer service system. Begin by asking yourself:
  JUST HOW GOOD DO I WANT MY SALON TO BE?

- Determine the information you need to collect from each client in order to improve service quality.

- Develop a customer service training program for all staff. Provide training on:
  CLIENT INTERACTION
  STAFF EMPOWERMENT
  SPECIFIC TECHNIQUES & TECHNICAL SKILLS TO ENSURE QUALITY SERVICE

- Implement a first-time client handling system. How will new customers be treated in your salon or spa?

- Build a loyalty-driven culture in your business by educating staff about the value of loyal clients.

- Review the seven-step game plan to team service on pages 376–378, and create a plan to implement them into your salon.

- Together, with the entire staff, develop team service contracts for the salon staff and clients.

- Develop a plan to educate salon clients on your new team service concept.

SALON & SPA NUMBERS MADE EASY

12

Understand your numbers...
and you'll never fly blind

Numbers can't lie. They will keep you honest. And they should tell a story — about the financial health of your business, its performance, and whether it's growing. Astute readers of financial statements can tell you volumes of information about your business, sometimes within minutes. They make the numbers "come alive."

Many salon and spa owners (and entrepreneurs collectively) find numbers difficult and challenging. Many despise accounting and recordkeeping, and avoid it like a contagion. Others find numbers boring and confusing, and nothing but a necessary evil. The end result is often frustration — so the business' operational numbers are either ignored or handed off to the accountant or another team member. Remember, you're *not* alone.

In their desire to avoid preparing the numbers, and the details of the process, salon and spa owners often miss the big picture and end up managing by the seat of their pants. *The more you know about the numbers of your business, the better your chances are for success.*

Internal versus external financial statements

Financial statements and other reports are necessary for both internal (management) and external (IRS, bankers, investors, etc.) purposes. It is therefore important to remember *why* you're preparing financial reports and *how* the information will be used.

EXTERNAL USERS HAVE SPECIFIC REQUIREMENTS for the format, style, frequency and content of financial reports. For example: Financial statements for tax filing and bank loans should adhere to generally accepted accounting formats.

INTERNAL REPORTS, ON THE OTHER HAND, can and should be customized to fit the unique needs of your business and the decision-makers using them. Internal reports should be user-friendly and help you quickly understand your financial performance in order to identify areas in need of adjustment and/or improvement.

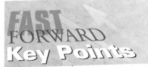

Numbers and financial reports keep you on top of your business. They help identify strong and weak performance areas. They are the key to making money and succeeding in business.

Cash versus accrual accounting methods

An accounting method is a set of rules which determines when and how to report the income and expenses of a business. You may use either the *accrual* or *cash* method for internal purposes. There are trade-offs with each: Accrual accounting will render a more accurate picture of the business, though cash accounting is simpler and less time-consuming.

You may not have a choice of which method to use for tax purposes. If you do, either method will have tax consequences...some of which may be significant. The IRS requires that you file tax returns using the same method each year. Changing methods will require IRS approval.

Cash basis

Under the cash-basis method of accounting, income (i.e., service, retail and gift certificate sales) is recorded when the money is received. Expenses are recorded when the bills are paid. It's simple: *Cash in...cash out.*

Accrual basis

Under the accrual basis, income is recorded when a sale is made, regardless of when the business receives payment. An expense is recorded when it is incurred, regardless of when the bill is paid.

THERE ARE TIMES WHEN BOTH METHODS YIELD THE SAME RESULT. For example: Because the majority of salon and spa sales are paid *upon delivery*, both methods will yield the same results.

GIFT CERTIFICATE SALES ARE AN EXCEPTION because payment is received prior to the actual delivery of the service or product. On an accrual basis, the income is not considered "earned" until the gift certificate is redeemed for a service or product, or when it expires. If gift certificate sales are a significant part of your business (as they are in many spas), the tax consequences can be dramatic.

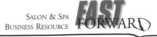
Gift certificates are not sales

The dollars a salon or spa receives for gift certificates are not service or retail sales, and should not be recorded as such when making deposits. Instead, they are best described as "loans" that clients make to your company — loans that have to be repaid. The proper term is *deferred income*. To illustrate:

■ A client comes in at the beginning of the day. She gives the coordinator $50 and says, "Keep this for me until later. I want to be sure to have $50 left for my hair and nail appointment at the end of my day."

Obviously, this money would be put aside until the client returned, and then used to pay for services at the time the sale actually occurs. If the client did not return, the money would be repaid rather than deposited because the salon did not earn it. It simply held the funds until the client reclaimed them. If the client did not return by the end of that first day, no entry would be made on the company's book for service or retail sales. *You cannot record the "sale" until the obligation is fulfilled.*

■ A gentleman comes in first thing in the morning and says, "I want to surprise my wife with a hair and nail appointment at the

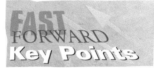

Key Points

A gift certificate purchase is an advance payment for services or products. The salon therefore incurs a liability and, under the accrual accounting method, gift certificate revenues should be recorded as a "liability" under the heading "Deferred Gift Certificate Income" on your balance sheet. When the gift certificate is redeemed, it becomes a "sale" and moves to the "Income" portion of your profit and loss (P&L) statement. Under a cash accounting method, it is considered a sale and recorded as income at the time of purchase. On a cash basis, you cannot defer taxes on unredeemed gift certificates. The accrual accounting method is best if you have an active gift certificate business.

end of the day. I cannot be here later; here is $50 to pay for her services." As in the preceding scenario, had the client not arrived for the appointment, the $50 given to the coordinator would not belong to the salon. You could not, in good conscience, deposit those funds and record that $50 as a service or retail sale.

This is exactly what happens with a gift certificate purchase. A client gives the salon money not for *services*, but for the *right to receive services* at a future date. This right is represented by the certificate, which the bearer may redeem for services or products. Consider it an IOU: The salon promises to provide services when the certificate is presented for redemption. There is no sale but, rather, a liability. The income is deferred until you earn it.

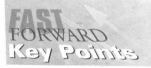

To avoid tax penalties, unredeemed gift certificate revenues should be moved from the "Liabilities" section of your balance sheet to the "Income" section on your financial statement after one year.

Using special accounts

For accounting purposes, it is imperative to show gift certificates as *liabilities* until they are redeemed. To record them properly:

- Meet with your accountant to discuss gift certificate sales, deferred income and setting up special accounts.
- Set up a special account (similar to accounts payable or taxes payable, which show the business' other liabilities) on the balance sheet of your financial statements. All gift certificates sold should be recorded in a special account called "Gift Certificates Outstanding" when they are deposited in the company's bank accounts. This is not a sales account, but a current liability.
- When the gift certificate is redeemed (i.e., services are rendered or products purchased) a *sale* occurs. The salon's income is earned, and its liability to the bearer of the certificate satisfied.
- A gift certificate is simply an alternate form of payment. When the transaction is posted, the company's books reflect the sale, and the "gift certificate outstanding" account is reduced.

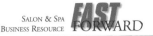

What about those unredeemed certificates?

UNREDEEMED GIFT CERTIFICATES MUST BE REPORTED UNDER "SALES" ONE YEAR AFTER THE ORIGINAL PURCHASE DATE. Leaving unredeemed certificates in the "outstanding" account for longer than one year puts the salon at risk for taxes due on unreported sales.

If an audit determines that the salon or spa should have recorded unredeemed certificates as sales, the salon may incur severe penalties and be held responsible for back taxes and interest. (The IRS has been known to seek interest and penalties for periods as far back as the original purchase date.) Proper accounting and compliance with IRS tax law is important for any salon or spa with a gift certificate business.

It is your business prerogative to honor gift certificates even after one year's time. But to make life simple, each should carry an expiration date of one year from the date of issue. Then a separate, in-house tracking system should be set up to monitor unredeemed gift certificates and record them as sales at the proper time.

Legally, you are obligated for only one year to honor gift certificates. Morally, however, many salons feel that outstanding certificates should be honored whenever they're redeemed. REMEMBER: If you honor outstanding gift certificates that are over one year old — and they have been recorded as sales for tax purposes — the redemption should *not* be deducted from the "outstanding" account.

Don't spend the money yet

GIFT CERTIFICATE MONEY IS NOT YOURS TO SPEND. Ideally, it should be held in reserve to defray the costs of providing services at the time of redemption. Remember, no cash will be generated at the time of service. Prudent cash managers put gift certificate proceeds aside in an interest-bearing account until they may be transferred back into the company's operating accounts for general bill paying.

HINT: Transfer, in advance, one-twelfth of the "gift certificate outstanding" account each month, in anticipation of redemptions and the variable costs of payroll and products.

Controlling your money

All you need is two simple things:
1. Understand the relationship between money and business activities.
2. Create and implement ongoing and straightforward money management tools and strategies.

A business is more than a money machine

Some people view business in strictly financial terms, as nothing more than a way to make money. But the financial side of business often intimidates others, who simply disregard finances as long as the bills get paid. While this may work temporarily, it ignores the great potential that lies within the business.

Each view is shortsighted, and both diminish the chances of achieving your strategic objective.

BUSINESS IS ABOUT MAKING YOUR LIFE BETTER...
NOT MERELY PAYING YOUR BILLS!

	Income Statement	Balance Sheet	Cash-Flow Statement
Describes	The financial **Performance** of the business	The financial **Health** of the business	The financial **"FUEL"** of the business
Time Period	Specific period of time (Mth., Quarter, Year)	"Snapshot"	Previous periods (Usually months)
Shows	Revenues and related expenses	Assets, liabilities, owner's equity	Receipts and disbursements

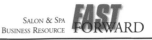
All you need to know about debits and credits

- Debit: recorded on the left side of a T-account.
- Credit: recorded on the right side of a T-account.
- Debits must always balance with credits.

How it works:

	Debit	Credit
Assets	Increase	Decrease
Liabilities	Decrease	Increase
Equity	Decrease	Increase
Revenues	Decrease	Increase
Expenses	Increase	Decrease

Some examples...

- The salon has revenues of $100.
- Cash (an asset) is debited $100 and Sales (Revenues) are credited $100.

- You borrow $100 from the bank.
- Cash (an asset) is debited $100 and Loans (a liability) is credited $100.

Financial statements

M any business owners rely on only one financial statement: the P&L (income statement). They do not understand or utilize two other primary financial statements: the balance sheet and cash-flow statement. The information provided by each is powerful. Combined, they are a series of business "report cards."

- **PROFIT AND LOSS STATEMENT**...shows business income and expenses over a period of time.
- **BALANCE SHEET**...a "snapshot" of the business for a specific date. The balance sheet is divided into three key parts:
  1. **ASSETS**: cash in bank accounts, accounts receivable (rare in salons), inventory, land and buildings, equipment and fixtures.
  2. **LIABILITIES**: accounts payable, deferred gift certificate income, mortgage payable, wages or commissions payable, notes payable, taxes payable.
  3. **OWNER'S EQUITY**: owners' or stockholders' stake in the value of the business. Ownership consists of the original amount the principal owners or stockholders invested to start or purchase the business, and any subsequent additions (called *capital* or *capital stock*); and any profits the company has accumulated and retained in the business since it began operation (called *retained earnings*). The owner's equity is the value that remains after all liabilities are met. The resulting "excess" is also known as the company's book value.
- **CASH-FLOW STATEMENT**...shows cash inflows and outflows over a period of time. This report will explain why an increase in profit does not necessarily equal an increase in cash.

Accountants have specific standards they must use in preparing business financials. These "rules" have been created to ensure that financial statements do not mislead their readers.

Data from financial statements can be used to create *ratios*. (We've included a number of key ratios at the end of this chapter.) Ratios compare various numbers from financial statements in order to reveal key relationships. Many are easy to create, and reveal important information regarding the financial performance and condition of your salon or spa.

What financial reports do for you...

- Give you an accurate, objective picture of your business.
- Reflect something real.
- Reflect something you do.
- Balance sheet: Describes the health of the business.
- Snapshot of what your business...
    1. Controls
    2. Owes
    3. And what is left over
- Income statement: The financial performance of your business; shows revenues and related expenses.
- Ratio analysis: Combines various line items and adds depth of understanding to financial dynamics.

Financial statements help you understand your business

- Help you quickly determine the health of the business.
- Allow you to easily measure performance.
- Are indispensable management tools: what's right and wrong.
- Help you with external reporting.
- Used for internal management purposes.
- Allow you to think about your business, the various parts of it, and how they work together to achieve a financial result.
- Help you make better decisions.
- A complete financial model of the vitality of the business.
- Give you objectivity and precision.
- Give you the whole view.
- Ratios provide insight into profitability/efficiency/solvency.
- Return on equity: Tells you if an investment is a good use of money.

Your cash plan: Managing the lifeblood of your business

- Gives you control of all activities that either receive or dispense cash.
- Gives you a reliable, accurate and all-inclusive source of financial information and documentation.
- Helps prevent cash-shortage surprises.
- Identifies strengths and weaknesses in your management systems (e.g., credit policies, payables).
- Helps anticipate cash needs in order to reach financial and business goals.
- Provides tools for communicating with lenders, suppliers and employees.
- Allows you to look at opportunities (e.g., money tied up).

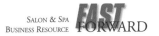

Calculating breakeven is easy

C osts and expenses must be recorded differently, depending upon whether they are *fixed* or *variable*. These differences can affect a salon or spa's income statement and may have a dramatic effect on the bottom line. NOTE: Few costs are entirely "fixed" or "variable." For example: Salaried or hourly technical staff, although paid a "fixed" wage, are variable costs because the cost of labor fluctuates with revenues. Administrative labor costs are always "fixed." Most of the costs of doing business have both fixed and variable components.

- *Fixed costs* remain constant from period to period, and are not influenced by changes in sales volume. General and administrative (G&A) expenses are predominantly fixed.

- *Variable costs* change from period to period, and *are* influenced by changes in sales volume. "Cost of Sales" expenses are variable costs. These include service payroll, service payroll taxes, retail product costs and professional product costs.

Breakeven calculations

1. CLASSIFY EXPENSES

    They are either fixed or variable. If your salon or spa uses a format similar to the model shown on the next page, it's easy to identify each. If your financial statements have all expenses grouped under one primary heading, you will need to specify each as either fixed or variable. The financial statement format shown here is the preferred model for salons and spas.

2. DETERMINE "VARIABLE PROFIT ON SALES"

    Subtract total variable costs from sales revenues:

$200,000	Total sales
−100,000	Total variable costs (cost of sales)
$100,000	Variable profit on sales

Continued on page 398

BREAKEVEN EXERCISE

MONTHLY PROFIT & LOSS STATEMENT

SALES

Service Sales	85.00%	$170,000
Retail Sales	15.00	30,000
TOTAL SALES	100.00%	200,000
COST OF SALES...	(Variable Costs)	
Service Payroll	34.00	68,000
Payroll Taxes	4.25	8,500
Retail Cost of Goods Sold	7.50	15,000
Professional Use Products	4.25	8,500
TOTAL COST OF SALES	50.00%	100,000
GROSS PROFIT MARGIN	50.00%	100,000

GENERAL & ADMINISTRATIVE EXPENSES...(Fixed Costs)

Admin. Payroll & Taxes	8.0	16,000
Advertising	5.0	10,000
Bank Charges	1.5	3,000
Benefits	2.0	4,000
Education	4.5	9,000
Interest	1.5	3,000
Maintenance & Repair	2.5	5,000
Miscellaneous	.5	1,000
Rent	6.5	13,000
Telephone	1.5	3,000
Utilities	1.5	3,000
TOTAL G & A EXPENSES	35.0	70,000
NET PROFIT	15.0%	$30,000

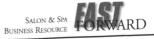
3. COMPUTE "VARIABLE PROFIT PERCENTAGE"
   Divide the variable profit on sales (step 2) by sales revenue:

   Variable Profit on Sales ÷ Sales Revenue = Variable Profit %

   $$\$100,000 \div \$200,000 = 50\%$$

4. CALCULATE BREAKEVEN
   Divide total fixed costs by variable profit percentage:

   Total Fixed Costs...$70,000 ÷ Variable Profit %...50% = $140,000

   If the salon in this model generates $140,000 in total revenues for the month, it will meet its breakeven requirement: Income will equal expenses, and there will be neither profit nor loss. Two significant conclusions may be drawn from this information:

   - There is a dramatic positive effect on profitability once the business' total sales revenue surpasses its breakeven point. In this model, sales exceeded breakeven by $60,000 ($200,000 – $140,000). This means that approximately 50% of every sales dollar beyond breakeven drops to the bottom line as *profit*. This is determined as follows:

   Net Profit...$30,000 ÷ Sales beyond breakeven...$60,000 = 50%

   - There is a converse effect on profitability when the breakeven point is *not* met. Assume that instead of achieving breakeven, the salon in this model generates only $135,000 in sales revenue. The following illustrates how this will result in a *loss* rather than a profit.

$135,000	Total sales
–67,500	Total variable costs (50%)
$67,500	Variable profit on sales
–70,000	Total fixed expenses
(2,500)	Loss

Proving your breakeven

To limit inaccuracies, it is prudent to "prove" your breakeven calculations by way of a confirming computation.

Breakeven sales revenue	$140,000
Less variable costs (50% of sales)	−70,000
Gross profit on sales	70,000
Less fixed costs	70,000
Net profit/(loss)	-0-

Forecasting and the cash-flow budget

The cost of doing business today leaves little room for error. Every expenditure must be planned, and realistic revenue goals set to ensure money is available when needed…and in the amount needed. Budgets alert business owners and managers that revenue and expenditures are either proceeding on course or are deviating from plan.

In this segment, we'll examine cash-flow budgets as a tool for monitoring operations and profitability. First, let's dispel a couple of myths about budgets.

■ MYTH #1: A BUDGET IS THE SAME AS A BUSINESS PLAN.

A business plan anticipates and provides for the future activities of an organization over a specific period of time (usually one, three or five years). It defines *what* a company will accomplish, and *how*. A business plan, however, does not detail costs, revenue or impact on the bottom line. That's where budgeting comes into play.

A budget should be an integral part of a business plan. It should separate the plan into specific sources of revenue and cost, and provide managers with a projection of the financial results of implementing the overall business plan.

■ MYTH #2: A BUDGET IS JUST ANOTHER FINANCIAL STATEMENT.

Not all financial documents are classified as financial statements. Financial statements are *after-the-fact* records of an organization's financial condition which may expose situations in need of management attention. The balance sheet and income statement are two such "historical" controls.

Cash-flow budgeting, on the other hand, looks forward in time. A budget is a projection of *future* revenue and expenses. Owners and managers generally use a budget in conjunction with financial statements in order to determine how well the business actually performed (financial statements) in comparison with its objectives (the cash-flow budget).

Creating your own cash-flow budget

To create a cash-flow budget for your salon or spa, you will need historical data on which to base assumptions. It's best to have financial statements for at least the last twelve consecutive months. These statements, combined with your revenue and spending objectives for the next twelve months, will provide the basis for "best guess" assumptions on the cash-flow budget.

Your cash-flow budget is your financial game plan, divided into twelve monthly "mini-games." The cash-flow budget shows revenue goals and spending budgets for each month. As you progress, revenues may be charted on a scoreboard to help the team remain focused on achieving objectives. Expenses should also monitored by comparing what has been (or is going to be) spent to what is planned in the cash-flow budget. This simple tool will enhance a salon or spa's bottom-line profits by helping the team reach target revenue goals and control expenses.

Cash-flow budget guidelines

- It's a "best guess." Some salon and spa owners labor over projections by over-analyzing, and trying to come up with an exact number. *Projections are simply best guesses.*
- If your best guess was too high or too low…guess again, and adjust the budget accordingly. Over time, your guesses will become more accurate. *Be patient.*
- Calculate G&A expense projections first. These are primarily fixed, and are easier to project.
- Calculate cost of sales projections second. These are variable costs, the biggest of which is service labor. Take your time in this area.
- Calculate service and retail revenue projections last. Consider seasonal fluctuations, staff availability, price changes, marketing efforts and other factors which may influence revenues.
- If you cannot justify the expense…*Cut it.*

SAMPLE SALON/SPA TWELVE-MONTH CASH-FLOW BUDGET

You can download this cash-flow budget template free from SALON BUSINESS STRATEGIES' *web site at www.strategiespub.com. Click on "Freebies." It is a Microsoft Excel® spreadsheet file. You will need Excel® in order to access and use the template.*

Developed by SALON BUSINESS STRATEGIES Magazine...800.417.4848					www.strategiespub.com				Copyright © 2000				
	Apr	May	Jun	Jul	Aug	Sep	Oct	Nov	Dec	Jan	Feb	Mar	TOTALS	%
Beginning Cash	1,000	5,541	10,158	17,085	26,673	32,623	40,107	46,766	53,743	69,905	67,952	72,189		
SALES&REVENUES														
Professional Services	44,000	42,000	46,000	49,500	48,500	48,500	48,000	50,000	54,000	46,000	46,000	50,000	572,500	75.15%
Retail	13,200	12,600	13,800	14,850	14,550	14,550	14,400	15,000	16,200	13,800	13,800	15,000	171,750	22.54%
Gift Certificates Sales	1,000	2,500	500	100	200	150	150	1,500	7,000	500	3,500	500	17,600	2.31%
TOTAL SALES	58,200	57,100	60,300	64,450	63,250	63,200	62,550	66,500	77,200	60,300	63,300	65,500	761,850	100.00%
Cost of Service/Retail Sales														
Service Payroll	19,152	19,152	19,000	19,000	21,000	21,000	21,000	23,000	23,000	23,000	25,000	25,000	258,304	33.90%
Team Bonus - Staff	0	908	923	1,385	1,918	1,190	1,497	1,332	1,395	3,232	0	847	14,628	1.92%
Professional Product (6% of Svc.)	2,640	2,520	2,760	2,970	2,910	2,910	2,880	3,000	3,240	2,760	2,760	3,000	34,350	4.51%
Retail Products	5,676	5,418	5,934	6,386	6,257	6,257	6,192	6,450	6,966	5,934	5,934	6,450	73,853	9.69%
TOTAL COST OF SALES	27,468	27,998	28,617	29,741	32,084	31,356	31,569	33,782	34,601	34,926	33,694	35,297	381,135	50.03%
GROSS MARGIN	30,732	29,102	31,683	34,709	31,166	31,844	30,981	32,718	42,599	25,374	29,606	30,203	380,715	49.97%
GENERAL & ADMINISTRATION														
Salaries: Admin & Support	1,536	1,536	1,536	1,536	1,536	1,536	1,536	1,536	1,536	1,536	1,536	1,536	18,432	2.42%
Officer's Salaries	6,000	6,000	6,000	6,000	6,000	6,000	6,000	6,000	6,000	6,000	6,000	6,000	72,000	9.45%
Accounting & Legal	240	100	100	100	100	100	100	100	100	100	100	100	1,340	0.18%
Advertising & Promotion	1,500	0	200	0	200	0	0	1,000	1,000	0	0	0	3,900	0.51%
Bank & Credit Card Fees	466	457	482	516	506	506	500	532	618	482	506	524	6,095	0.80%
Debt Payments (Loans-Credit Cards)	1,300	1,300	1,300	1,300	1,300	1,300	1,300	1,300	1,300	1,300	1,300	1,300	15,600	2.05%
Dues & Subscriptions	125	125	125	125	125	125	125	125	125	125	125	125	1,500	0.20%
Education	0	200	200	200	200	200	200	200	200	200	200	200	2,200	0.29%
Insurance - Employee Group	266	266	135	135	135	135	135	135	135	135	135	135	1,882	0.25%
Insurance - General	249	249	249	249	249	249	249	249	249	249	249	249	2,988	0.39%
Insurance - Workmans Comp	624	624	624	624	624	0	0	0	0	1,020	624	624	5,388	0.71%
Lease Payments	202	500	500	500	500	500	500	500	500	500	500	500	5,702	0.75%
Loan Payment	3,132	3,132	3,132	3,132	3,132	3,132	3,132	3,132	3,132	3,132	3,132	3,132	37,584	4.93%
Maintenance, Repairs & Cleaning	260	260	260	260	260	260	260	260	260	260	260	260	3,120	0.41%
Meals & Entertainment	75	75	75	200	75	75	75	75	150	2,000	75	75	3,025	0.40%
Office & Facility Supplies	500	500	500	500	500	500	500	500	500	500	500	500	6,000	0.79%
Rent	3,256	3,256	3,256	3,256	3,356	3,356	3,356	3,356	3,356	3,356	3,356	3,356	39,972	5.25%
Taxes - Payroll	2,535	2,535	2,521	2,521	2,711	2,711	2,711	2,901	2,901	2,901	3,091	3,091	33,130	4.35%
Taxes - Other	500	0	0	0	0	0	0	0	0	0	0	0	500	0.07%
Telephone	225	225	225	225	225	225	225	225	225	225	225	225	2,700	0.35%
Travel & Lodging	0	0	0	100	0	0	0	0	0	0	0	0	100	0.01%
Utilities	290	290	320	320	320	290	290	290	290	290	290	290	3,570	0.47%
Salon Savings Account	2,910	2,855	3,015	3,223	3,163	3,160	3,128	3,325	3,860	3,015	3,165	3,275	38,093	5.00%
Total General & Admin.	26,191	24,485	24,755	25,121	25,216	24,360	24,322	25,741	26,437	27,326	25,369	25,497	304,820	40.01%
Gross Net	4,541	4,617	6,927	9,588	5,949	7,484	6,659	6,977	16,162	-1,953	4,237	50,994	122,183	16.04%
ENDING CASH	5,541	10,158	17,085	26,673	32,623	40,107	46,766	53,743	69,905	67,952	72,189	123,183	123,183	
Seasonality	7.64%	7.49%	7.91%	8.46%	8.30%	8.30%	8.21%	8.73%	10.13%	7.91%	8.31%	8.60%	100.00%	

Key ratios

Profitability ratios

- RETURN ON REVENUES (also return on sales, net profit ratio)... shows how much net income is derived from every dollar of net revenues.

    RETURN ON REVENUES = NET PROFIT ÷ NET REVENUE

- RETURN ON EQUITY (also net worth, or return on owner's profit and owner's investment)...shows the relationship between net profit and owner's equity.

    RETURN ON EQUITY = NET PROFIT ÷ OWNER'S EQUITY

Efficiency ratios

- CONTRIBUTION MARGIN RATIO...a percentage of net revenues; tells you how well the business is generating funds to cover fixed expenses and make a profit.

    CONTRIBUTION MARGIN RATIO =
    CONTRIBUTION MARGIN ÷ NET REVENUES

- BREAKEVEN REVENUES...the dollar amount of revenues that exactly covers all variable and fixed costs, with nothing left over for profit.

    BREAKEVEN REVENUES =
    FIXED EXPENSES ÷ CONTRIBUTION MARGIN RATIO

- INVENTORY TURNOVER...the number of times in the accounting period inventory is sold, or "turns over."

    INVENTORY TURNOVER =
    COST OF GOODS SOLD ÷ TOTAL INVENTORY

Solvency and liquidity ratios

- CURRENT RATIO...measures the company's ability to use current assets to pay off current liabilities. Generally, a current ratio of 2:1 is considered reasonable.

    CURRENT RATIO = CURRENT ASSETS ÷ CURRENT LIABILITIES

■ QUICK RATIO...measures the company's ability to pay its short-term liabilities. Strive for a quick ratio of at least 1:1.

QUICK RATIO = CASH + MARKETABLE SECURITIES + ACCOUNTS RECEIVABLE ÷ CURRENT LIABILITIES

■ WORKING CAPITAL...the short-term resources available to maintain normal business operations.

WORKING CAPITAL = CURRENT ASSETS − CURRENT LIABILITIES

■ DEBT-TO-EQUITY...indicates how much the owners have at stake in the company, compared to how much creditors have at stake.

DEBT-TO-EQUITY = TOTAL LIABILITIES ÷ OWNER'S EQUITY

Glossary of financial terms

Asset...something of value that the company owns.

Accounts payable...the total dollar amount of money owed by a company, generally due within thirty days.

Accrual method of accounting...under accrual, sales and expenses are recorded when they occur. (i.e., a gift certificate becomes a sale when it is redeemed.)

Backbar...an all-inclusive term for all professional products and supplies consumed in rendering services. It includes dispensary, station use and all other items that become depleted when rendering services.

Balance sheet...reports company assets, liabilities and equities (the owner's ownership portion of the company's holdings) at the end of the accounting period.

Book value...the "worth" of a business, calculated by subtracting total liabilities from total assets. Also called owner's equity.

Bottom line versus top line analysis...the comparison of the retained earnings of a company versus the top line of the balance sheet or internal cash flow, which is cash and marketable securities.

Breakeven analysis...the analysis of "at what point" a company will make a profit. One way of analyzing breakeven is to consider at what point *revenues* will equal *expenses*. Another method of determining the breakeven point is to subtract cost of service and retail from selling price, and divide this amount into your fixed costs. This will give you the total number of units (service/retail) needed to reach breakeven.

Budget...a financial plan of all the company's anticipated or planned expenses for a given period of time. Budgets are helpful in properly running a company and planning its day-to-day operations, as well as in financing and expansion.

Capital...money invested or available for use by the company.

Cash flow...a financial worksheet that demonstrates the inflows (revenues) and outflows (expenses) of cash within an organization, and the resulting cash balances. It is usually prepared for future (i.e., projected) time periods.

Cash method of accounting...under cash basis, sales and expenses are reported when cash is received or paid. (i.e., A gift certificate is recorded as a sale when it is purchased.)

COGS...Cost of Goods Sold. COGS is the cost, at purchase price, of all items resold to the public.

Credit...an entry on the right side of an account ledger sheet. It is usually an amount of money earned by the company.

Debit...an entry on the left side of an account ledger sheet. It is usually an amount of money paid by the company.

Equity...the ownership of a company, usually through shares of common stock.

Fixed costs...expenses whose amount is not influenced by the salon's production level.

Gross profit margin...total revenues minus variable costs.

Income statement... reports revenues and expenses, and resulting profit or loss, throughout an accounting period.

Liability...money the company owes. Liabilities can be payable to suppliers, vendors, employees, government agencies or banks.

Net profit margin...gross margin minus fixed costs. It may also be expressed as revenue minus total costs.

Net worth...equal to total assets minus total liabilities. It is also referred to as stockholder equity.

Overhead...fixed costs.

Owner's equity...the owner's residual interests in assets after liabilities have been deducted. It's the part of the balance sheet that reflects the "net worth" of the company. It consists of the owner's or stockholders' investments, plus any profits retained to date. Also called book value.

Ratios...financial measurements of a company's performance or good standing according to varied criteria.

Retained earnings...profits accumulated since the formation of the company which have not been distributed as dividends.

ROI..."return on investment," or after-tax profit divided into the original investment.

Service payroll…the payroll of all service providers, excluding any administrative or sales support personnel.

T–Accounts…used to illustrate the debit and credit entries made in an account's ledger sheet.

Variable costs…expenses whose amount is influenced by, and varies according to, the salon's production level.

13

COMPENSATION STRATEGIES

Thinking outside the box

Compensation is a complex puzzle whose pieces are part of a comprehensive program that should motivate and inspire employees to perform at consistently high levels. Designing the best pay program for your salon or spa will take time, research, plenty of planning — and adjusting and fine-tuning as you go. There is no one-size-fits-all pay program for salons.

Why is the salon industry's standard approach to compensation out of sync with today's business thinking? Consider the behaviors it rewards. Commission pay, in all its variations, rewards employees for *individual sales performance.*

And it endures because it's easy for owners, managers and employees to understand. (For example: If a technician is paid a 50% commission and her chair, station or treatment room produces $1,000 in one week, she will earn $500.) It's also *safe* for those with weak cash-flow management skills because, unlike the fixed expense of salary and/or hourly wages, a commission payroll simply rises and falls with the level of sales. But are employees truly motivated by commission, even if it represents an extraordinarily high percentage of their sales?

Most of the on-site consulting we do at STRATEGIES results in conversions from commission to team-based (i.e., salary plus team bonus incentive) pay programs. The reason is simple: Many salons and spas are paying commission rates which, even after product-cost deductions and service charges, guarantee such a high percentage of sales revenues to technicians that profit, if ever achieved, is impossible to maintain.

Commission rates which hover around 50% have changed little since the '60s and '70s, but other costs of business have increased dramatically. Consequently, the commission rates of the past no longer fit the costs of doing business. They are therefore the primary force behind the chronic cash-flow crises — and eventual collapse — of many salons. (They are especially dangerous considering the extensive build-out costs and related debt service of a well-equipped day spa.)

Payroll costs must be managed. Guaranteeing a fixed percentage of sales to employees in the form of commission *before* factoring in the other costs of doing business is a proven "kiss of death" in this industry.

Compensation must reward the right behaviors

What *exactly* does commission pay reward, and does it complement your salon or spa's vision and culture? If your business rules state that "the higher your sales, the more you make," and "the higher your request rate, the higher your value," what message are you sending to staff — and which behaviors are you rewarding? The messages employees hear are, "sell more to clients" and "build your following" before *anything* else gets done.

Prescribing additional services to clients may be good for sales, but what happens when a staff member, pushed on by commission, attempts a service he or she doesn't have the skill to perform? ANSWER: Quality is compromised and client retention rates suffer. What if, due to a lack of technical or selling skill, a technician chooses not to recommend a service that would benefit a client?

ANSWER: The client, business and staff all *lose,* simply because no formal system exists to efficiently move that client to another chair or treatment room. In such instances (and they occur countless times each day in salons and spas), employees are *rewarded* for *poor* performance.

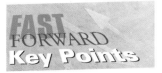

The strongest message commission pay delivers is: *Build a following.* Yet in the new age of teamwork and empowerment, individual followings are an anomaly. They are a dusty relic that don't fit into today's fast-paced, customer-driven business thinking.

Why would a technician who is paid commission and rated by his or her individual request rate encourage clients to visit other technicians?

Followings and full books

Clients want access to salon and spa services when they need them. Unfortunately, they often encounter stylist and technician gridlock because compensation and other traditional operational systems discourage team service. After all, why would a technician who is paid commission and rated by his or her individual request rate encourage clients to visit other technicians?

No other element of the salon business is more worshiped than followings and full books. For most technicians, they are prestigious indicators of success. But they are universally *feared* by salon owners and managers because they are used as leverage to hold management hostage. They also are the "walk-out bombs" that devastate many otherwise successful salons.

As individual followings build, loyalty and income security gradually shift from the employer to the employee's column in the appointment book. The employee's mode of thought then becomes: *"I'm* paying *you* 50% of what I bring in." This is a sure sign that your salon culture has been compromised.

Aftermath marketing to a technician's client list will never make up for the missed opportunities to direct client loyalty to the salon and the team. Likewise, non-compete agreements cannot reverse the damage inflicted by a poorly designed pay program. Employees will do what your pay program rewards them for doing. Your compensation system must encourage the behaviors and culture your business needs to grow.

What vision- and culture-specific behaviors does your current compensation system reward and/or discourage? Because commission rewards individual sales, performance behaviors such as client retention, productivity, skill development and referrals go unacknowledged. If these and other performance factors are not tied into your compensation plan, employees will regard them as nothing more than superficial intrusions. Remember, they will receive their sales commission whether or not they adopt the salon's vision and culture.

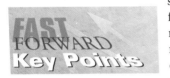

FAST FORWARD Key Points

Employees will do what your pay program rewards them for doing. Your compensation system must encourage the behaviors and culture your business needs to grow.

How can you address a myriad of behavior problems such as lateness and absenteeism; poor attitude, communication, image and appearance; non-team play, etc…if your pay program lacks the muscle to impact employee paychecks? Your compensation system must reward overall performance.

What gets rewarded gets repeated.

Everyone is responsible for growth

There was a time when the salon which offered the best haircuts or color was the hottest place in town. Those with the latest technical skills had "the magic." But time, technology and training soon rendered that competitive advantage commonplace. Even the addition of a day spa no longer offers the competitive edge it was just a few short years ago.

Just like the rest of the business world, salons and spas are finding that delivering a good product or service guarantees neither success nor customer loyalty. To stand out from the crowd, you must focus on fundamental competencies which reach far beyond technical skill. The business' vision and culture, and its operating and compensation systems, must be engineered to meet the new and demanding expectations of today's client.

EVERYONE MUST TAKE RESPONSIBILITY FOR GROWING THE BUSINESS. Barriers created by old pay programs must be destroyed. The new mantra is: If it's good for the client, it must be done…and associated employee behaviors must be rewarded. It no longer matters "whose" client it is, as long as quality is maintained, and customer satisfaction and retention are high.

TODAY'S EMPLOYEES ARE DEMANDING. They want to see career growth paths. They want to know their income can continue to grow, even when their appointment book is gridlocked. They want to know the rules of the game. If they are rewarded for building a following, they'll build it…and take it with them when they leave. If they are rewarded for overall performance and for growing business, they'll grow it faster and bigger than you can ever imagine.

Commission-based pay:
A piece for me, a piece for you

Most salons and spas pay technicians on a commission basis, rewarding them primarily for the volume of work they perform. Because commission is the predominant compensatory structure for the industry, it has become part of the culture of the modern salon.

There are many reasons why commission is the most common pay method in salons, but they can be summed up in one thought: *The professional salon industry loves to celebrate the individual.* Everything else is predicated on that idea. Clients are loyal to stylists and technical staff rather than the salon or spa that employs them. And management in many salons is best described as *laissez-faire,* resulting in a culture which allows employees to "do their own thing" with work schedules, customer service, technical competency and overall performance.

So why does the industry celebrate the individual through the legacy of commission? The three primary causes are:

■ THE CLIENT OWNERSHIP FACTOR. In the old days of weekly wash-and-sets, there was a much closer bond between stylists and clients. (Seeing someone every week can do that to a person.) Clients wanted to be "owned," especially when encouraged by a stylist with whom they had developed a close, personal relationship.

■ THE MOTIVATION FACTOR. Most owners and managers have long reasoned that technical staff would be motivated if they received a "piece of the action." The commission incentive is meant to motivate stylists to

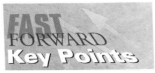

Key Points

Personal clienteles are often used as leverage against management. And yet, many owners and managers continue to judge technical staff's value by the size of their followings.

produce more. But in reality, commission is not a sales and productivity driver in salons.

■ THE MANAGEMENT FACTOR. Many owners never gain practical human resource experience in the salon environment. The necessity for most owners and managers to work as technicians within their businesses encourages the laissez-faire management so prevalent today.

Commission pros

■ COMMISSION DOES MOTIVATE MANY STYLISTS. By paying staff on commission, the salon or spa owner effectively says, "Your value to this salon and the client base is directly proportional to how hard you work." This is particularly effective with staff who have a strong work ethic and career drive. They're the ones who stay to service the last customer who walks through the door.

■ COMMISSION MAKES IT EASY FOR MANY STYLISTS TO OPEN THEIR OWN BUSINESSES. Without a commitment to a fixed payroll, new owners can hire all the people they need. (Incidentally, this approach also spawned the practice of looking for technicians with large followings. Stealing stylists and trading clients has long been a by-product of commission.)

■ COMMISSION OFFERS AN EQUITABLE MEANS TO DISTRIBUTE INCOME. Most technical staff understand the concept of working harder to earn a higher wage, and few find inequality in the administration of commission.

■ IT'S SIMPLE. A given percentage is all you need to determine payroll for any period. Many salons pay 50% commission, which makes splitting sales right down the middle the basic calculation. (Interestingly, 50% has always seemed the magic number. Unfortunately, few owners calculate its impact on profitability.)

Commission variations include *sliding scales, service charges, product-cost deductions* and *multi-level pricing*. Deductions and service charges lower commission payouts by giving the illusion that commission rates have not been reduced. Multi-level pricing, though it may be used to reward years of experience, is simply another tool to increase pay without increasing commission rates.

Commission cons

- COMMISSION TENDS TO TRAP OWNERS AND TOP PRODUCERS IN PRO-DUCTION ROLES. These people are so busy making a living that they cannot find the time to teach new stylists or help them become productive. Thus, the salon's greatest asset — the skill of senior staff — is lost to each new generation.

- IT CAN RESTRICT SALON AND SPA PROFITS. Often, up to 60% or more of all service income is consumed in payroll and related taxes. It's difficult to make money when only forty cents of each dollar is left for overhead, taxes and reinvestment in the business. The difference between successful and unsuccessful salons and spas can often be traced directly to their commission percentages. Those with staying power have *lower* commissions and *stronger* management.

- COMMISSION LIMITS PRODUCTIVITY. It can actually demotivate a significant segment of technical staff because it tells them that they can make as much or as little as they choose. Many settle for less, and avoid the "pressures" of being busy.

- COMMISSION IS PURELY SALES-DRIVEN. When technical staff are paid for the amount of work they do — with no regard for how well they do it — quality and quality-related behaviors suffer. The underlying assumption is that if a technician does good work, he or she will become more popular and "do better." However, many believe it doesn't really matter if a client comes back, as long as their station or treatment room is busy.

- STAFF AREN'T REWARDED FOR RETAINING CLIENTS. Client retention is the single most important growth indicator of any salon, and should be the focus of any compensation system.

- COMMISSION BURNS OUT MANY NEW TECHNICIANS BEFORE THEY GET THE CHANCE TO BECOME SUCCESSFUL. Many leave the profession after only one or two years because it's difficult to build a following and earn a living.

Other considerations

- Perhaps the greatest flaw in commission compensation, by modern business management standards, is its inherent tendency to promote individualism. Teamwork is a hot topic for salons today, yet their dominant compensation system rewards *individual* performance, without regard to *team* contributions.

■ By design, commission encourages service providers to build personal clienteles which are often used as leverage against management. And yet, many owners and managers continue to judge technical staff's value by the size of their followings. Even the most experienced and competent stylists, nail technicians, massage therapists and estheticians find that when they relocate to a new town, they command little or no income security and must start all over simply because they don't have a following.

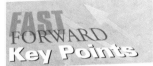

Commission pay can work effectively in a sales environment — but a salon business is a service environment. The main reason commission presents so many problems for salons is that its structure doesn't fit the industry.

■ Commission pay can work effectively in a sales environment. *But the salon business is a service environment.* The main reason commission presents so many problems for salons is that its structure doesn't fit the industry. Stylists are not professional salespeople and receive little or no sales training, yet they are paid via a commission system which simply doesn't match their nature. The industry's dominant method of compensation therefore contributes to many of the problems that hold it back.

Salary: Only one part of the solution

S alary guarantees a specific level of compensation for a specific period of time. All compensation systems which reward employee time without regard to production fall into this category (e.g., an hourly wage, weekly rate of pay or annual salary). It's the way most of the world works, and the most prevalent compensation system used in American industry.

In salons and spas which pay salary, technicians generally earn an hourly wage or weekly guarantee. Compensation levels may be set according to a number of criteria, including technical ability, sales performance, seniority and other factors. (In many salary-based salons and spas, pay is based on sales performance. Although a valid criterion, this simply transforms salary into a "deferred commission.") Some owners consider the number of services rendered, rather than their dollar value, while others define production as units of time purchased by clients.

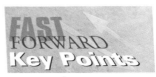

Key Points

Regardless of how pay is determined, the most distinguishing feature of a salary-based compensation program is that pay is generally fixed over long periods of time.

Regardless of how pay is determined, the most distinguishing feature of a salary-based compensation program is that *pay is generally fixed over long periods of time* (i.e., does not fluctuate with service sales to the same degree as commission).

Salary pros

- FLUCTUATION IS LIMITED. Salary is more stable than the volatile ups and downs of commission, and creates income security for staff. Knowing in advance what their take-home pay will be simplifies personal budgeting for them and payroll for the salon. HINT: This makes cash-flow management easier.
- PAYROLL DOES NOT INCREASE WITH SALES. Well-managed salary-

based salons and spas can be quite profitable. A fixed payroll enables owners to establish a sound financial footing by alleviating the burden of fixed-percentage disbursements to employees. Payroll increases only at the discretion of management.

- NEW TEAM MEMBERS EARN A FAIR WAGE. During the first weeks and months of employment, new staff must learn the business' procedures, systems, culture and True Quality programs. A properly structured and managed salary program provides the opportunity to develop a true team-based environment.

- VETERAN TECHNICAL STAFF CAN GROW BEYOND THE LIMITATIONS OF COMMISSION. For example: A successful stylist paid on salary has a vested interest in developing the skills of his teammates. Because salary is not tied directly to sales, he can get away from the chair or treatment room periodically to focus on education, training and building a successful business. Attention shifts from building a personal following to building salon clients.

- SALON AND SPA OWNERS HAVE MORE CONTROL. Every system, such as recruiting, training, retention and cash management, is directed by the leadership team. There is less "free-form" activity than in most commission salons. Salary is a good choice for owners who desire structure and operational control.

Salary cons

- SALARY CAN SQUELCH STYLIST MOTIVATION AND ENCOURAGE COMPLACENCY. If the salon is not proficient at keeping people motivated, they can stagnate. Owners fear the attitude: *I'm going to get paid anyway, so why work harder?*

- DELAYED GRATIFICATION. Many owners and managers depend on raises and bonuses to ward off complacency. But for technicians accustomed to instant gratification, these incentives come few and far between. Stylists, especially younger ones, like to see immediate results. The situation is further complicated by owners' struggles (due to unfamiliarity with cash-flow planning and control) to determine criteria on which to base raises.

- BUDGETING IS PROBLEMATIC IF SALES CANNOT SUSTAIN PAYROLL THROUGH SEASONAL TRENDS OR SEVERE WEATHER. Owners of salaried salons and spas must exercise cash management skills to overcome seasonal sales fluctuations and remain prepared for slow periods. This is where many falter.

- SALARIED SALONS ARE THE MINORITY. Owners must often overcome the preconceptions of employees and fellow owners. Yet many prevail and operate successful businesses.

The bottom line

Some believe that salaried salons and spas are superior to commissioned ones because they offer owners more structure, control and organization. These same people believe they are also superior for employees because they offer security, income stability and career opportunities. But is the system really a better design for the salon industry?

Certainly, many struggle with the notion of a fixed payroll. Most stylists and technical staff have been taught that they can *earn more* by *working harder*, and resent growing busier without receiving a corresponding pay increase. Increasing income by *working smarter* instead of harder is a foreign concept in this industry.

Implementing salary compensation in salons is difficult because it differs so significantly from traditional commission pay. Some view salary as too long-term, structured or difficult for team members to follow. Salary does control payroll, however, which is the largest expense at any salon or spa. For this reason alone, the system is a financially superior choice.

CONCLUSION: Certain truths must be established in a salary discussion. The most important is where client loyalty lies. Owners and technical staff who believe clients belong to individual service providers, and that it is the service provider's responsibility to build sales, find it difficult to make salary work. The owner who builds the salon or spa's client list through marketing, merchandising and broad-based retention programs is a far better candidate to manage, and flourish under, a salary compensation system.

Ten sobering pay questions

The following questions will indicate the ability of your present compensation system to contribute to the salon or spa culture you want to create. Use the accompanying "quiz keys" to assess your responses.

1. Where did your current pay program come from?
2. Which vision- and culture-specific behaviors was it designed to reward?
3. Which negative behaviors was it designed to discourage?
4. If you pay a commission percentage on sales, how did you arrive at the percentage rate(s)?
5. How did you integrate the compensation system into the business' overall financial plans?
6. Are controls designed into the program which will allow the business to adjust to increased operating costs?
7. What strategies did you include to offer continued income growth to senior staff, who are typically booked solid?
8. How is the compensation system meant to encourage staff to develop their skills?
9. What strategies did you include to encourage teamwork?
10. How does the program benefit clients?

Quiz keys...
- QUESTION 1: Most pay programs are mirror images of the ones salon owners previously worked under at other salons and spas. If not, they typically are still commission-based designs. Consequently, the commission rates selected seldom allow for the other operational costs of the business.
- QUESTION 2: If client retention, productivity, skill development, communication, attendance and other performance elements are not addressed through compensation, the salon's culture can be compromised. Most commission-based programs do not encourage these behaviors.

- QUESTION 3: If the current pay program does not address negative behaviors such as tardiness, absenteeism, attitude and failure to recommend retail products…they *will* continue.

- QUESTION 4: Most commission rates reflect "the going rate" (i.e., what the other guy is doing), or the rate paid in the salon where the current owner was previously employed. But if the original template was poorly designed, its inefficiencies will exist in all cloned versions.

- QUESTION 5: Few commission programs are designed around the financial realities and operational costs of a salon business.

- QUESTION 6: When the largest operating expense is a fixed percentage of sales allocated to payroll (usually 50% or higher), any other cost increases will compromise profits.

- QUESTION 7: When commission employees are booked solid and their individual service prices cannot be increased, their income is gridlocked.

- QUESTION 8: "If you want to earn — you've got to learn." What could be more important to one's earning potential in a service business than skill development?

- QUESTION 9: In a team-based business, everyone is responsible for every hour available for sale, and focuses on achieving the company's sales and service goals. Commission pay focuses on individual sales, and therefore delivers a mixed message in a team-based environment.

- QUESTION 10: Clients serviced by the collective skills of the entire team can truly experience world-class service. A team-based pay program makes it possible.

The mechanics of team-based pay

There are many indicators that it's time to reassess a business' structure. In salons and spas, the most common are shrinking profits, less-than-motivated staff, lack of a clear direction for growth, marginal client retention and low productivity figures. But can skill- and team-based pay, and open-book management, resolve such deep-rooted problems? Certainly…if owners also implement strategies to change the underlying behaviors which traditionally contradict the teamwork message of the salon's new management and compensation systems.

Understanding the differences

Commission and team-based pay directly conflict in three ways:

1. COMMISSION IS DRIVEN ENTIRELY BY INDIVIDUAL SALES…
   TEAM-BASED PAY IS DRIVEN BY OVERALL PERFORMANCE.

For example: Consider a salon paying 60% commission and falling steadily deeper into debt because payroll is out of control. A decision is made to implement a new compensation system which is based on overall performance, both as individuals and as a team.

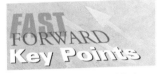

The first step of the conversion process is to calculate each technician's starting salary by examining their previous year's earnings, gross pay for the last four to six months, and overall performance. HINT: It's time to stop tracking request rates, and start tracking retention. *(See chapter 7.)* For our model, assume the salon scored only 37% on first-time client retention. In the time frame assessed, only fifty-eight of 158 first-time clients returned.

During the pay calculation process, red flags may go up for technicians with low client retention rates. Particularly if they have

The importance of a technician's "busy factor" pales beside his or her retention numbers. It's impossible to calculate the costs of lost and dissatisfied clients.

been with the business for a number of years, they can be paid quite a bit of money via commission, yet lose 70%–80% of the new clients assigned to them. The importance of a technician's "busy factor" pales beside his or her retention numbers. It's impossible to calculate the costs of lost and dissatisfied clients.

A popular conversion strategy — and one that works well for a low-retention salon, such as our model — is to compensate technicians at their income level of the previous year…with a ninety-day window from the date of conversion in which to improve their retention and other performance factors. The owner's role is not to *dictate* improvement, but to coach and encourage specific and measurable results. Discrepancies between compensation *earned* and *paid* are erased in a performance-based framework.

2. COMMISSION PUTS PRODUCTION CONTROL IN EMPLOYEES' HANDS… TEAM-BASED PAY AWARDS CONTROL TO OWNERS.

Most salons and spas cannot continue to fund their present commission rates if they hope to keep pace with rising operating costs. Product cost deductions and service charges are not the answer; they simply cannot keep pace with increasing overhead expenses, and often cause significant staff upheaval.

The recession of the early '90s forced businesses of all shapes and sizes to "reengineer" their systems and cultures. Those that succeeded quickly realized they could not expect new behaviors and levels of performance if they didn't also reengineer compensation.

- REENGINEERING RULE #1: You cannot reengineer halfway.
- REENGINEERING RULE #2: Don't expect new behaviors and team performance if your pay program still rewards the old behaviors you are trying to change. You'll only confuse staff and stall the reengineering effort.

Recently published studies state that 30% of all U.S. companies now use the "new pay" (i.e., skill-based pay with team incentives for overall performance). That number was zero percent in 1990. The "new pay" and reengineering phenomena are driven by efficiency, productivity, quality, value and customer service.

3. COMMISSION DOES NOT INSPIRE TEAM PERFORMANCE...
   TEAM-BASED PAY IS DEFINED BY IT.

Commission rewards individual sales and creates natural roadblocks to team service and performance. Team-based incentives are perhaps the most powerful new performance-driven tools to arrive on the management scene in the last half century. They focus employee energy on *growing the business.* Few if any commission programs can make that claim. Since many salons already pay out more in commission than they can afford, there's no room left for team incentives. For most salons, reengineering the entire pay program is the only logical alternative.

Shifting into "new pay" thinking

There is no "red badge of courage" for reengineering your pay program. It will not solve all your business woes, or instantly inspire staff to raise the performance bar. A *compensation system* is a *reward system* and nothing more. How efficiently you manage the program will determine its success or failure.

The most common mistakes business owners who are "new" to the "new pay" make are...

- INTRODUCING IT WITHOUT A VISION (i.e., goal, objective and purpose). Employees must understand the vision in order to understand the changes that must take place to achieve it.

- FOCUSING ON THE PROGRAM ITSELF rather than the behaviors and results it is meant to inspire and reward. The new pay program will drive your business forward only if you steer it toward your vision. The team must know the weekly and/or monthly targets for sales, retention, productivity, average ticket, etc.

- THINKING THE PROGRAM WILL MANAGE ITSELF. Commission is a simple program because the burden of building sales rests with the employee. Commission says, "If they're hungry, they'll produce." The new pay says, "You and the team must meet these standards of performance." If one or more team members drops the ball the entire team, and the client, pays the price.

It's like learning to walk again.

Communicating your new pay program

As you move forward with your new pay program, it is vital to remain focused on the objectives of the transition. *A conversion to salary is not:* a ploy to force pay cuts or take anything away from staff. *It is not:* another smoke-and-mirrors, variable commission, product cost/service charge, multi-level pricing, request-driven, inefficient, hostage-management pay program. *It is:* a modern, efficient, True-Quality driven program which is spreading like wildfire through the business community.

The team-based pay program presented in here in FAST FORWARD SALONS & SPAS was developed by Neil Ducoff, publisher of SALON BUSINESS STRATEGIES Magazine. It excels in the service environment because it focuses the imagination and energies of an entire team on a single goal: growing the salon. Nothing is more powerful than the united and focused efforts of an inspired team. *Nothing.*

As discussed earlier, most efforts to implement new programs which alter the culture of a business through improved productivity and efficiency quickly run aground because the *behaviors* necessary to navigate the process are not defined or rewarded. MENTAL TICKLE: What gets rewarded gets repeated.

If one continues to reward only sales (i.e., pay stylists and techni-

FAST FORWARD NAVIGATION KEY

REVIEW AND CHECKLIST

Before introducing and launching a new pay program, complete the following:

- Research current compensation trends in business.

- Compile a detailed list of every performance requirement and behavior that is important to growing your salon. Staff participation is a must.

- Determine your breakeven point and prepare a twelve-month revenue and expense projection to guide your selling efforts and control expenses.

- Calculate the average paycheck for each employee.

- Define the standards of overall performance you want the program to reward.

cians via commission), sales will occur with varying degrees of success. But the accompanying counterproductive behaviors and independent attitudes will go unchecked. The new pay program taught here will not allow pay to increase unless overall individual and team performance meets the salon's established standards. At the heart of the program is the *team-based incentive* which unites the efforts of the entire staff to move the numbers in the right direction: revenues up and costs down.

TEAM-BASED PAY IS NOT A QUICK-FIX OR PANACEA. It will not solve all your operational, financial or growth problems. It requires planning and constant attention to detail. It requires leadership, honesty, teamwork and open communication. It is simply a compensation system...but one which rewards the behaviors that enable a business to grow. It will unleash truly staggering growth opportunities.

Broadbanding

Broadbanding establishes concise performance guidelines for employee groups, based on their contribution to salon growth. Although there is no fixed or "proper" number of bands, the trend today is toward as few as possible, or one for each staff group. The following example shows one band for professional technical staff and another for the leadership team. You may label the bands, but do not use names that imply superiority...focus on *performance*, not titles or status. You may construct broadbands for any staff group (e.g., junior stylists or spa specialists), as long as their overall performance criteria are clearly *defined* and *understood*.

The broadband process will likely be completely new to your staff. To avoid the natural fear and uncertainty of new pay programs, communicate and explain its purpose thoroughly and patiently. Employees need to know exactly how their pay is determined...and how they can advance.

Planning the pay program launch

Confidentiality is a part of every salon and, in many instances, is best. Salon and spa owners often worry that if word of major

Continued on page 430

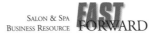
TEAM-BASED BROADBAND PAY SCALE

This model of a team-based broadband pay scale details six skill levels, and their corresponding pay ranges and performance criteria. Individual and team performance bonus structures are clearly identified. The model also shows how growth potential is tied to all key areas of performance.

TEAM-BASED BROADBAND PAY SCALE...SKILL SETS 1 – 3

	Skill Set 1		Skill Set 2		Skill Set 3	
	Minimum	Maximum	Minimum	Maximum	Minimum	Maximun
Year	$15,000	$19,999	$20,000	$39,999	$40,000	$59,999
Month	1,250.00	1,666.58	1,666.67	3,333.25	3,333.33	4,999.92
Week	288.46	384.60	384.62	769.21	769.23	1,153.83
Hour	7.21	9.61	9.62	19.23	19.23	28.85

◄─── Pay based on Hourly Rate ───►

◄─── Individual Performance Bonus = 5% of Service/Retail Sales ───►

◄─── TEAM PERFORMANCE BONUS (Monthly) = 5 % of Net] ───►

◄─── SUPER TEAM PERFORMANCE BONUS (Monthly) = Team Bonus jumps [───►

PERFORMANCE REQUIREMENTS	PERFORMANCE REQUIREMENTS	PERFORMANCE REQUIREMENTS
• 1st Visit Retention…40% • Existing Retention…70% • Productivity Rate…60% • Ave. Svc. Tkt…$50 • Ave. Retail Tkt…$18 • Retail = 35% of Service	• 1st Visit Retention…45% • Existing Retention…75% • Productivity Rate…70% • Ave. Svc. Tkt…$60 • Ave. Retail Tkt…$21 • Retail = 35% of Service	• 1st Visit Retention…45% • Existing Retention…75% • Productivity Rate…75% • Ave. Svc. Tkt…$65 • Ave. Retail Tkt…$23 • Retail = 35% of Service

TECHNICAL SKILL DEV.	TECHNICAL SKILL DEV.	TECHNICAL SKILL DEV.
• Shampoos • Draping • Basic haircuts/finish • Color mix & application - No formulation	• Shampoos • Draping • Intermediate haircuts/finish • Color formulation • Foil Highlighting	• Shampoos • Draping • Intermediate haircuts/finish • Color formulation • Foil Highlighting

NON-TECHNICAL SKILL DEV.	NON-TECHNICAL SKILL DEV.	NON-TECHNICAL SKILL DEV.
• 1st Visit Consultation • Escorting/Salon/Spa Tours • Retail Product Knowledge • Service Descrip./Pricing • Phone skills/scripts • Towel/sanitation engineer • '3 products' on paper • Svc. completion Procedures • Learn Cust. Svc. Scripts	• 1st Visit Consultation • Escorting/Salon/Spa Tours • Retail Product Knowledge • Service Descrip./Pricing • Phone skills/scripts • Towel/sanitation engineer • '3 products' on paper • Svc. completion Procedures • Learn Cust. Svc. Scripts	• 1st Visit Consultation • Escorting/Salon/Spa Tours • Retail Product Knowledge • Service Descrip./Pricing • Phone skills/scripts • Towel/sanitation engineer • '3 products' on paper • Svc. completion Procedures • Learn Cust. Svc. Scripts

BONUS DISQUALIFIERS	BONUS DISQUALIFIERS	BONUS DISQUALIFIERS
• Less than 70% of Goal • Less than 35% retail/svc. • Two or more 'You're Late' • Two or more Absent • Less than 90% '3 Products'	• Less than 80% of Goal • Less than 35% retail/svc. • Two or more 'You're Late' • Two or more Absent • Less than 90% '3 Products'	• Less than 90% of Goal • Less than 40% retail/svc. • Two or more 'You're Late' • Two or more Absent • Less than 90% '3 Products'

TEAM-BASED BROADBAND PAY SCALE...SKILL SETS 4 – 6

Skill Set 4		Skill Set 5		Skill Set 6	
Minimum	Maximun	Minimum	Maximun	Minimum	Maximun
$60,000	$79,999	$80,000	$99,999	$100,000	$120,000
5,000.00	6,666.58	6,666.67	8,333.25	8,333.33	10,000.00
1,153.85	1,538.44	1,538.46	1,923.06	1,923.08	2,307.69
28.85	38.46	38.46	48.08	48.08	57.69

Pay based on Salary

Individual Performance Bonus = 7% of Service/Retail Sales

Profit...*Total sales must be 90% or higher of monthly goal.*

to 1 0 % of Net Profit...When total sales equals 100% or more of monthly goal

---

PERFORMANCE REQUIREMENTS
- 1st Visit Retention...50%
- Existing Retention...80%
- Productivity Rate...80%
- Ave. Svc. Tkt...$70
- Ave. Retail Tkt...$28
- Retail = 40% of Service

TEAM RESPONSIBILITIES
- Mentoring
- Skill Trainer

TECHNICAL SKILL DEV.
- Shampoos
- Draping
- Advanced haircuts/finish
- Color formulation
- Foil Highlighting

NON-TECHNICAL SKILL DEV.
- 1st Visit Consultation
- Escorting/Salon/Spa Tours
- Retail Product Knowledge
- Service Descrip./Pricing
- Phone skills/scripts
- Towel/sanitation engineer
- "3 products" on paper
- Svc. completion Procedures
- Learn Cust. Svc. Scripts

BONUS DISQUALIFIERS
- Less than 90% of Goal
- Less than 45% retail/svc.
- Two or more "You're Late"
- Two or more Absent
- Less than 90% "3 Products"

PERFORMANCE REQUIREMENTS
- 1st Visit Retention...55%
- Existing Retention...80%
- Productivity Rate...85%
- Ave. Svc. Tkt...$75
- Ave. Retail Tkt...$30
- Retail = 40% of Service

TEAM RESPONSIBILITIES
- Mentoring
- Skill Trainer

TECHNICAL SKILL DEV.
- Shampoos
- Draping
- Advanced haircuts/finish
- Color formulation
- Foil Highlighting

NON-TECHNICAL SKILL DEV.
- 1st Visit Consultation
- Escorting/Salon/Spa Tours
- Retail Product Knowledge
- Service Descrip./Pricing
- Phone skills/scripts
- Towel/sanitation engineer
- "3 products" on paper
- Svc. completion Procedures
- Learn Cust. Svc. Scripts

BONUS DISQUALIFIERS
- Less than 90% of Goal
- Less than 45% retail/svc.
- Two or more "You're Late"
- Two or more Absent
- Less than 90% "3 Products"

PERFORMANCE REQUIREMENTS
- 1st Visit Retention...60%
- Existing Retention...85%
- Productivity Rate...90%
- Ave. Svc. Tkt...$80
- Ave. Retail Tkt...$32
- Retail = 40% of Service

TEAM RESPONSIBILITIES
- Mentoring
- Skill Trainer

TECHNICAL SKILL DEV.
- Shampoos
- Draping
- Advanced haircuts/finish
- Color formulation
- Foil Highlighting

NON-TECHNICAL SKILL DEV.
- 1st Visit Consultation
- Escorting/Salon/Spa Tours
- Retail Product Knowledge
- Service Descrip./Pricing
- Phone skills/scripts
- Towel/sanitation engineer
- "3 products" on paper
- Svc. completion Procedures
- Learn Cust. Svc. Scripts

BONUS DISQUALIFIERS
- Less than 90% of Goal
- Less than 45% retail/svc.
- Two or more "You're Late"
- Two or more Absent
- Less than 90% "3 Products"

change gets out, their staff will "abandon ship." But communication is essential when implementing a new compensation structure. Optimum results can only be achieved by placing the details right in the open, for all to see. Keeping the details under wraps can engender harmful rumors and may even encourage skepticism when the program does eventually surface.

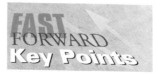

FAST FORWARD Key Points

In the case of a new pay program filled with incentives, bonuses and reward systems, employees must know the details. Otherwise, they will have no idea what their goals are, or what the rewards will be for meeting them. With a team-based pay system, goals and objectives are the foundation of the entire program. Staff must be clued in to what's happening or goals will never be met.

Breaking with tradition

Traditionally, people don't talk much about pay, except to complain about it. In fact, compensation systems and formulas are a great mystery in many companies: Management keeps details from employees, and employees don't ask questions because they have no details. It's a frustrating cycle that breeds rumors and discontent. If compensation guidelines are not articulated in a way everyone understands, trouble can erupt.

In the case of a new pay program filled with incentives, bonuses and reward systems, employees *must* know the details. Otherwise, they will have no idea what their goals are, or what the rewards will be for meeting them. With a team-based pay system, goals and objectives are the foundation of the entire program. Staff must be clued in to what's happening or goals will never be met.

The faith factor

Your team depends on you for information. They have faith that you will make decisions in their best interest — and in the best interest of the salon or day spa. Only when they suspect foul play do they begin to lose faith. Owners must maintain the integrity of their actions, and alleviate staff fear of change through *education*.

Communications research reveals that employees typically

receive more than 50% of their information through "the grapevine" (i.e., fellow workers, rather than team leaders). Pertinent facts and details are often omitted, changed or even falsified as they travel through the salon. This of course results in a less-than-accurate view of the real picture. As a result, staff can draw untrue conclusions even before the leadership team has an opportunity to tell the real story.

Strong communication can eliminate the grapevine effect by beating the rumor-mill to the punch. Leadership announcements and personal contact with staff must start well before the program is implemented and last long after. Once the staff hears about it from the source — team leaders and management — rumors will be snuffed out.

Tie it all together

During times of dramatic change, people become overly sensitive. The communication process must ensure a clear and concise message, which is understood by everyone.

- THE MEANS OF COMMUNICATION SHOULD AGREE WITH THE CURRENT SALON OR SPA CULTURE. If the culture is: *I lead, you follow,* and you suddenly announce a completely new pay program, skepticism and unrest will follow. Thoroughness, detail and a willingness to listen are key. If the salon's culture is self-directed (i.e., hostage management), your communications must define a new vision and commitment from the top. No matter how well-managed a salon appears on the surface, changing the way people are paid will always create unrest.

- COMMUNICATION MUST ENCOMPASS EVERYONE: STAFF, MANAGEMENT, LEADERS. It's the only way a new compensation system will succeed. Every team member wants to have a voice in change. *Give it to them.* You'll be surprised at the ways different ideas and opinions can improve the outcome.

- ANY SIGNIFICANT CHANGE IN SALON OPERATIONS MUST COMPLEMENT THE SALON VISION. Compensation must be discussed in terms of changes already made, as well as those to come. Why? Compensation is the true force behind most successful change initiatives. For example: If the pay system is designed to improve productivity, staff must be kept fully informed of progress, both personal and salon-wide.

■ THE MESSAGE OF ANY NEW COMPENSATION SYSTEM MUST BE CLEAR. Teach the team to play a new game with new rules. Focus on the growth opportunities the new program offers. Explain new terminology, performance criteria, skill certification and team-based incentives. Employees' fears stem from what they *don't* comprehend. Help them understand.

Ultimately, communication should address and link every part of the salon. It should clarify roles: Who is responsible? Why must things happen a certain way? Without proper communication, a pay program may never reach its true potential.

To Learn More...

Converting from commission to a team-based pay program requires attention to detail and plenty of planning and preparation. Because it requires well-designed business systems, sound cash-flow management and excellent team communication, it is not for every salon or spa.

SALON BUSINESS STRATEGIES has created a TEAM-BASED PAY VIDEO & CD TOOLS KIT (Cost: $249 plus S/H). It contains a 68-minute video for owners and managers, a 38-minute video for staff, and a CD which contains manuals, conversion guides, compensation/cash-flow templates, and performance evaluation forms.

To order your kit, call STRATEGIES toll-free at: 800.417.4848, Ext. 114.

Things to do:

■ Evaluate your current pay program.

DOES IT REWARD THE RIGHT BEHAVIORS?

DOES IT REWARD OVERALL PERFORMANCE — OR JUST SALES?

DOES IT ENCOURAGE TEAM SERVICE?

IS IT MANAGEABLE AND AFFORDABLE?

DOES IT OFFER EMPLOYEES INCOME GROWTH?

IS IT TRUE-QUALITY DRIVEN?

■ List all the performance behaviors you want your pay program to reward. Here are some to get you started:

QUALITY AND CONSISTENCY

CLIENT RETENTION

PRODUCTIVITY RATE

MINIMAL ABSENTEEISM/TARDINESS

CONTINUED SKILL DEVELOPMENT

TEAMWORK

SERVICE AND RETAIL SALES

■ Construct a twelve-month cash-flow budget to determine the financial impact of your current pay program on future growth.

USE THE CASH-FLOW PLANNING BUDGET IN CHAPTER 12.

■ Explore all of your pay program options.

IS COMMISSION GIVING YOU THE RESULTS YOU WANT?

IS CHAIR RENTAL GIVING YOU THE RESULTS YOU WANT?

IS TEAM-BASED PAY A VIABLE ALTERNATIVE?

TAXES: A FACT OF BUSINESS LIFE

Taxes are not an option

14

Over the past few years, the Internal Revenue Service (IRS) has focused attention on proper tip reporting in the restaurant industry. One of the catalysts that spawned their interest was credit card processing. Every time you add a tip to a credit card charge receipt, you provide tracking data for tip income. Consequently, the IRS has worked hard to create education and reporting programs to bring restaurant workers into compliance with tip-reporting regulations. *The word to emphasize is* COMPLIANCE.

Another goal of the IRS is to bring salons into tax compliance. Since, according to the IRS, mass auditing of the salon industry would be both inefficient and costly, agents will depend on spot-checks and educational programs. Though the focus is more on bringing salons into compliance than on chasing yesterday's unreported wages, we urge readers to remember that the IRS never forgives back taxes. If your salon is audited, the IRS will seek all past and present taxes owed.

The stress of cheating

Paying wages under the table cuts right to the core of how you choose to run your business. The consequences are far-reaching. Here are just some of the business compromises you make:

- Every day, you must falsify sales records in order to hide cash.
- All payroll records are falsified.
- The revenue and payroll expense data your accountant needs to prepare accurate financial statements is falsified, and therefore useless.
- Borrowing money on the merits of your business is virtually impossible. No lending institution will loan money to a business with two sets of books.
- If you use a point-of-sale software system, you either record every transaction (therefore documenting all revenues), or contaminate data by not recording sales or making false end-of-day adjustments.
- As willing participants, your staff are exposed to personal audits, back taxes and stiff penalties.
- Your staff knows you are willfully falsifying revenue and payroll records for the specific purpose of tax evasion. This knowledge can come back to haunt you.
- Employees are unable to use their true income to secure auto loans, home mortgages and other forms of credit.
- Bank accounts (business and personal), your home and all personal assets can be attached or seized by the IRS.

Which path to choose?

As we inch closer to a cashless society via credit and debit cards, online banking and the ever-expanding capabilities of the internet, paying wages under the table will become increasingly difficult. People don't carry cash like they used to, and this leaves less cash in the drawer. Without that cash, it's difficult to dole out under-the-table pay without creating an incriminating paper trail.

The decision to own and operate a legitimate, ethical business is yours to make. Likewise, the decision to falsify sales and payroll records, and to compromise the integrity of the business, is also

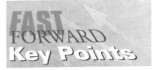

Of all the negative practices the salon industry has conjured up, this one takes the cake. Its casual name is "paying under the table." The federal government and the Internal Revenue Service (IRS) call it "failure to report income"; "tax evasion"; "willful violation of federal law"; "tax fraud" and other not-so-pleasant names. Simply put, failure to report wages is against the law.

The practice is so widespread in this industry that it can only be described as "out of control." And when under-the-table pay gets out of control…the IRS steps in.

yours. But no matter how hard salon owners try to justify their habit of tax evasion, they will never have the sense of security and peace of mind that come with a properly run business.

To all who read this chapter — it's time to play the business game according to the rules. The risks are just too great. Enough damage has already been done.

An ounce of prevention...

T he salon industry is cash-oriented and highly artistic. Though the entrepreneurial spirit runs deep, many salon owners and staff are much more comfortable with creative design than with rigid numbers. And this lack of comfort with numbers often precludes reliable recordkeeping. Consequently, the records are often incomplete when the IRS audits a salon.

Each examination is challenging and unique for both agent and salon owner. The initial interview is not comprised entirely of reconciling the books to the return, evaluating internal systems and testing general operations.

Additional considerations are:

- Reconciling the reported tax return to the taxpayer's financial records.
- Evaluating the cash situation to determine that all cash is reported.

The following is an outline for an initial IRS interview. As a business owner, you are responsible for this information, regardless of whether you have a degree in business.

Keep in mind that this is simply a general outline of what to expect during an audit. There may be additional and more complex questions to answer. The best way to prepare for an audit is to conduct business correctly from the beginning. If your salon is not in compliance, you must turn it around.

Required documentation
- Appointment book(s)
- Individual schedules or worksheets
- Cash box receipts
- Copies of cash service slips
- Lease agreements for stations (booths)
- Franchise fee agreements
- Tip diaries

Retail revenue

- Are there retail sales?
- What is the mark-up percentage on products?
- What is the gross product percentage?
- What percentage is sold to "walk-through" traffic?
- Is commission paid on product sales? What percentage?
- Who supplies the retail product?
- Does the salon have its own product line?

Salon owner

- Is the owner a technician, or strictly a manager?
- How many days per week does the owner work behind the chair? What specific days?
- Which services does the owner provide?
- How often are the appointments booked?

Service revenue

- How many employees are in the salon?
- What are the appointment procedures?
- How are employees compensated?
- How is compensation determined?
- Do you have a tanning bed? How many?
- Do you have a facial table? How many?
- What are the sources of shop revenue?
- Which are your busy months? Slow months?
- What types of services does the salon offer? Time allotments and procedures?
- How many clients make appointments?

Operational questions

- What is your customer tracking system?
- How are walk-ins, cancelations and no-shows designated in the appointment book?
- Do you maintain customer cards?
- Is there a daily/weekly report for each operator?
- What is the procedure for handling inventory?

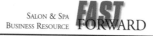
Rental revenue — Booth rentals

- If more than one, what is the total number of locations?
- How many stations are in the salon? What types?
- Are the stations leased? If so, what was the occupancy rate for the year(s) under audit?

Employee versus independent contractor

- Are front desk services provided? Is there a fee charged for these services?
- How is the rental rate determined (i.e., is it fixed or a percentage of sales)?
- What is the daily/weekly/monthly rental rate?
- Does the individual rent a particular space?
- Who is responsible for equipment damage?
- Is there a maintenance charge for the lease?
- Who determines service pricing? Hours of operation?
- Who maintains the renter's appointment book?
- Who collects sales money from clients: the salon or the renter?
- Who pays for the renter's supplies? Who provides tools and equipment?
- Who maintains the books and records of the renter?
- Who pays for the phone system? How many lines? Do renters have their own phones?
- How many phone lines are in the salon?
- Do renters receive any form of compensation on sales? Are they issued 1099s?
- Are renters expected to meet specific standards of performance?
- Are there assistants for renters? Who pays the assistants?
- Is there a contract that identifies the renter as an independent contractor?

Independent contractor or employee?

If a salon directs or controls individuals — or possesses the right to — it's an employer/employee relationship.

The IRS uses several measures to determine how much *control* a business has over an individual. If any element of the relationship indicates that the business can direct and control the individual, an employer/employee relationship exists. Even if the salon doesn't actually control or direct the individual, it's sufficient if the salon has the *right* to do so.

When determining worker status, the presumption of correctness and compliance is always in the hands of the IRS. If the IRS decides the relationship is employer/employee, the salon owner and individual must present evidence to prove otherwise. Generally, borderline situations favor employer/employee status.

The relevant factors of employment status fall into three main categories: *behavioral control, financial control,* and *relationship of the parties.*

Behavioral control

A worker is an employee when the business has the right to direct and control the worker. The business does not have to actually direct or control the *way* the work is done, as long as the employer has the right to direct and control the *work.*

- INSTRUCTIONS: A worker who is required to comply with another person's instructions about when, where and how he or she works is ordinarily an employee. Examples include determining tools or equipment used; which assistants to hire; where to purchase supplies and services.
- TRAINING: Training a worker indicates that the employer exercises control over the means by which the result is accomplished. In other words, when the business provides a worker with training, it suggests that the business wants the work done in a certain way. Consequently, the worker may be an employee.

Financial control

Is there a right to direct or control the business *part of the work?*

- SIGNIFICANT INVESTMENT: A worker is an independent contractor if he or she invests in facilities that are not typically maintained by employees (such as the maintenance of an office rented at fair value from an unrelated party). An employee depends on the employer for such facilities.

- EXPENSES (E.G., TOOLS/MATERIALS, OR BUSINESS TRAVEL): If the employer furnishes significant tools, materials and other equipment, an employer-employee relationship usually exists. Payment of the worker's business and/or traveling expenses is indicative of an employer-employee relationship.

- POTENTIAL FOR PROFIT OR LOSS: A worker who can realize a profit or loss (in addition to the profit or loss ordinarily realized by employees) is an independent contractor. The worker who cannot is generally an employee.

Relationship of the parties

How do the business and the worker perceive their relationship?

- EMPLOYEE BENEFITS: Benefits indicate an employee/employer relationship. If a worker does not receive benefits, he may be an employee or independent contractor.

- WRITTEN CONTRACTS: A contract may be significant if it is otherwise difficult to determine worker status.

Other considerations...

- INTEGRATION: When the success or continuation of a business depends on the performance of certain services, the worker performing those services is subject to a certain amount of control by the owner of the business.

- CONTINUING RELATIONSHIP: A continuing relationship between the worker and the employer indicates that an employer-employee relationship exists.

- SET HOURS OF WORK: The establishment of set hours of work by the employer indicates control.

- FULL-TIME REQUIRED: If the worker must devote full-time hours to the employer's business, the employer has control over the worker's time. An independent contractor is free to work when and for whom he chooses.

- DOING WORK ON THE EMPLOYER'S PREMISES: Control is indicated if the work is performed on the employer's premises.
- ORDER OR SEQUENCE SET: Control is indicated if a worker is not free to choose his or her own pattern of work, but must perform services in the sequence set by the employer.
- ORAL OR WRITTEN REPORTS: Control is indicated if the worker must submit regular oral or written reports to the employer.
- PAYMENT BY HOUR, WEEK OR MONTH: Payment by the hour, week or month points to an employer-employee relationship, provided that this method of payment is not just a convenient way of paying a lump sum agreed on as the cost of a job. An independent contractor usually is paid by the job in an agreed-upon lump sum.
- WORKING FOR MORE THAN ONE FIRM AT A TIME: If a worker performs services for a number of unrelated firms at the same time, he/she is usually an independent contractor.
- MAKING SERVICES AVAILABLE TO THE GENERAL PUBLIC: A worker is usually an independent contractor if he or she makes his or her services available to the general public on a regular and consistent basis.
- RIGHT TO DISCHARGE: The right of the employer to discharge a worker indicates that he or she is an employee.
- RIGHT TO TERMINATE: A worker is an employee if he or she has the right to end the relationship with the principal at any time without incurring liability.

The computer conundrum

M any salon reporting and paperwork problems can be eased by a computer and a good software package at the front desk. A computer can process standing appointments or coordinate a day of beauty in just seconds — alleviating the necessity of telling clients that things are "just too hectic," but you will be "happy to call them back." The ease with which a computer changes appointment times or dates and adjusts employee schedules is not even comparable to the use of pencil and paper. Yet many salon owners refuse to automate, choosing instead to use unwieldy and unreliable paper appointment books. Why?

Walking on water

A point-of-sale system on your computer records every transaction entered. If the cash drawer can only be opened by inputting amounts of sales, the system will record the dollar amount, the computer operator, the technician to whom the sale is credited and the time of day. It's all there. Therefore, you expose yourself to a number of tax evasion charges by continuing to pay wages "off-the-books." There are also considerable risks to your staff: Accepting money under the table is just as dangerous as paying it. One misstep can affect the whole salon.

There are many salon owners who operate with computers, but continue to disburse unreported income. If you are in this situation, consider how much of a risk you are willing to take. You don't have to be an agent of the IRS to see that the income you report on tax returns does not match the bank deposits and computer records of service and retail sales. If the issue ever arises, there is no way to explain away the discrepancies between the computer records and the bank records.

Walking on broken glass

Operating a salon in this manner is dangerous. There must be a method of calculating the salon's gross and net income in order to ensure continued profitability. With no books at all, a salon owner can easily drive himself out of business. And it's nearly as bad with two sets of books — what happens when someone gets confused?

There is no doubt that computers bring order to the quagmire of many salon operations. They offer a beautifully efficient way to obtain accurate reports and statistics. Yet this is precisely why they are so intimidating to many salon owners. The uneasiness of change often stems from the fear of acknowledging former duplicity. Like children worried that their parents will discover the bald spot on the cake, salon owners cringe at the idea of shedding light on incomplete and inaccurate records.

For salon owners who routinely pay under the table, a computer may represent an unwanted intrusion — an ever-vigilant "big brother" to be feared and hated. Many owners' sole reason for not automating is the computer's efficiency at recording appointments and financial information.

Consider this instead: How many unproductive hours slip by, *wasted,* because the desk staff are scrambling to keep up with client and staff requests?

Business as usual

Hiding services and "forgetting" to record retail sales simply should not be an option for today's salon owner. Business ethics and integrity apply to every industry, and the salon industry should not set itself apart. The fact is, one of the greatest favors a salon owner can do himself and his staff is to realize that a salon is a professional business, and treat it as such.

Of course, it is possible (with some effort) to operate without a computer, and many salon owners will continue to do so. If you are one of these, make yourself aware of the dangers of incomplete or inaccurate records. And if you do use a computer, take steps to ensure that all sales are recorded properly and completely. Whatever your method of recordkeeping, do it right.

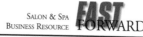
Just the facts: What are your responsibilities?

Though complex, the process of filing tax returns is not as difficult as you might think — and it's the law.

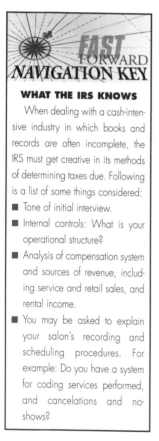

WHAT THE IRS KNOWS

When dealing with a cash-intensive industry in which books and records are often incomplete, the IRS must get creative in its methods of determining taxes due. Following is a list of some things considered:

■ Tone of initial interview.

■ Internal controls: What is your operational structure?

■ Analysis of compensation system and sources of revenue, including service and retail sales, and rental income.

■ You may be asked to explain your salon's recording and scheduling procedures. For example: Do you have a system for coding services performed, and cancelations and no-shows?

Ben Franklin spoke truthfully: There are few things certain in life, but you can rest assured that taxes will always be one of them. Keeping up with income and payroll taxes certainly isn't most people's idea of fun. It may often seem that the amounts withheld from your checks are much too high — but there is no escaping the fact that United States law requires taxes to be paid. If you are receiving unreported cash tips, or are paying or being paid a portion of your salary under the table, you are not playing it smart — you're playing with fire.

The following pages contain an in-depth listing of the forms and procedures the IRS expects every business owner to fill out completely and follow. These records provide the paper trail which is essential to prove compliance with current tax codes. If the need arises, you should be prepared.

Worker responsibilities in reporting wages

Definition of taxable income: Taxable income includes wages, payments for services, rents received and tips. All of these items are applicable to the beauty industry.

What and how to declare
- For employees of salons: All funds paid (by check or cash) by the salon to the employee, with or without a Form W-2 or Form 1099, are includable as income on the employee's tax return.
- All tips received from patrons are includable as income on the Form 1040 tax return of the employee, whether or not the employee properly reports these tips to the employer. Tips not reported to the employer should also be included on Form 4137 to correctly compute applicable employment tax due.
- For salon workers who rent chairs or booths from a salon owner and are independent contractors: All funds for services received from patrons (including tips) are includable on Schedule C of Form 1040 as gross income.

Penalties for failure to report
- Failure to report all income and to pay all respective taxes on filed returns is subject to a failure-to-pay penalty of up to 25% of the tax not paid.
- Failure to file a return is subject to a penalty of up to 25% of the tax required to be filed, in addition to the full payment of delinquent taxes.
- When both penalties are asserted, the total penalty cannot exceed payment of taxes due, plus 25%.
- If failure to file or pay is due to reasonable cause, the penalties will not be asserted. If, however, it is due to willful neglect or fraud, penalties as high as 75% of taxes due (in addition to the payment of all delinquent taxes) may be asserted, with the potential for criminal prosecution.

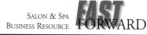
Independent contractors

- Rent payments of at least $600 per year, paid by booth or chair renters to a non-corporate salon owner, must be reported on Form 1099. Failure to file this form can result in a $50 penalty. Backup withholding may be required if payments were not filed on Form 1099 or were reported on Form 1099 without a proper Taxpayer Identification Number (TIN). Backup withholding rate: 31% of gross earnings.

Salon owner responsibility in reporting wages

All requirements for reporting taxable income, and the penalties for not reporting, which are applicable to salon employees are also applicable to salon owners.

What and how to declare

- The employer must report all payments (cash or check) made to the employee for work performed, as well as all tips reported to the employer. These reports must be made on Form W-2 at the end of the year and on Form 941 on a quarterly basis.
- The employer must withhold federal income tax and the employee's share of employment taxes from the employee's pay; the employer also must report the employer's share of employment taxes on Form 941 each quarter.

Penalties for failure to report

- Failure to pay or file is subject to the same penalties mentioned previously and, additionally, may be subject to a failure-to-deposit penalty of up to 15%.
- Failure to furnish Form W-2 or file a correct Form W-2 can subject the salon owner to a $50 penalty per violation.

Independent contractors

- Salon owners must report all income received via rent from either booth or chair rentals on the appropriate income tax schedule.
- Salon owners must report all income received from patrons for services provided by the salon owners themselves.
- Carefully consider agreements with booth or chair renters. Improperly characterizing a worker as a renter or independent contractor may result in a determination by the government that the salon owner is liable for employment taxes on income received by the worker. Carefully consider the common law factors mentioned in Publication 1779.

The tip factor

- The salon owner should provide a means for employees to report tips in order to ensure proper employment taxes are paid and income tax withholding is paid by the employer.

- The government has developed the Tip Reporting Alternative Commitment agreement to encourage employers and employees to properly report tips. Through this program, the employer agrees to provide a means for reporting charge and cash tips received by the employees and to file all proper tax returns. The government agrees, with certain exceptions, to assess the employer share of employment taxes only on tips reported by employees on their Form 1040, on Form 4137 or as discovered through an employee tip examination on Form 885-T. Experience in the restaurant industry (also a cash-intensive industry) shows that this program can increase tip reporting by at least 30%.

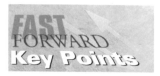

The IRS has compiled an MSSP (Market Segment Specialization Program) Audit Guide for Beauty and Barber Shops which "focuses on issues that arise in auditing cash-intensive businesses."

Download a copy of the MSSP from the IRS web site at www.IRS.ustreas.gov at "Tax Info for Business."

Or write:
Superintendent of Documents
Government Printing Office
P.O. Box 371954
Pittsburgh, PA, 15250-7954

Or call:
202.512.1776
(from 8.00 a.m. to 4.00 p.m., EST)
You will be asked to leave a fax number, and will receive a list of all MSSP guides and their stock numbers.

IRS tips on tipping

W hat can you do to better conform to IRS regulations on tipping, and better protect your business in the event of an audit or tip examination? Unless your salon is in complete compliance with IRS regulations on tipping, and you can prove it, you may end up in an unpleasant situation. Others' mismanagement of money can affect you.

SUGGESTION: Simply, and with purpose, educate your team about IRS tip regulations. Obtain copies of applicable tax codes and share them with team members, along with Publication 1244, the "tip diary." Many salon owners are already aware of the tip diary and encourage their employees to use it.

Present these documents to all team members at the first of the year (perhaps at a staff meeting). Staff should sign and date a form stating they received a copy of the tax law and Publication 1244. This document will become a valuable part of the salon's records, and proof of your compliance with the law.

A helping hand from the IRS

For a truly impartial look at tipping and the way it should be handled (as opposed to the way it often is), where better to turn than the Internal Revenue Service? Too often, salon owners and employees ignore the proper channels for reporting tips and neglect to calculate and pay applicable taxes. It's a game of Russian roulette played with no discernable rules — and it's dangerous.

There are two methods of discovering under-reported tips and discrepancies in tip reporting between employers and employees: an audit of either employer or employee. Candidates for personal and business audits are usually selected through the normal course of business (i.e., your name comes out of the computer). Occasionally, however, information received from one individual will spur an investigation of another. A salon owner's best course of action is to take no chances, and report tips correctly from the beginning.

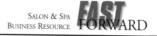

The purpose of the IRS' current tip project in the salon industry is to achieve voluntary compliance from as many salons as possible. The goal is to educate all directly and indirectly tipped employees on tip-reporting requirements. However, salon owners and employees should not disregard the fact that the IRS is fully aware of the potential for under-reporting earnings in the industry, and they do look deeply into industries with such potential.

Who has to do what?

Ensuring that tips are properly reported is not the burden of a single individual. It is a responsibility shared by employers and employees alike. There are some pretty basic "rules of thumb":

- Employees must report all tips in excess of $20 per month to their employer so that the employer may properly report them as income and withhold appropriate employment tax.
- Any tips less than $20 per month should still be reported on the employee's personal return, though they are not required to be reported to the employer. Salon owners should also bear in mind that if an employee reports tips on a personal tax return (even though the tips are not reported to the employer), the employer may still be assessed his share of employment tax.
- Contract laborers should include all tips as a portion of their income on Schedule C of their returns. (Technically, contract laborers aren't receiving "tips"; it's all considered income from their business.) Regardless of the labor status of a worker, if it is determined that an employer did not properly withhold FICA, the owner will have to pay it.

How to do it

All salon employees who receive tips should record them daily in a "tip diary," IRS Publication 1244. The diary contains Form 4070A, the Employee's Daily Record of Tips, and Form 4070, the Employee's Report of Tips to Employer. The salon owner should receive Form 4070 from employees monthly.

Records of amounts recorded on Form 4070 are essential for filing a complete and accurate Form 941. Form 941 is required quar-

Department of the Treasury
Internal Revenue Service

Publication 1244
(Rev. July 1996)

Employee's Daily Record of Tips
and
Report to Employer

This publication contains:
Form 4070A, Employee's Daily Record of Tips
Form 4070, Employee's Report of Tips to Employer

For the period

beginning ...., 19 ...

ending ...., 19 ...

Name and address of employee

Form **4070**
(Rev. July 1996)
Department of the Treasury
Internal Revenue Service

Employee's Report
of Tips to Employer
▶ For Paperwork Reduction Act Notice, see back.

Employee's name and address

Employer's name and address (include establishment name, if different)

Form **4070A**
(Rev. July 1996)
Department of the Treasury
Internal Revenue Service

Employee's Daily Record of Tips
This is a voluntary form provided for your convenience.
See instructions for records you must keep.

Employee's name and address

Employer's name

Establishment name (if different)

Date tips rec'd.	Date of entry	a. Tips received directly from customers and other employees	b. Credit card tips received	c. Tips paid out to other employees	d. Name

terly of employers who withhold income tax on wages. Tips are considered wages, and should be included.

If there are tip amounts not reported to employers, but included by employees on personal returns, those employees must file Form 4137, Social Security and Medicare Tax on Unreported Tip Income.

To obtain further information or necessary forms and publications, call the IRS toll-free at 800.829.3676 or visit the web site at *www.IRS.ustreas.gov.*

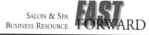
Employee responsibilities in reporting tips

E mployees who receive a large portion of their income from tips often have many questions about how and even why tips should be reported. Here are some *answers.*

ANSWER: Yes, all tips must be reported. If your tips total $20 or more in a given month, all tips must be reported to your employer so that appropriate taxes can be withheld. Even indirectly paid monies (e.g., from "tip-outs") should be reported. A monthly total less than $20 should be included on your personal return.

ANSWER: Adequate and accurate records should be kept on an ongoing basis. Free copies of an IRS "tip diary" are available through their toll-free number (800.829.3676). In the event of an examination, you will need one.

ANSWER: If tips are underreported, you may be liable for back taxes, penalties and interest.

Dealing with taxes is far from the top of most people's "happy" list, including those who work for the IRS. But, the IRS was created to ensure compliance with federal tax statutes. Salon employees not accustomed to paying taxes on tip income will question the necessity of doing so. Here's why it's necessary:

Why it should matter to you
- Social security benefits.
- Unemployment compensation benefits.
- Increased employee pension, annuity or 401(k) participation.
- Better credit standing (think about home and/or car loans).
- Compliance with the law prevents increased taxes and interest in the event of a tip audit.

Salon owner responsibilities in reporting tips

Business owners in tip-intensive industries have more than one tip reporting option: the Tip Rate Determination Agreement (TRDA), the Tip Reporting Alternative Commitment (TRAC), or status quo. If an employer decides to enter either TRDA or TRAC, the IRS will assist him or her in understanding and meeting all requirements for participation.

The main objective of the TRDA and TRAC programs is to make it easier for employers bound by statutory tip provisions to comply with federal tax regulations. One benefit of enrollment for your employees is that the IRS will conduct no tip examinations as long as the provisions of the TRDA or TRAC agreement are met and all tips are reported.

The TRAC agreement is accepted in every district. All eligible employers will be assisted in understanding and meeting the requirements for participation. Through the TRAC agreement, the IRS district director and the salon owner agree to jointly resolve disputes and establish procedures to prevent future problems. An employer's TRAC application may only be rejected if he does not comply with tax regulations (i.e., does not file or does not pay taxes due), cannot fulfill his obligations under the agreement, or is the subject of a federal action or investigation.

TRAC...Commitment of salon owner

- Maintain a quarterly education program, emphasizing cash tip procedures.
- File all applicable forms in a timely manner, including Forms 941 and W-2.
- Pay and deposit all federal taxes in a timely manner.
- Maintain accurate tip records (cash) and receipts (charge).
- Make all tip records available to the district director upon request.
- Establish a procedure and devise a written statement for reporting cash and charge tips.

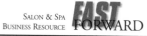
TRAC...Commitment of IRS district director

- With exceptions, a notice and demand shall be based solely on amounts shown on Form 4137 (Social Security and Medicare Tax on Unreported Tip Income, filed by employee with Form 1040), or on form 885-T (Adjustment of Social Security Tax on Tip Income Not Reported to Employer).

- The district director may revoke the agreement only if the salon owner fails to maintain his obligations as outlined under the agreement, substantially underreports tip income for two continuous calendar quarters or becomes the subject of a federal action or investigation. The salon owner may terminate the TRAC agreement at any time by notifying the district director, in writing, of his desire.

To enter either program, salon owners need only submit a letter of application to the tip coordinator in their local examination/ compliance division. Call 800.829.1040 for the phone number of your local tip coordinator; he or she can provide detailed information on each arrangement.

Why it should matter to you

It's always better to play by the rules than to gamble and lose. To many salon owners and staff, running a business by the numbers can be harrowing. To some, it's unfamiliar and intimidating territory. But no matter how you look at it, the law is still the law. You'll be better off in the future if you play fair today.

For your information...

This is a partial list of available IRS publications and forms. Publication 1779 is also available at this number. Each form listed here relates to tip income reporting. Call toll-free: 800.829.3676.

- Pub 505: Tax Withholding and Estimated Tax
- Pub 551: Reporting Tip Income
- Pub 1244: Employee's Daily Record of Tips and Report to Employer. (Includes Form 4070, Employee's Report of Tips to Employer, and Form 4070A, Employee's Daily Record of Tips.)
- Form 941: Employer's Quarterly Federal Tax Return
- Form 1040ES: Estimated Tax for Individuals
- Form 4137: Social Security and Medicare Tax on Unreported Tip Income
- Form W-2: Wage and Tax Statement

15

PERSONAL AND INTERPERSONAL MOTIVATION

Creating a values-based business that will flourish and prosper

GUEST CHAPTER BY:
> *Andrew Finkelstein, President*
> BEAUTY MATTERS, LTD.

Have you ever dreamed of creating a salon unlike anything that has ever existed, radically different from anything you have previously experienced? A place that looks special, behaves a certain way, acts in a particular manner, even smells distinctive? Was that only a fantasy, or did you really have a glimpse of something you considered extraordinary? If you are like thousands of other salon owners, chances are that (at one time or another) you had a certain idea in mind about the business you set out to create. And you wanted something great, not mediocre.

Intent is an important part of a visionary leader's goal achievement process. Through intent, a vision is transformed from a mere fleeting moment in the owner's mind into a reality, a place where people — clients, employees, lenders and vendors — can experience something different, something extraordinary that did not exist before in the present form. Your business, as well as your life, is special, and its uniqueness distinguishes it from every other business in the world.

Vision originates in the owner's mind or, perhaps more correctly, in the heart. (If vision is at the heart of motivation, let us say that it comes from the heart.) And vision begins with the knowledge that what one is about to create will serve a purpose that transcends the monetary, and has a greater value than financial means. If the salon one creates is only about dollars and cents, then the owner will never be satisfied.

The magic begins with the leader and her willingness and courage to explore herself, to understand what drives her. The process is about self-knowledge. Dr. Steven Covey, author of *The 7 Habits of Highly Effective People,* lists habit number 5 — "Seek first to understand, then to be understood" — as a guiding principle for communication. Does not this concept begin with you, and your commitment to personal and business growth? It is this sense of self, and one's ability to maintain a commitment to a vision and its attendant accountabilities, that gives a leader the fortitude to do what must be done.

Daniel Goleman, Ph.D. and author of the books *Emotional Intelligence* and *Working with Emotional Intelligence,* makes a case for the role of emotional intelligence in achieving excellence in virtually any field. Emotional intelligence has been discussed for decades, referred to by such names as *character, personality, soft skills* and *competence.*

Dr. Goleman writes: "We now have twenty-five years' worth of empirical studies that tell us with a previously unknown precision just how much emotional intelligence matters for success." In his research in psychobiology, he tracks cutting-edge findings in neuroscience which make it crystal clear *why* emotional intelligence matters so much: "The ancient brain centers for emotion also harbor the skills needed for managing ourselves effectively and for social adeptness. Thus these skills are grounded in our evolutionary heritage for survival and adaptation."

Moving beyond ordinary

T rue leaders move beyond what is considered ordinary into the realm of the extraordinary. If one's business creations are truly a reflection of one's thinking, then one is enabled to take actions consistent with that thinking. This convergence of thought and action paves the way for a business to do ordinary things in an extraordinary way.

After all, salon owners create businesses that cut and color hair, perform beauty treatments and sell retail...and these activities are rather ordinary. They are no different than delivering a box from one city to another, which is what FEDERAL EXPRESS *really* does; no different than having a theme park with rides and food, which is what WALT DISNEY *really* does. And is MCDONALD'S *really* anything more than a hamburger stand serving, at best, adequate food?

So when a visionary salon owner looks at what she does in its most basic form, of course it's just a bundle of beauty services. The real question, which requires the *thinking* is: How can we create a place where ordinary people can do what they do in an extraordinary fashion?

HOW CAN WE DESIGN A COMPANY THAT DOES ORDINARY THINGS
IN AN EXTRAORDINARY WAY, AND...

WHAT IS THE ONE UNIQUE THING WE COULD ACCOMPLISH
THAT WOULD TRANSFORM OUR BUSINESS AND DISTINGUISH IT
FROM EVERY OTHER?

These questions are essential because the vision of the company revolves around the answers, and everything the company does moves it closer to actually accomplishing that *one* nearly impossible but definitely achievable thing.

Fred Smith, founder of FEDERAL EXPRESS, posed this question in a business school thesis which described the company he would create. His question was: What would it take to create a company to deliver packages anywhere in the world overnight, on time, every time? As the story goes, Fred Smith got a grade of C on this paper. Yet FEDERAL EXPRESS is now a FORTUNE 500 company. *IT IS BY ASKING THE QUESTION THAT WE ARE ABLE TO FIND WHAT WE SEEK.*

Another component of the art of leading others via your vision is highlighted by James M. Kouzes and Barry Z. Posner, authors of *The Leadership Challenge*, who write: "The mastery of the art of leadership comes with the mastery of the self." In other words, it requires one to work on a deeper level within oneself.

The art of leadership

A s a business leader, you have great impact on employees. This impact is either positive or negative, depending upon your behavioral characteristics. Following is a number of vital leadership characteristics. The list is by no means complete, but will serve as a starting point for assessing your abilities.

- Honesty
- Strength
- Thoroughness and persistence
- Willingness to listen
- Patience
- Desire for learning
- Resiliency
- Calmness
- Compassion
- Vision and the ability to dream
- Systemic thinking
- Lack of cynicism

These characteristics may be learned by anyone with the desire to do so. It is no secret that if the will is present, the rest will follow. But there is work involved in learning to lead, and in the creation of leadership qualities. The process does not happen overnight; it requires the systematic cultivation of a particular mindset, which can be accomplished by completing the following steps. Think of this as a long-term project, and give it the energy and vital importance you would any major project.

Learning to lead: A six-step method

First, a few ideas to facilitate the process: REMOVE yourself from outside distractions and other influences. It may be wise to leave your office and find a quiet place. EVALUATE yourself according to your own standards, not other people's. TRUST yourself. You have feelings as well as thoughts. If it feels right, pay attention.

1. PERFORM A SELF-EVALUATION using each of the qualities bulleted on the previous page. (Also include additional qualities you feel a leader possesses.) Consider where you presently stand with each. Which are major strengths or weaknesses, true most of the time, or in need of attention? Record your answers.

2. SELECT ONE OR TWO CHARACTERISTICS you consider most important and want to develop.

3. REMEMBER SITUATIONS FROM THE PAST in which you behaved *positively* — the way you envision a true leader would.

4. REMEMBER SITUATIONS IN THE PAST when your behavior was *not* up to the leadership standards you want to achieve. Recast them in your mind, as you would *like* to see yourself in those situations. This is simply a mental practice of rehearsing positive behavior and eliminating the negative.

5. PAY ATTENTION TO YOUR BUSINESS; SEEK REAL-LIFE SITUATIONS in which you can practice leadership behavior. Be careful not to *create* a situation just to do this, as it would ring false to employees. They know the difference! Simply be aware of the multitude of opportunities that present themselves, and behave with *intent.* As noted author and business consultant Tom Peters says, "Each day in business a manager is presented with a thousand opportunities to reinforce the culture of her company, whether she chooses to use them or not."

6. KEEP AT IT, AND PERIODICALLY REVIEW your behavior until you notice the habits you have been working on are fully cultivated.

On a practical note, you may find that developing new behavior takes some time; however, employees will notice and appreciate what you are doing. You are now consciously working on something of benefit to them, and they will see a leader who truly knows how to lead.

REMEMBER: Leadership is about finding the confidence and strength necessary to lead. Only the belief that one does not possess a leader's qualities, or that leaders are only born and cannot created, will stop you from becoming what your company needs.

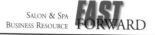

Identifying values and beliefs

T he next stop on this magical mystery tour lies in the ability to recognize one's values and beliefs. Once these are known, they can be put to work.

- Values are ideals (such as freedom), qualities (such as kindness or generosity) and entities (such as education) that people consider desirable. They are those things most important to us.
- Beliefs are ideas that have come to be accepted as true, though they cannot be proven. A belief can be argued strongly by one person, while another argues its opposite.

While your values and beliefs may not exactly coincide, they are reflected in one another. Both affect the way you see the world around you, and how you interpret and judge what you see in that world. This in turn affects the way you act, respond to others and make both business and personal decisions.

Identifying beliefs and values is also important because they offer insight into the motivations which drive your actions. These motivations provide a clearer perspective on happenings in the business, which enables clearer communication with staff. This clarity then enables one to carry on in a calm and self-assured manner rather than behaving impulsively — a quality that stems primarily from an oblivion toward what is going on inside oneself.

Likewise, it is important to be aware of *assumptions* — things taken for granted or believed to be true, though not known for certain. An assumption is similar to a belief, in that people are also sometimes unaware of the assumptions under which they operate. The difference is that beliefs can be far-reaching, and an assumption is generally specific to a particular situation.

Consider a sales representative who requests a meeting with a salon owner to show her new product offerings. The owner politely refuses. The sales representative might take the owner's refusal at face value without any assumptions, or he may assume a number of things: that the owner is not interested in the line, that she is busy and does not want to be disturbed, even that she does not like him. Most likely, the assumption he chooses will affect what he does next.

- If he assumes the owner is not interested in the line, he might suggest they meet to discuss ways to build business with the lines the salon carries.
- If he assumes she is too busy, he might suggest another time for the meeting.
- If he assumes the owner does not like him, he may feel reluctant to work with her.

When an incorrect assumption is acted upon, it can set off a chain of events resulting in problems, wasted time and negative feelings. The effects of such behavior can be far-reaching. Acting on assumptions leaves others "in the dark" instead of "in the know." And "in the dark" is not the place to be.

A leader's challenge is to realize when actions or reactions are based on assumptions. If so, are the assumptions valid? One must learn the difference between what one *assumes* to be true and what one *knows* to be true. Deciphering assumptions enables one to see others differently, and to be more competent and compassionate in everyday business dealings.

The force of impact

Impact is defined as the way one makes others feel. Too often people make decisions, only to discover afterwards that they had no idea how these choices would impact others. This occurs because people have no idea of how *they* impact others. There are any number of ways to create impact: by the way one looks, talks, listens, responds and, yes, even through reputation. Impact can occur in the immediate vicinity or a thousand miles distant, and in a million different ways.

But *your* responses tell only half the story of impact; there is also the half that resides with others. People are impacted in different ways — one may think you a role model, while another feels threatened. Learning about your impact on others will make you a better leader, and create more fruitful relationships. Most people picture themselves quite differently than others do.

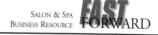
- Consider the impact you *think* you have on your team. How does this compare with the impact you would *like* to have?

- Discover the impact you truly have, this time from the team's perspective. Do not simply think about it yourself; ask them what *they* think. Encourage honesty by creating an environment safe from recrimination. Some responses may surprise, disappoint or even hurt you…but constructive criticism is necessary for change and growth. And, on the flip side, you'll also hear positive things.

- Don't let emotion interfere with what you want to accomplish. Objective feedback will ultimately translate into better leadership skills, a more successful business and a positive impact on the business overall. It will help you recognize the way people see you, and understand their reactions.

Mirror, mirror

In the pursuit of greater self-understanding one must be honest with oneself. Are you able to observe yourself in the mirror and pinpoint those things that are hard to look at? Once found, one must also recognize the methods habitually employed to avoid them; only then can you take steps to change from within in order to achieve a more favorable external impact. Call them weaknesses, natural tendencies or even character defects, but always consider them opportunities for improvement.

WHAT ARE THESE AREAS? Consider delegation. Many salon owners continue to do things that others could and *should* be doing. They continue to exist in a comfort zone. Consider indirect communications. Instead of saying "I am unhappy and this is why," owners only hint at situations.

You may wonder what is wrong with having these unaddressed traits. The answer? These "difficult" areas nearly always prevent people from getting what they want, from achieving their vision. When employees do not know "the score" and do not respect leadership, morale suffers and the business is incapable of attaining the best possible results.

Not recognizing and dealing with individual problem areas creates an atmosphere of negativity — and a pattern of habitual evasion often results. After a time, the aspiring leader no longer recognizes the effects of this pattern and loses the ability to choose. *But the ability to choose is fundamental to leadership.* Avoiding the "tough stuff" results in missed opportunities to make the simplest choices, and to discover the great possibilities inherent in one's business and in oneself.

Exploring the unknown

The next item to address on the path to self-knowledge is the *unknown*. It is not unusual for people to feel uncomfortable about being in the unknown, partly because they must admit to being inexperienced. It takes away the "expert" label. It means there is someone out there who knows more, and therefore creates a position of vulnerability.

There is irony in the way many people respond to the unknown. Rather than embracing it and humbly admitting (to themselves at least) that they don't know what is going on, they resist and fall back into an even more emphatic position. They believe that acting more self-assured, more certain, will convince others that they really *do* know what's going on — when precisely the opposite is true. They even rationalize that it's good for their team if they appear "strong" and confident.

Today, the new concept of leadership states that it is alright not to know, that the leader doesn't always have to be the expert. She need not have all the answers. As a matter of course, it is often preferable *not* to have all the answers because team members can otherwise be adversely affected. They may feel devalued, and think, "If you have all the answers, why ask me?…You really don't value my thinking." But your team has a great deal to contribute, and such negative thinking encourages a loss of helpful information.

Embracing the unknown provides an opportunity to let go of the inhibitive feeling that you always need to be the expert. It allows you to be open to the endless choices and possibilities in front of you. Fully embracing the unknown enables you to be yourself, which in turn opens new horizons for your business and all associated with it.

Getting a grip — On yourself

How do you proceed to understand more about yourself so that you can *be* yourself and, in turn, a more effective leader? It requires a great deal of intuition, but there are steps that you can follow.

- UNDERSTAND THE IMPORTANCE OF SELF-KNOWLEDGE. Acceptance and self-knowledge are at the heart of leadership ability. As you become more self-confident, you'll further appreciate the importance of self-knowledge for your team members.
- CREATE A SELF-KNOWLEDGE "BASELINE" by writing down your values and beliefs, then ranking them in order of importance. The process is simple. List them in no particular order, numbered 1–15. Compare #1 to #2 by considering which you value more. Compare the "winner" to #3 in the same manner. Work your way through the list; then consider the remaining items and repeat the process. Eventually, all fifteen will be ranked in order of their importance to you. Completing this exercise will help you more fully understand yourself, and put your experiences into a standard context.
- IDENTIFY YOUR NEXT PERSONAL STEPS. Consider a current situation, and reframe it to reflect your new perspective. For example: Assume you have a belief which states, "I need to have all the answers. If I don't, it's a sign that I'm really not a leader." You can reframe the belief to state: "When I don't have all the answers, I have the opportunity to approach people and involve them in the business, which is a sign of strong leadership."
- SET UP A PERSONAL TRACKING SYSTEM AND PRACTICE EVERY DAY. Stop throughout the day and ask yourself insightful questions. "What belief is underlying my experiences in this situation? Am I being as open as possible in this unknown area? Is there another approach to solving this problem?"
- BE A ROLE MODEL. PRACTICE SELF-KNOWLEDGE IN YOUR BUSINESS. As you become more comfortable with what you are doing, share it with the team. Tell them about the impact it has had on you. Share experiences and techniques, and ask questions to help them learn more about their internal experiences.

THERE ARE TANGIBLE BENEFITS OF SELF-KNOWLEDGE LEADERSHIP WORK:
- A feeling of greater inner strength follows the learning process.
- The ability to make better decisions, and an increased willingness to turn decisions into action.

- The increased ability to inspire trust and confidence in others.
- The ability to find and implement better ways to get results.
- A way to see your business and the world around you more clearly.
- Better and more authentic relationships with others.
- More willingness to relinquish control (delegate) to others.
- Increased ability to handle change and uncertainty in ways that are productive and reassuring to others.

Sharing your vision of the future

How do you draw the salon team into your vision? How do you harness the energies of the team to achieve the desired results — the ones contained in your vision for the business? First and foremost, put your vision in writing, in the form of a *strategic objective* (see *The E-Myth Revisited,* HarperCollins, 1995). It need not be elaborate. The strategic objective is a one- or two-page document which describes your vision of the future of the business: how it will look, act and perform when complete. It always contains vital indicators such as sales and profits, retention rate, percentage of retail to total business, or other quantifiable indicators important to your salon.

THE STRATEGIC OBJECTIVE WILL SERVE AS A CORNERSTONE for the work you and the team perform. Simply constructing this document may represent a change in your business thinking. But you are working on your leadership skills — and dealing with the unknown is one of them.

Change is a constant in business. Harnessing change — viewing it as a resource instead of a stumbling block — creates the opportunity to develop an environment that will generate the results outlined in the strategic objective. The most desirable type of environment is a *high-performance* environment.

Shifting your salon into high gear

A high-performance environment requires vision, structure and tools. Once the *vision* (i.e., the strategic objective) is in place, one must develop a structure designed to actualize the business' purpose and goals, and provide employees the tools they need to achieve the vision. To accomplish this, change must be used as a resource, as an opportunity to test assumptions and systems, add to the collective knowledge of the business and grow the business. This frees people to look at the business through a new filter, and drives creativity and innovation.

More than anything, this requires persistence on the owner's part. It takes time. But moving in this direction allows you to create a game worth playing, for yourself *and* the team. It draws in customers, motivates vendors and reassures lenders. In short, it energizes all those who play a part in the business. With this energy, confidence in the business builds, which spurs further energy and leads to increased confidence. It's an *upward* spiral.

How does one design a high-performance environment? *Systemically,* of course!

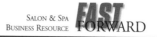
Creating a high-performance environment

STEP ONE: Integrate your vision into the culture of the business

Build a strategy designed specifically for this purpose. Remember, it all starts with the leader. A leader is responsible for articulating, reinforcing and protecting the *vision*. She may accomplish this through various methods, all of which are designed to achieve the same result: driving the vision into the company.

- HOLD REGULARLY SCHEDULED ONE-ON-ONE BUSINESS DEVELOPMENT MEETINGS (as well as other scheduled meetings) with team members. Face-to-face interaction is the best way to achieve a positive impact. Remember, you are not "selling" your vision — you want to enroll the team members and encourage them to enhance your vision with their own objectives. You are creating a common goal and spirit. There is no substitute for face-to-face communication at the beginning of this journey. Since you have been developing your leadership skills, you know your presence can be powerful. *Be the leader* whose attributes you have been developing. Make your vision a shared creation.

- CREATE INFORMAL OPPORTUNITIES TO BE WITH YOUR TEAM. A breakfast or informal celebration of a particular accomplishment, with an open agenda, helps encourage conversation.

- MODEL THE VISION. Since you have identified values important to the company, reinforce them at every opportunity. Catch people doing something right, something that is a positive example of what you are looking for. Praise them in the presence of other staff. You may be surprised at the positive impact.

- USE PRINTED MATERIALS TO REINFORCE THE VISION. While they are not as powerful as face-to-face contact, there is a focused method of using printed materials to positively impact customers, vendors and lenders. For example: A general vision statement could be included in virtually every document the business distributes or shows its team members. The employee handbook should highlight the impact you want to have on your customers. Review all printed materials; innovate ways to integrate your vision into them.

- BE CONSCIOUS OF YOUR ATTITUDE toward employees and their role in the business. A leader, by definition, is someone who has followers. One cannot exist without the other. Viewing team members as active rather than passive participants will move you closer to accomplishing your vision. It also sets a tone that says to team members, "Yes, she really can lead." If they think you can lead, they will align themselves with you. If you think of the team as co-creators, the vision will materialize. They will innovate, once taught to do so — and this innovation will propel your business toward its strategic objective.

STEP TWO: Remove the roadblocks

The structure of your company goes beyond an organizational chart. *Structure* consists of everything in the business that influences, directs and controls its activities, including its formal and informal relationships. For example: Your vision may promote an environment in which the customer feels comfortable visiting any stylist. But the compensation system may reinforce the "my client" syndrome. The desired action is more strongly implied in the compensatory reward than the simple verbal representation of the salon's vision. *This* is why the team's behavior is what it is.

There are many components of a company structure:

- YOUR VISION will have a strong positive effect on the everyday decision-making of team members.
- YOUR HIERARCHY should make sense for your business. It will not necessarily follow industry tradition. The hierarchy should *reflect the needs* of the business as opposed to attempting to *shape* the business.
- "THE WAY WE DO IT HERE" is the culture of your company: the habits, standards, rules and practices that shape its behavior. Some of it is ritualized, and will become part of the company's *myth*. There is also a "parallel" culture, which surfaces when the company's actions are not aligned with its professed values. For example: A company professes that employees are its most

important resource, but with a downturn in business, those employees are immediately laid off. Viewing problems as opportunities, as a leader does, offers the chance to evaluate assumptions, and discover a better way to integrate them into one's vision and business practices.

■ YOUR BELIEFS ABOUT WHAT IS TRUE can shape a high-performance environment. If one believes people are a certain way, they will be. If one believes people have nothing to contribute, they won't contribute anything. If a business owner believes people can make useful contributions, she will create a system to encourage it. As with the preceding bullet point, continually evaluate assumptions — especially as part of a decision-making process.
Another underlying characteristic of a business leader that generally goes unacknowledged is one's attitude toward risk. While today's buzz words and management techniques promote the virtues of risk-taking, the truth is organizations put a greater premium on the virtue of compliance.

Because creating a high-performance environment sometimes means venturing into the unknown (and that means risk), one needs a way to coach team members on how to create a system to quantify risk. This means they must know a great deal about systemic business operations and the way each area impacts others. The more they know, the better they can quantify the impact of their decisions upon other areas of the business. Assessing these consequences will enable them to evaluate the risk.

In incorporating a system into a company, one takes a quantifiable risk, which may be regarded in an objective manner. And if one rewards risk-taking, because now the risks are controlled, one has successfully created a system that honors innovation. Remember, there are only two ways to fail: by not trying or by believing that one has failed.

STEP THREE: Training and training tools

To create a high-performance environment, all players need to know not only their own accountabilities, but also how the business works. They need to see the big picture, how their role fits into the business' overall goals, and how to take actions that will lead the company to success.

Many companies offer or require training, yet withhold information pertaining to the results. Training gives your team members *tools,* including information to help them fulfill their responsibilities. It is first and foremost about teaching job skills — methods adopted by a business to accomplish necessary tasks. This applies not only to the technical arena, but also to management, where training in documentation, systems development and innovation are but a few of the required job skills. Training teaches "how to do it."

Once "how to do it" is mastered, the team needs tools with which to get the job done. One tool is *information.* With information, one can steer a course toward the goal, evaluate early signs of trouble, even change a course of action. Some businesses recognize the power and value of sharing information, and have gone "open-book." The Springfield Remanufacturing Company, led by Jack Stack, who writes about it in *The Great Game of Business,* is a shining example of the power of open-book management.

In addition to financial information, your team needs organizational skills — tools to help them "get it done" with the help of others. Teamwork skills and conflict resolution, for example, can be taught. Also, the team may benefit from self-knowledge and self-management tools, which do not have to cost a great deal of money. Personality-typing systems such as *Managing Interpersonal Relationships* (from JOSSEY-BOSS, INC.), and MYERS-BRIGGS systems can be found in your local bookstore or library.

As with any other business system, you'll want to track the results of the systems you use to create a high-performance environment. Ask yourself: "What would indicate that we have a high-performance environment in our salon?" Indicators can be either measurable or intangible. Each should be tailored to fit your particular salon. Examples include:

MEASURABLE INDICATORS
- Number of hours of training per team member.
- Number of awards given for risk-taking.
- Percentage of performance goals met.
- Number of business development meetings held.

INTANGIBLE INDICATORS
- Overall employee satisfaction.
- Manager's/owner's satisfaction with employee and salon performance.
- Team member satisfaction with company training.

Today's leader does best if she is flexible, but absolutely certain of her purpose. One trait without the other will lead, at best, to inconsistent results. A well-considered vision expresses your hopes and dreams for the future, and helps create the energy necessary to reach them. Purposefully designing a culture that promotes teamwork and group learning will allow you to change course if the path taken proves to be undesirable.

A high-performance environment allows the creation of a game that is truly worth everyone's while to play; encourages interpersonal engagement of the highest order; and allows everyone to reach new levels of personal and professional competence. It's a game in which the fun is not only in winning, but in playing. And that's what all this is about…the magic of leadership that keeps your team in your game.

Andrew Finkelstein is President of New York City-based BEAUTY MATTERS, LTD., *a consulting firm specializing in salon leadership, management and marketing development. Mr. Finkelstein is a CEC (Certified E-Myth Consultant). For additional information, contact* BEAUTY MATTERS, LTD. *directly…*
Phone: 212.831.2421
E-mail: beautym@mail.idt.net

Things to do:

■ Learn to lead: Use the six-step method on page 465.

■ Identify your values and beliefs. Write them down.

■ Share your vision of the future with your entire staff.

■ Follow the steps on pages 474–478 to create a high-performance environment in your salon.
Write down how you will accomplish each step.

Books of interest:

Ken Blanchard, with John P. Carlos and Alan Randolph, *The 3 Keys to Empowerment* (BERRETT-KOEHLER, 1999)

Charles D. Brennan, *Proactive Customer Service: Transforming Your Customer Service Department Into a Profit Center* (AMACOM, 1997)

Stephen R. Covey, *The 7 Habits of Highly Effective People: Personal Lessons in Personal Change* (SIMON & SCHUSTER, 1989)

Clare Crawford-Mason and Lloyd Dobbins, *Quality or Else: The Revolution in World Business* (HOUGHTON MIFFLIN COMPANY, 1992)

Kenneth Delavigne and J. Daniel Robertson, *Deming's Profound Changes: When Will the Sleeping Giant Awaken?* (PRENTICE HALL, 1994)

Dr. W. Edwards Deming, *The New Economics for Industry, Government and Education* (Massachusetts Institute of Technology, Center for Advanced Engineering Study, 1993)

Michael Gerber, *The E-Myth Revisited* (HARPERCOLLINS, 1995) and *The E-Myth Manager* (HARPERCOLLINS, 1998)

Daniel Goleman, *Working with Emotional Intelligence* (BANTAM BOOKS, 1998)

Jill Griffin, *Customer Loyalty: How to Earn it, How to Keep It* (JOSSEY-BASS, INC., 1997)

Michael Hammer and Steven A. Stanton, *The Reengineering Revolution: A Handbook* (HARPERCOLLINS, 1995)

Beverly Kaye and Sharon Jordan-Evans, *Love 'Em or Lose 'Em* (BERRETT-KOEHLER, 1999)

Alfie Kohn, *Punished By Rewards: The Trouble with Gold Stars, Incentive Plans, A's, Praise and Other Bribes* (HOUGHTON MIFFLIN COMPANY, 1999)

James M. Kouzes and Barry Z. Posner, *The Leadership Challenge* (JOSSEY-BASS, INC. 1995)

Lawrence L. Lippitt, *Preferred Futuring: Envision the Future You Want and Unleash the Energy to Get There* (BERRETT-KOEHLER, 1998)

Don Peppers and Martha Rogers, *The One to One Future: Building Relationships One Customer at a Time* (DOUBLEDAY & COMPANY, INC., 1996) and *Enterprise One to One: Tools for Competing in the Interactive Age,* (DOUBLEDAY & COMPANY, INC., 1999)

Don Peppers and Martha Rogers, with Bob Dorf: *The One to One Fieldbook: The Complete Toolkit for Implementing a 1 to 1 Marketing Program* (BANTAM DOUBLEDAY DELL PUBLISHING GROUP, 1998)

Tom Reilly, *Value-Added Customer Service: The Employee's Guide for Creating Satisfied Customers* (CONTEMPORARY BOOKS, INC., 1996)

Jack Stack, with Bo Burlingham, *The Great Game of Business* (CURRENCY DOUBLEDAY, 1992)

Mary Walton, *The Deming Management Method* (BERKLEY PUBLISHING GROUP, 1986)